# Essentials of Pathology

# Essentials of Pathology

Editor: Hans Affleck

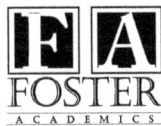

FA
FOSTER
ACADEMICS

www.fosteracademics.com

www.fosteracademics.com

**FA**
FOSTER
ACADEMICS

Cataloging-in-Publication Data

Essentials of pathology / edited by Hans Affleck.
    p. cm.
Includes bibliographical references and index.
ISBN 978-1-63242-507-2
1. Pathology. 2. Diseases. 3. Medicine. I. Affleck, Hans.
RB111 .E87 2017
616.07 --dc23

Foster Academics,
118-35 Queens Blvd., Suite 400,
Forest Hills, NY 11375, USA

ISBN 978-1-63242-507-2 (Hardback)

Printed and bound in the United States of America.

# Contents

# Preface

Over the recent decade, advancements and applications have progressed exponentially. This has led to the increased interest in this field and projects are being conducted to enhance knowledge. The main objective of this book is to present some of the critical challenges and provide insights into possible solutions. This book will answer the varied questions that arise in the field and also provide an increased scope for furthering studies.

Pathology is the study of disease or poor health and it comprises the systematic diagnosis of illness. This book on pathology discusses the medical principles that help to determine disease and the subsequent health-care that is to be provided. Pathology itself comprises of anatomical pathology or screening and clinical pathology that requires chemical assistance. Topics in this book deal with clinically relevant aspects of pathology. It strives to provide a fair idea about this discipline and to help develop a better understanding of the latest advances within this field. A number of latest researches have been included to keep the readers up-to-date with the global concepts in this area of study. This book is an essential guide for both academicians and those who wish to pursue this discipline further.

I hope that this book, with its visionary approach, will be a valuable addition and will promote interest among readers. Each of the authors has provided their extraordinary competence in their specific fields by providing different perspectives as they come from diverse nations and regions. I thank them for their contributions.

**Editor**

# Implant based differences in adverse local tissue reaction in failed total hip arthroplasties

Giorgio Perino[1]*, Benjamin F Ricciardi[2], Seth A Jerabek[2], Guido Martignoni[3], Gabrielle Wilner[4], Dan Maass[4], Steven R Goldring[4] and P Edward Purdue[4]

## Abstract

**Background:** Adverse local tissue reaction (ALTR) is characterized by periprosthetic soft tissue inflammation composed of a mixed inflammatory cell infiltrate, extensive soft tissue necrosis, and vascular changes. Multiple hip implant classes have been reported to result in ALTR, and clinical differences may represent variation in the soft tissue response at the cellular and tissue levels. The purpose of this study was to describe similarities and differences in periprosthetic tissue structure, organization, and cellular composition by conventional histology and immunohistochemistry in ALTR resulting from two common total hip arthroplasty (THA) implant classes.

**Methods:** Consecutive patients presenting with ALTR from two major hip implant classes (N = 54 patients with Dual-Modular Neck implant; N = 14 patients with Metal-on-Metal implant) were identified from our prospective Osteolysis Tissue Database and Repository. Clinical characteristics including age, sex, BMI, length of implantation, and serum metal ion levels were recorded. Retrieved synovial tissue morphology was graded using light microscopy and cellular composition was assessed using immunohistochemistry.

**Results:** Length of implantation was shorter in the DMN group versus MoM THA group (21.3 [8.4] months versus 43.6 [13.8] months respectively; p < 0.005) suggesting differences in implant performance. Morphologic examination revealed a common spectrum of neo-synovial proliferation and necrosis in both groups. Macrophages were more commonly present in diffuse sheets (Grade 3) in the MoM relative to DMN group (p = 0.016). Perivascular lymphocytes with germinal centers (Grade 4) were more common in the DMN group, which trended towards significance (p = 0.066). Qualitative differences in corrosion product morphology were seen between the two groups. Immunohistochemistry showed features of a CD4 and GATA-3 rich lymphocyte reaction in both implants, with increased ratios of perivascular T-cell relative to B-cell markers in the DMN relative to the MoM group (p = 0.032).

**Conclusion:** Our results demonstrate that both implant classes display common features of neo-synovial proliferation and necrosis with a CD4 and GATA-3 rich inflammatory infiltrate. Qualitative differences in corrosion product appearance, macrophage morphology, and lymphocyte distributions were seen between the two implant types. Our data suggests that ALTR represents a histological spectrum with implant-based features.

**Keywords:** Adverse local tissue reaction, Corrosion products, Revision arthroplasty, Synovial inflammation

* Correspondence: perinog@hss.edu
[1]Department of Pathology, Hospital for Special Surgery, 535 East 70th Street, New York, NY 10021, USA
Full list of author information is available at the end of the article

## Background

Modifications in bearing surface modularity and stem designs in total hip replacement (THA) were introduced in the past two decades with the goal of reducing the incidence of aseptic loosening and instability [1,2]. One of these modifications included the metal-on-metal (MoM) bearing surface, which was combined with a metallic adapter sleeve for large heads in the early 2000s. The rationale for the revival of this bearing surface included a reduction in volumetric wear and osteolysis compared to conventional metal-on-polyethylene bearings (MoP), decreased impingement throughout range of motion, and decreased rates of dislocation [1]. A second modification to increase modularity in THA was the introduction of the dual-modular neck. This provided surgeons with increased reconstructive options to potentially match each patient's anatomy and permit the use of a MoP or ceramic-on-polyethylene (CoP) bearing surface [2].

The unintended consequence of these implant modifications has been an increasing number of new interacting surfaces of different biomaterials, subject to short-term mechanical and no biologic testing before worldwide marketing and use [3]. This has resulted in increased MoM implant failures due to a distinct type of cellular/tissue reaction, originally reported as aseptic lymphocyte dominated vasculitis-associated lesions (ALVAL), now collectively referred in the literature as adverse local tissue reactions (ALTR) or adverse reaction to metallic debris (ARMD) [4-12]. Previous histological analyses of retrieved periprosthetic tissue have shown evidence of corrosion products, metallic debris generated by abrasion and/or surface fatigue, extensive soft tissue necrosis, combined macrophagic and lymphocytic infiltrate with variable plasmacytic and eosinophilic components, and vascular wall changes [5,13-19]. A comprehensive review describing features of periprosthetic inflammation to wear debris has been addressed in a recent review article by Gallo et al. [20]. The constellation of pathologic findings observed in response to MoM implants was encompassed under the acronym ALVAL by Willert et al. to illustrate the unique lymphocytic component and probable vascular changes not seen in other typical modes of THA failure such as osteolysis or infection [14]. Failure due to ALTR has predominantly been attributed and described for MoM bearing surfaces, but evidence of head-neck and neck-stem corrosion in modular implants has been reported to result in ALTR [4,9-12,21-23].

We hypothesized that corrosion products, as previously described in the literature, generated at different contact surfaces of THA implants could be the defining factor of ALTR irrespective of the bearing surface, and these differences would be reflected in the histologic and immunohistochemical profiles of retrieval tissue between different implant types [5,7,11]. In order to investigate this hypothesis, we compared the morphologic and immunohistochemical characteristics from retrieved periprosthetic tissue using two separate classes of implants: 1) MoM bearing surface and a metallic adapter sleeve at the head-neck taper junction and 2) conventional bearing surface (metal-on-polyethylene or metal-on-ceramic) with a dual-modular neck with tapers at the head-neck and neck-stem junctions. The purposes of this study were to analyze implant-based similarities and differences in: 1. Periprosthetic tissue structure, organization, corrosion product morphology, and cellular composition by conventional histology; and 2. Cellular composition by immunohistochemistry.

This is the first study to describe the morphologic and immunohistochemical similarities and differences between ALTR associated with different implant classes. Our results demonstrate that implant design can affect corrosion product morphology and the periprosthetic tissue pathology, and indicate that the interaction between implant design and host biology can have important clinical consequences in surveillance and outcomes of hip orthopedic implants in the future.

## Methods

### Patients

Between April 2012 and June 2013, all patients with the diagnosis of ALTR based on histological analysis were identified retrospectively from the Osteolysis Tissue Database and Repository at the Hospital for Special Surgery. This prospective database collects demographics, selected clinical data, periprosthetic tissue, and biological fluid (serum, synovial fluid) from all consenting patients undergoing revision THA with suspected ALTR. Ethical committee approval was obtained prior to this study (Institutional Review Board, Hospital for Special Surgery, Protocol Number 26085). Two groups of patients were selected, representing the two major implant classes resulting in ALTR: the Dual-Modular Neck group (DMN) had a MoP or CoP bearing surface with a dual-modular neck (cobalt-chromium-molybdenum, CoCrMo) and TMZF (titanium, molybdenum, zirconia, iron) stem (Stryker, Rejuvenate) [N = 55 hips, 54 patients], and the MoM THA group had a MoM bearing surface (CoCrMo) with a metallic adapter sleeve (CoCrMo) at the head-neck junction and titanium stem (Smith & Nephew, Birmingham THA) [N = 18 hips, 14 patients]. All polyethylene used in the DMN implant was second-generation highly cross-linked polyethylene (X3, Stryker Corporation). Exclusion criteria included previous revision arthroplasty, positive intraoperative cultures, and insufficient tissue retrieval for comparative pathologic examination (less than 5 tissue sections and more than 75% tissue necrosis at light microscopy examination on all slides examined). These two implants were selected because they are examples of recently marketed modular implants with a sufficient number of cases in our institution to allow an in-depth morphologic and immunohistochemical analysis. Preoperative serum cobalt and chromium levels were obtained by quantitative inductively coupled plasma-mass spectrometry at the operating surgeons' discretion (ARUP Laboratories, Salt Lake City, Utah). Acetabular and stem components were recorded for each implant.

### Tissue collection and sampling

All patients suspected of having ALTR at our institution undergo magnetic resonance imaging (MRI) with multi-acquisition variable-resonance image combination (MAVRIC) scan to further reduce susceptibility artifact [24]. Findings suggestive of ALTR include bulky synovitis, extracapsular disease, tendon/intramuscular edema, and capsular avulsion [24]. Periprosthetic tissue sampling in revision cases for the implants included in the database has been standardized in our institution since September 2011, when the first cases of the two series of patients described in this report were observed. Areas of inflammation were identified preoperatively on MRI, and used as guidance for tissue sampling by the operating surgeon. Samples were taken from multiple regions around the hip joint including the periprosthetic pseudocapsule, bursal synovium, and adjacent skeletal muscle when necessary and labeled accordingly. The use of cautery was minimized to avoid compromising the tissue for histologic and molecular analysis. Additionally, acetabular and femoral bone samples, core biopsies of osteolytic areas, and/or reamings were sent separately to evaluate possible bone marrow involvement when suitable. Separate tissue samples identified by location were sent to the microbiology laboratory to rule out infection and, if sizable, retrieved after culture preparation for further histological analysis.

The project research coordinator (DM, GW) harvested biological samples with presence of the pathologist (GP) to assure consistency among all the surgeons contributing cases to the database. The tissue was retrieved fresh in labeled tissue cups from the sterile area as soon as possible and kept on ice. One pathologist (GP) performed frozen section by sampling of the fresh tissue in order to assess viability and cell composition and when feasible, a representative tissue sample was processed for RNA isolation for future investigations. Remaining tissue samples were provided between two and six sites surrounding the implant. Extensive sampling was performed at macroscopic examination with care to the orientation of the specimens, including necrotic areas and/or friable, loose material. Acetabular reaming was also collected, osteolytic areas were sampled when present, and cancellous bone was also scraped from the femoral stem and/or the acetabular shell when possible. The number of paraffin blocks containing one or two tissue sections processed per case varied from 7 to 14, to minimize sampling error due to necrosis and to ensure valuable representation of the viable tissue. Photographs of each implant and selected gross tissue specimens were taken.

### Histologic analysis

All sections were processed and embedded with standard procedures, stained routinely with hematoxylin-eosin, and examined by an experienced musculoskeletal pathologist (GP) to assess the presence of ALTR. A range of 7 – 14 sections were examined per case depending on tissue availability. Cases were scored by one investigator experienced in examining periprosthetic tissue from revision THA (GP), one experienced surgical pathologist (GM), and a third investigator trained for three months on 100 archival hip revision cases with a full spectrum of adverse reactions (BR). Investigators were blinded from clinical patient characteristics. Discrepancies in scoring were resolved by consensus agreement. The ALVAL scoring system proposed by Campbell et al., which was previously used at our institution as correlative index with MRI imaging analysis, was recorded for each case [16,25-27].

Histological sections were examined for the presence (Y) or absence (N) of synovial lining loss/hyperplasia, partial or full thickness necrosis of the neo-synovial membrane and subsynovial soft tissue, cell exfoliation, vascular wall changes, high endothelial cell venules (HEV), granulomas (sarcoidosis-like with or without central necrosis), and skeletal muscle inflammatory infiltrate (Table 1). Semi-quantitative evaluation was undertaken for grading of the macrophages [28]. Macrophages were graded on a 0–3 scale (absent, occasional, clusters, diffuse/sheets). Total lymphocytes were graded as interstitial (band-like) and/or perivascular. Perivascular lymphocytes were graded according to average lymphoctic cuff thickness using a Zeiss Axioskop 40 calibrated reticule and scored as described by Natu et al. on a 0–4 scale with absence or presence of germinal centers [17]. Neutrophils were graded on a 0–2 scale [(absent, occasional, focally numerous (>5 cells x 10 HPF)]. Plasma cells were graded on a 0–2 scale [(absent, occasional, or numerous (>10 cells per HPF)]. Eosinophils were graded on a 0–1 scale (absent or present), stromal cell cellularity was graded on a 1–3 scale (slight, moderate, marked). Results were expressed as the percentage of samples containing the selected feature.

Macrophage content (polyethylene, metal, and ceramic particles) was graded according to the method used for metallic particles by Natu et al. [17] (Table 1). Presence of intracellular corrosion products was recorded and extracellular aggregates were graded on a 0–1 scale (absent or present). Presence of hemosiderin deposits and/or suture material was recorded.

**Table 1 Morphologic comparison of synovial structure, cellularity, macrophage content, and bone marrow involvement between the Dual-Modular Neck and the Metal-on-Metal (MoM) total hip arthroplasty (THA) groups**

| Morphologic characteristic | Dual-Modular Neck THA (N = 55 hips) | MoM THA (N = 18 hips) | P value |
|---|---|---|---|
| **Synovial structure** | **Cases (%)** | **Cases (%)** | |
| Synovial layer loss | 96.4 | 100.0 | |
| Synovial layer hyperplasia | 78.2 | 77.8 | |
| Cell exfoliation | 87.3 | 94.4 | |
| Necrosis | 65.5 | 61.1 | |
| Vascular wall changes | 18.2 | 16.7 | |
| High endothelial cell venules | 14.5 | 16.7 | |
| Granulomas | 18.2 | 11.1 | 0.482 |
| **Cellularity** | | | |
| Macrophages | | | 0.016* |
| Grade 1 | 16.4 | 5.6 | |
| Grade 2 | 30.9 | 5.6 | |
| Grade 3 | 50.9 | 88.9 | |
| Lymphocytes | | | 0.066# |
| Grade 1 | 1.8 | 16.7 | |
| Grade 2 | 9.1 | 5.6 | |
| Grade 3 | 52.7 | 61.1 | |
| Grade 4 | 34.5 | 16.7 | |
| Stromal Cells | | | 0.593 |
| Grade 1 | 27.3 | 38.9 | |
| Grade 2 | 50.9 | 44.4 | |
| Grade 3 | 16.4 | 11.1 | |
| Neutrophils | 10.9 | 11.1 | |
| Plasma cells sparse | 32.7 | 38.9 | |
| Plasma cells numerous | 20.0 | 22.2 | |
| Eosinophils | 32.7 | 33.3 | |
| **Macrophage content** | | | |
| Polyethylene particles | 1.8 | 0.0 | |
| Metallic particles | 1.8 | 33.3 | <0.005* |
| Corrosion products | 100 | 100 | |
| Intracellular distribution | Sparse | Diffuse | |
| Intracellular morphology | Irregular | Globular + Irregular | |
| Extracellular corrosion aggregates | 72.7 | 66.7 | 0.662 |
| **Bone/bone marrow** | | | |
| Necrosis | 47.1 | 28.6 | |
| Macrophage infiltration | 47.1 | 100.0 | |

**Table 1 Morphologic comparison of synovial structure, cellularity, macrophage content, and bone marrow involvement between the Dual-Modular Neck and the Metal-on-Metal (MoM) total hip arthroplasty (THA) groups** (Continued)

| | | | |
|---|---|---|---|
| Benign lymphocytic aggregates | 35.3 | 28.6 | |
| Germinal centers | 17.6 | 0.0 | |

*Statistically significant at p < 0.05 for Dual-Modular Neck versus MoM THA.
#trend towards statistical significance p < 0.10 for Dual-Modular Neck versus MoM THA.
Morphologic Characteristics of Synovial Tissue from Dual-Modular Neck and MoM THA Groups.

Bone marrow sections were evaluated for the presence (Y) or absence (N) of necrosis of bone and marrow cellular elements, macrophage infiltration, and benign lymphocytic aggregates with or without presence of germinal centers. Results were expressed as a percentage of patients displaying each morphologic feature.

### Immunohistochemistry

Fifteen cases for each of the DMN and MoM THA groups were analyzed by immunohistochemistry. The cases from the larger DMN group were selected to be representative of the spectrum of histological patterns observed as described in the results section. Conventional immunohistochemistry was performed using standard techniques on consecutive sections (GM). Heat-induced antigen retrieval was performed using a microwave oven and 0.01 mol/L of citrate buffer. All samples were processed using a sensitive 'Bond polymer Refine' detection system in an automated Bond immunohistochemistry instrument (Vision-Biosystem, Menarini, Florence, Italy). Antibody dilutions and source are shown in Table 2. Commercially available monoclonal antibodies were used and each batch was tested by titration for optimal dilution on both internal and external controls. Macrophage markers were CD68 (all macrophages) and CD163 (M2 macrophages) [29,30]. The lymphocytic response was assessed by expression of CD20 for B cells and CD3, CD4, and CD8 for T cells. Expression of T-bet, GATA3, and FOXP3 was used as marker for transcription factors for Th1, Th2, and Treg cells to sub-classify the T cell distribution [31-33]. High endothelial cell venules were identified as CD123 positive cells. Mast cells were identified as CD117 positive cells [34].

Semiquantitative analysis was performed for evaluation of macrophage, mast cell, and HEV distributions. Evaluation of CD68 and CD163 stained sections were graded as +, ++, and +++ by three investigators (GP, GM, BR) blinded to the clinical data. CD117 staining was assessed from 0–2 [absent, occasional, numerous (>5 forms per HPF)]. Granzyme immunohistochemistry and the presence

**Table 2 Description of antibodies and dilutions utilized for immunohistochemistry**

| Antibody | Clone | Source | Dilution |
|----------|-------|--------|----------|
| CD3 | SP7 | THERMO SC. | 1:150 |
| CD4 | 4B12 | NOVOCASTRA | 1:150 |
| CD8 | C8/144B | DAKO | 1:200 |
| CD20 | L26 | NOVOCASTRA | 1:100 |
| CD68 | PG-M1 | DAKO | 1:50 |
| CD123 | 7G3 | BD Phamingen | 1:100 |
| CD163 | 10D6 | NOVOCASTRA | 1:200 |
| GATA-3 | L50-823 | BD Phamingen | 1:150 |
| FOXP3 | 221D/D3 | SEROTEC | 1:200 |
| T-bet | 4B10 | SANTA CRUZ | 1:100 |
| Granzyme | GrB-7 | MONOSAN | 1:100 |
| CD117 | T595 | NOVOCASTRA | 1:10 |

Antibody Sources and Dilutions for Immunohistochemistry.

of CD123 positive HEVs were assessed by the presence (Y) or absence (N) of positive cells.

A quantitative analysis (Bioquant Osteo, Bioquant Image Analysis Corporation, Nashville, TN) was performed on all sections to evaluate lymphocytic distributions in both perivascular and interstitial regions. Two perivascular and two interstitial areas on each slide were randomly selected and evaluated at high power ($\times 400$), and lymphocytes with positive stain were counted manually by two investigators blinded to the clinical characteristics (BR, GP). The results were expressed as percentage of positive cells per mm$^2$. The same areas from consecutive sections were chosen for each stain, ensuring consistency in area of evaluation. The ratios between CD20:CD3, CD4:CD8, and GATA3:T-bet on the same sections were then calculated. The CD20:CD3, CD4:CD8, and GATA3:T-bet were described as a > 2:1, 1:1, or > 1:2 ratio.

A comparison control group of periprosthetic tissue was used for immunohistochemistry. For the control group (N = 17), average age was 63.5 years (standard deviation 14.0) and 71% were females. These included three cases (N = 3) of osteoarthritis with variable amount

of lymphoplasmacytic infiltrate without clinical diagnosis of rheumatic disease, three cases of periprosthetic osteolysis from polyethylene/metallic wear debris in standard THA, and three (N = 3) cases of MoM implants not examined in our series (1 resurfacing, 2 MoM THA). Average time of implantation was 30 months in these patients. Additionally, we examined all cases of preoperative native synovial tissue (time zero) available for patients in our series with ALTR and identified five cases (N = 5) with variable perivascular lymphoplasmacytic infiltrate to provide a baseline comparison. These cases underwent the same pathologic and immunohistochemical evaluation as the ALTR cases in this study. Two archival cases of pelvic lymph nodes in patients with history of total hip replacement served as negative and positive immunohistochemistry controls.

## Statistics

Categorical variables were reported as frequencies and percentages and compared between the DMN and MoM THA groups by chi-square tests. Continuous variables were summarized as means and standard deviations and compared between groups with independent samples t-tests. In cases where data was not normally distributed, a Mann–Whitney $U$ test was utilized. All statistical tests were two-sided and p-values less than 0.05 were considered statistically significant. Statistical analyses were performed with SAS version 9.3 (SAS Institute, Cary, NC).

## Results

### Clinical demographics

Demographics for patients that met study criteria are summarized in Table 3. Patients were older in the DMN group (N = 55 hips in 54 patients) versus the MoM THA group (p = 0.03) (Table 3). Mean time to revision was earlier in the DMN group versus MoM THA group (21.3 [8.4] months versus 43.6 [13.8] months respectively; p < 0.005) (Table 3). Serum cobalt and chromium levels were increased in the MoM THA relative to the DMN group, however, only the chromium level in unilateral cases reached statistical significance (Table 4).

**Table 3 Demographic data for the Dual-Modular Neck and Metal-on-Metal (MoM) total hip arthroplasty (THA) groups**

| Demographic factor | Dual-Modular Neck THA N = 54 patients N = 55 hips | MoM THA N = 14 patients N = 18 hips | P Value |
|--------------------|---------------------------------------------------|-------------------------------------|---------|
| Age (years) | 67.3 (range 47 – 87) | 58.6 (range 31–75) | 0.03* |
| Female (%) | 59.3 | 64.3 | 0.79 |
| BMI (mean [SD]) | 27.1 (4.8) | 26.6 (4.3) | 0.72 |
| Time to revision (mean [SD]) | 21.3 (8.4) | 43.6 (13.8) | <0.005* |
| Campbell score (mean [SD]) | 8.1 (1.9) | 7.4 (1.6) | 0.15 |

SD: standard deviation. *statistically significant at p < 0.05 for Dual-Modular Neck versus MoM THA.
Demographic Factors in the Dual-Modular Neck and MoM THA Groups.

**Table 4 Preoperative serum cobalt and serum chromium levels in patients with unilateral or bilateral arthroplasties in the Dual-Modular Neck or Metal-on-Metal (MoM) total hip arthroplasty (THA) groups**

|  | Dual-Modular Neck THA | MoM THA | P value |
|---|---|---|---|
| Serum Cobalt (ng/mL) | | | |
| Unilateral (N = 43, N = 6) | 7.5 (5.6) | 29.0 (54.4) | 0.581 |
| Bilateral (N = 3, N = 5) | 16.8 (1.5) | 23.8 (21.2) | 1.0 |
| Serum Chromium (ng/mL) | | | |
| Unilateral (N = 43, N = 6) | 1.2 (1.4) | 11.0 (16.4) | 0.004* |
| Bilateral (N = 3, N = 5) | 2.9 (1.5) | 14.6 (14.2) | 0.142 |

Data represented as mean (standard deviation) for all values.
Preoperative Serum Ion Levels in the Dual-Modular Neck and MoM THA Groups.
*statistically significant at p < 0.05 for Dual-Modular Neck versus MoM THA.

### Histological analysis

Histologic examination of the retrieved tissues showed similar development of ALTR in both implants (Figures 1 and 2). Development of a reactive neo-synovial membrane ranging from flat/micropapillary, especially in bursal specimens, to florid papillary hypertrophy, ranging from coarse to polypoidal configuration, with a variable amount of stromal cell proliferation and hyperplasia of the lining layer was observed in both series (Figures 1A and 2A). The lining layer of the neo-synovium was predominantly formed by macrophages with exfoliation of viable and necrotic elements with occasional formation of a distinct eosinophilic border of coagulative necrosis, previously described in the literature as adherent fibrinous exudates (Figures 1B and 2B). An underlying band of dense sclerosis/fibroplasia and abundant macrophagic exfoliation was more commonly seen in the MoM THA (Figures 1B and 2B). Superficial perivascular lymphocytic infiltrate associated with particle-laden macrophages was commonly observed (Figures 1C and 2C). Detachment of the superficial layer or of cell contents with macrophages at different stages of degeneration (foamy elements) of the papillary projections was also observed in the MoM THA, contributing to the formation of a dense creamy fluid occasionally filling the groove of the metallic femoral head (Figure 2D). Florid papillary hypertrophy with a distribution of the inflammatory infiltrate similar to those seen in rheumatologic disorders was occasionally seen in the DMN group (Figure 1D). Tissue necrosis/infarction of variable thickness of the neo-synovial membrane, possibly reflecting more advanced stages of the reaction, was observed in 61.1% and 65.5% of cases in the MoM THA and DMN groups respectively (Table 1; Figures 1E and 2E). A deep layer of mixed macrophagic and lymphocytic infiltrate with variable number of plasma cells and eosinophils was seen in both implants (Table 1; Figures 1F and 2F). Deep perivascular lymphocytic infiltrate with formation of germinal centers and CD123 positive tall endothelial cell venules containing lymphocytes was also seen in both implants (Table 1; Figure 2G with inset). Other vascular changes were observed: the most frequent was a variable amount of non-specific myointimal proliferation of vessels with stenosis of the lumen but without identifiable luminal fibrinous exudate, thrombi, and wall damage. Occasionally onion skin pattern was present, albeit focal without evidence of a diffuse distribution in any case. Formation of sarcoidosis-like granulomas with giant cells with distinct positivity for CD123 (interleukin-3) and lymphoctic cuffing associated with the presence of corrosion products was observed in both groups (Figure 1G with inset). Higher grades of macrophagic infiltrate were seen in the MoM THA (p = 0.016) (Table 1). In contrast, higher grades of lymphocytic infiltrate were seen in the DMN group, and this trended towards significance (p = 0.066) (Table 1).

Bone marrow involvement was observed in both implants when sampled, with cell necrosis and macrophagic-lymphocytic infiltrate with associated osteoclastic activity (Figures 1H) or with benign lymphocytic aggregates associated with particle-laden macrophages (Table 1 and Figure 2H).

### Evaluation of corrosion products

Corrosion products with morphologies similar to those described in previous studies were seen in many cases in both implant types, with the exception of retrieved tissues with extensive necrosis of the superficial neo-synovial layer, in which case it was not possible to adequately assess the samples [5,11,35,36] (Figure panel 3; A-D, DMN implant; E-H. MoM THA implant). Large aggregates of corrosion products were seen in the soft tissues in both implants (66.7% versus 72.7% for MoM THA and the DMN groups respectively). A crystal-like appearance of the corrosion products with formation of flat sheets in both implant types was seen, often with alternating green and red layers on H-E staining (Figures 3A,B,E). In other areas, these larger aggregates were fragmented, and these irregular particles of variable size were engulfed within multi-nucleated giant cells and mononuclear macrophages either in soft tissue (Figure 3C) or bone marrow (Figure 3D). We confirmed the origin of these corrosion products from the implants by embedding loose black

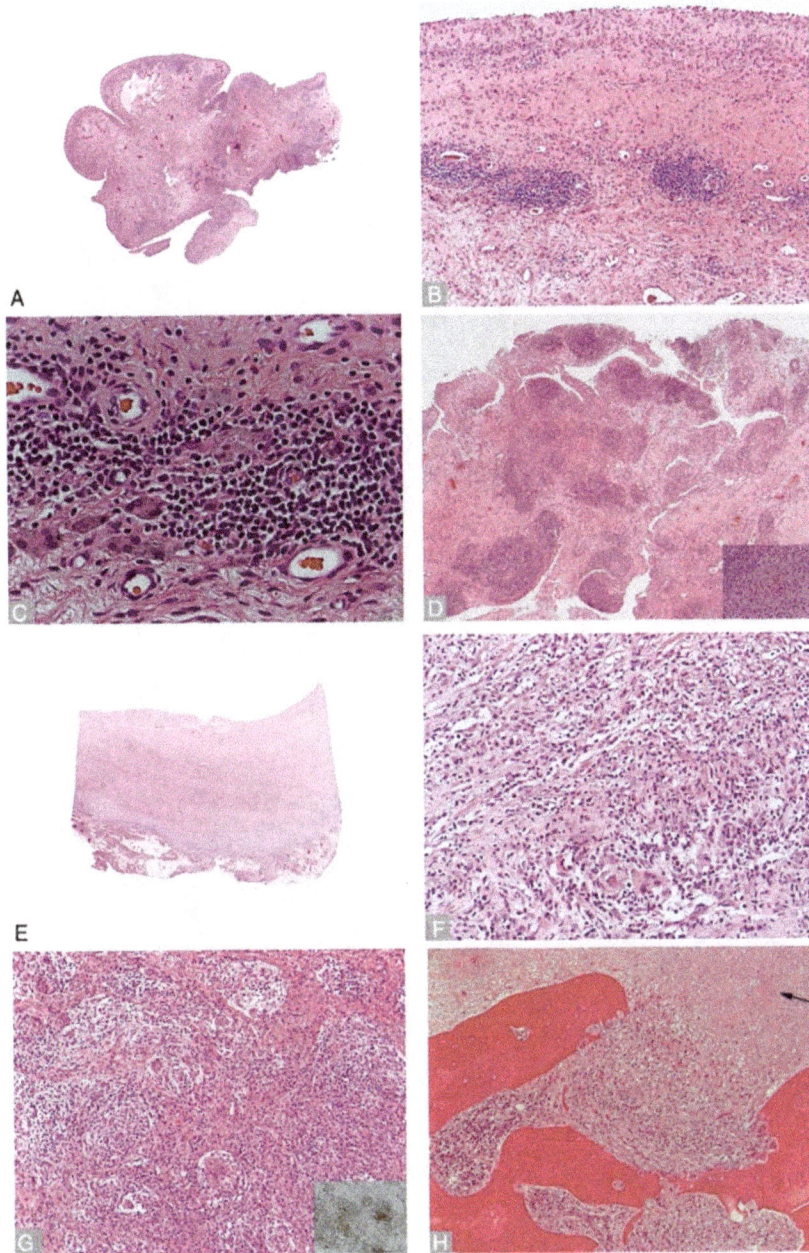

**Figure 1 Histopathologic images from Dual-Modular Neck group. A)** Periprosthetic neosynovium with polypoid hypertrophy (whole mount). **B)** Neo-synovial membrane with lining layer composed of macrophages, marked stromal sclerosis, and perivascular lymphocytic infiltrate (x100). **C)** Perivascular lymphocytic infiltrate associated with particle-laden macrophages (x400). **D)** Papillary synovium with marked perivascular lymphocytic infiltrate (x40) associated to giant cells containing corrosion products (inset x400). **E)** Late stage of adverse reaction with thick layer of necrosis/infarction and deep seated inflammatory infiltrate (whole mount). **F)** Band-like inflammatory infiltrate composed of macrophages, lymphocytes, plasma cells, and eosinophils (x400). **G)** Granulomatous pattern composed of small granulomas with multi-nucleated giant cells and lymphocytic cuffing (x100). **H)** Bone marrow involvement with area of necrosis (black arrow) and mixed macrophagic and lymphocytic infiltrate with resorptive osteoclastic activity (x100).

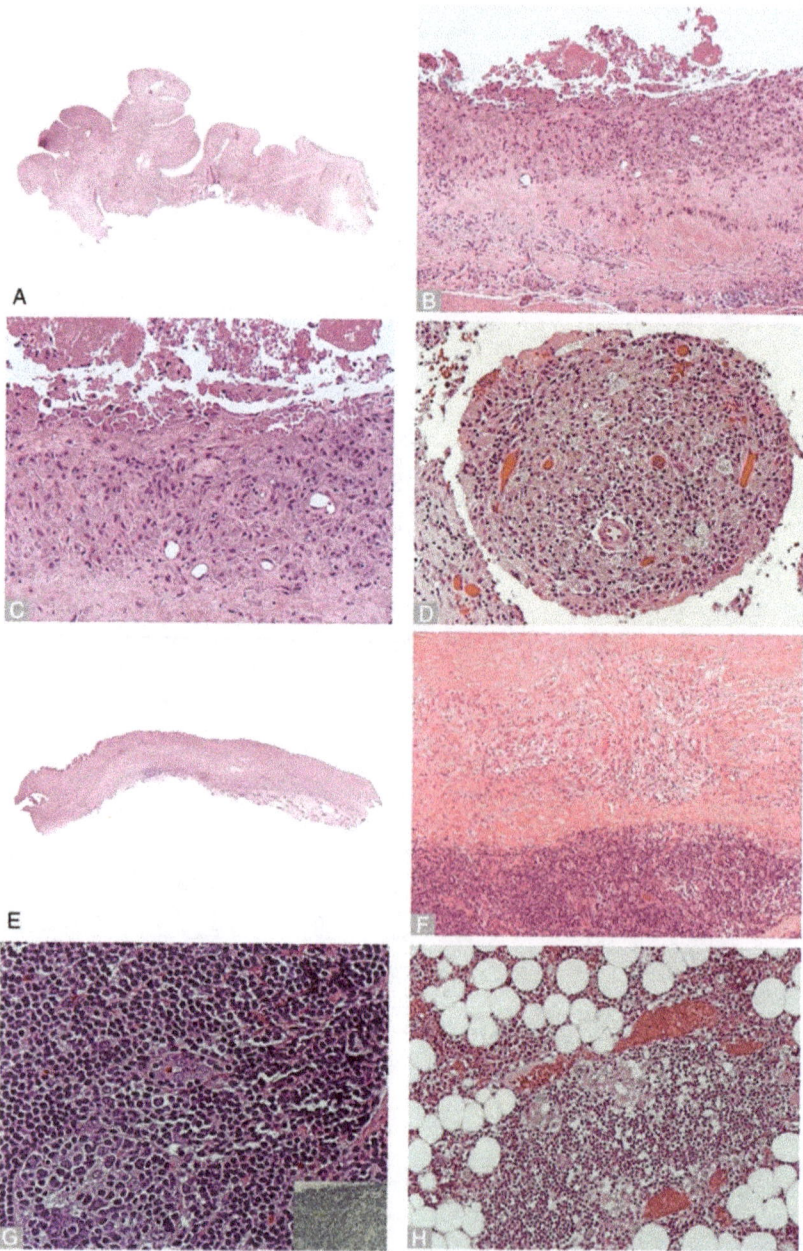

**Figure 2** Histopathologic images from MoM THA group A) Periprosthetic neo-synovium with polypoid hypertrophy (whole mount).
**B)** Superficial macrophagic infiltrate with exfoliation of necrotic elements without significant lymphocytic response (x100). **C)** Corrosion product-laden macrophages with exfoliation of viable and necrotic elements (x200). **D)** Synovial papilla with particle-laden macrophages at different stages of degeneration with foamy elements (x200). **E)** Late stage of reaction with thick layer of necrosis and deep seated inflammatory infiltrate (whole mount). **F)** Band-like mixed inflammatory infiltrate and deep perivascular lymphocytic infiltrate (x100). **G)** Evidence of germinal center formation (lower left corner) and tall endothelial cell venule (x400) with positive staining for CD123 (inset x400). **H)** Bone marrow with benign reactive lymphocytic aggregate mixed with particle-laden macrophages (x200).

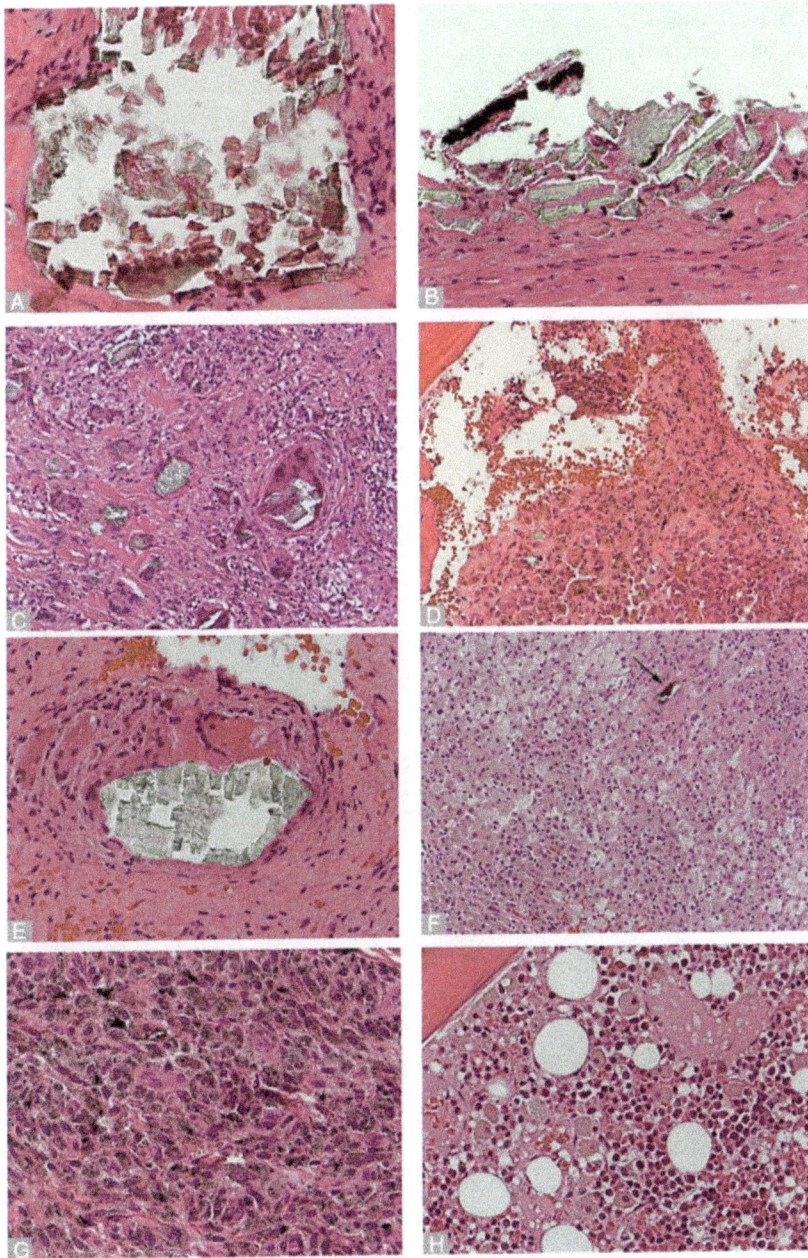

**Figure 3 Histopathology of corrosion products in Dual-Modular Neck and MoM THA groups.** Dual Modular Neck : **A)** Large fragments of layered corrosion products with crystal-like configuration (x400). **B)** Large aggregate of green oxidized corrosion product with plated crystal-like configuration (x400). **C)** Fragmentation of corrosion material from **(B)** engulfed into multinucleated giant cells (x200). **D)** Macrophages containing small and large particles of corrosion products infiltrating the bone marrow. MoM THA: **E)** Large aggregate of green crystal-like corrosion material surrounded by giant cells (x400). **F)** Macrophages containing corrosion products with many foamy elements and one giant cell containing larger aggregate, black arrow (x200). **G)** Macrophagic infiltrate containing predominantly globular particles of corrosion products and irregular black particles of metallic abrasion debris (x400). **H)** Hematopoietic marrow infiltrated with many macrophages containing green particles of corrosion products of variable size (x200).

debris from the taper junctions of both implants in paraffin and obtaining H-E sections, which revealed similar morphology to those observed in the periprosthetic soft tissue of the same cases.

In contrast to these irregular extracellular aggregates, the intracellular content of the macrophages showed distinct differences between the two groups: in the DMN group the cells contained scattered irregular greenish particles which were present in large amount only in areas close to the large aggregates (Figure 3C); moreover particles were difficult to identify in the deep inflammatory layer in the cases with marked necrosis. In the MoM THA group, larger macrophages were observed, containing cytoplasmic globular particles ranging from golden brown to greenish, similar in morphology to cases of resurfacing with the same bearing surface, and scattered irregular particles. Additionally, in the MoM THA, black, irregular metallic particles were seen along

with green corrosion products within the macrophages, suggesting different origins and/or compositions of metallic debris being produced in this implant type (Figure 3G). In contrast, the DMN implant did not have a metal-on-metal bearing surface, and abrasion metallic particles were not identified at light microscopy (Table 1). Bone marrow involvement of these larger aggregates and corrosion product-containing macrophages was observed in cases of both implant types if bone samples were available (Figure 3D,H).

### Immunohistochemistry

Both implant types had significant macrophagic infiltrates expressing CD68 and CD163 in all samples examined, with higher intensity of the latter (Figures 4A and B). Both implants displayed a mixed perivascular lymphocytic infiltrate, with increased T cell to B cell ratios in the DMN group relative to the MoM THA (Table 5; $p = 0.032$). In

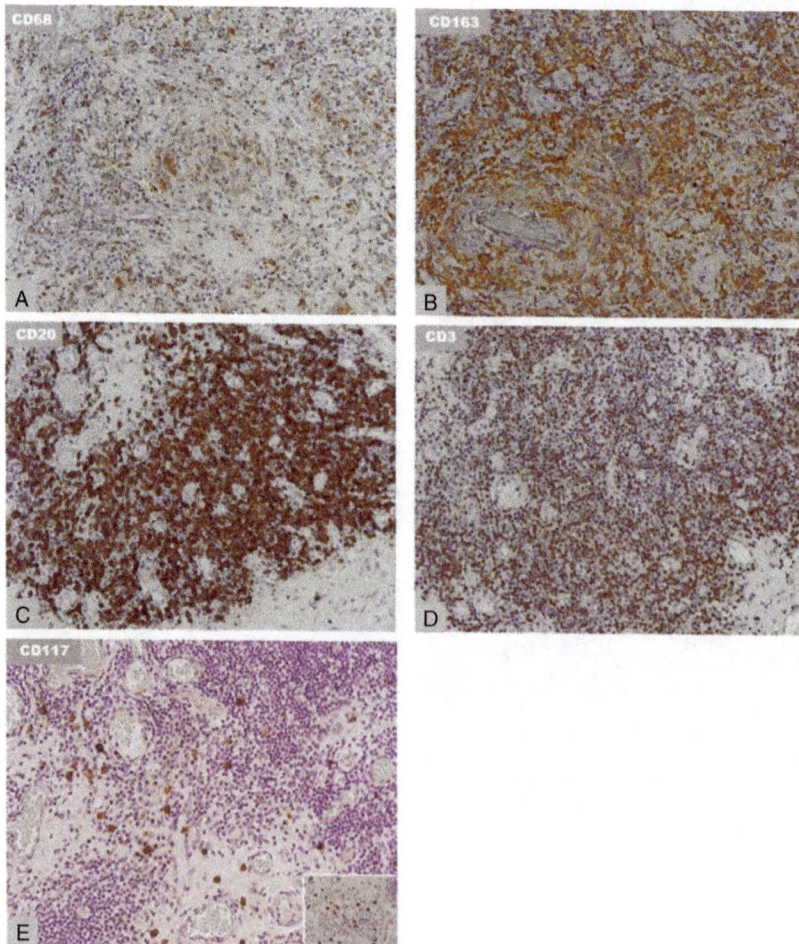

**Figure 4 Immunohistochemistry in the Dual-Modular Neck and MoM THA groups (all 200X magnification).** Macrophage positivity for **A)** CD68 and **B)** CD163. Perivascular lymphocytic infiltrate with **C)** CD20 positivity, **D)** CD3 positivity, and **E)** interstitial CD117 positive mast cells.

**Table 5 Immunhistochemistry comparison between Dual-Modular Neck and the Metal-on-Metal (MoM) total hip arthroplasty (THA) groups**

| | Perivascular region | | | Interstitial region | | |
|---|---|---|---|---|---|---|
| | Dual-Modular Neck THA (N = 15) | MoM THA (N = 12) | P value | Dual-Modular Neck THA (N = 15) | MoM THA (N = 12) | P value |
| CD20:CD3 | | | *0.032 | | | 0.35 |
| 1:2 | 46.1% | 0% | | 85.7% | 66.7% | |
| 1:1 | 30.8% | 25.0% | | 14.3% | 25.0% | |
| 2:1 | 23.1% | 75.0% | | 0% | 8.3% | |
| CD4:CD8 | | | | | | |
| 1:2 | 15.4% | 14.3% | 0.964 | 50.0% | 16.7% | 0.189 |
| 1:1 | 23.1% | 28.6% | | 35.7% | 66.7% | |
| 2:1 | 61.5% | 57.1% | | 14.3% | 16.7% | |
| GATA3:Tbet | | | | | | |
| 1:2 | 0% | 0% | 1.00 | 0% | 0% | 0.42 |
| 1:1 | 0% | 0% | | 38.5% | 22.2% | |
| 2:1 | 100% | 100% | | 61.5% | 77.8% | |

All values listed as percentage of cases representing qualitative grade for each antibody. *statistically significant at p < 0.05 for Dual-Modular Neck versus MoM THA.
Immunohistochemistry Characteristics of Synovial Tissue from Dual-Modular Neck and MoM THA Groups.

the interstitial regions, both implants had T cell predominant lymphyocytic infiltrates. The majority of patients had a mixed population of CD4 and CD8 positive T cells, with CD4 cells being more numerous in most cases in perivascular regions (Figures 5A and B; Table 5). In interstitial regions, a subset of patients in both implant types had increased CD8 positive cell density relative to CD4, however, there was no significant difference between the implant types in CD4 to CD8 ratio (p = 0.189). Further lymphocytic sub-classification showed increased number of GATA3 positive expression relative to T-bet in all samples examined (Figures 5C and D; Table 5). FOXP3 positive lymphocytes were frequently present in lymphocyte-rich regions in both implant groups, and were graded as numerous in 47% and 25% of cases in the DMN and MoM THA respectively (Figure 5E). Immunohistochemistry for granzyme showed increased presence of positive cells in the DMN group relative to the MoM THA (27% versus 0% of cases respectively), and this trended towards significance (p = 0.053). Staining for CD117 showed a variable number of mast cells, ranging from occasional to numerous (>5 cells per HPF) in interstitial and perivascular regions in both implant groups (Figure 4E).

Examination of control samples of retrieved revision tissues from patients with polyethylene-induced osteolysis showed no lymphocytic infiltration in any cases and a similar staining pattern for the macrophagic markers CD68 and CD163. A similar distribution of CD20:CD3, CD4:CD8, and GATA3:T-bet was seen in perivascular regions in the synovium from patients with osteoarthritis with excessive synovial chronic inflammatory infiltrate. We had the unique opportunity to evaluate native,

preoperative synovial tissue from five patients in our series who subsequently developed ALTR after their total hip arthroplasty. A comparison of their native synovium with synovium after revision for ALTR showed similar lymphocytic distributions, including the presence of a CD4, GATA3 predominant perivascular lymphocytic infiltrate. Synovial necrosis was not identified in these pre-operative groups, although mild hyperplasia of the lining layer was observed. Similarly, in cases of ALTR with other MoM implants, a similar CD4 and GATA3 predominant lymphocytic infiltrate was seen.

### Histologic patterns

Three distinct histologic patterns were identified at light microscopy in this series: 1) a predominantly macrophagic pattern with absent or minimal lymphocytic response, 2) mixed inflammatory pattern, macrophagic and lymphocytic with variable presence of plasma cells, eosinophils, and mast cells, and 3) granulomatous pattern, predominant or associated with the inflammatory pattern. The predominantly macrophagic group represented a group of patients with an adverse soft tissue reaction resulting in implant failure with minimal lymphocytic activation [16,18,37]. The mixed inflammatory pattern was subdivided into those with (A) or without (B) germinal centers because this may stratify patients based on variation of the immune response [15,17,19]. The third group had prominent formation of sarcoidosis-like granulomas in the presence of a mixed or macrophagic infiltrate, and this may represent a subset of patients with particular macrophage characteristics [15,17]. In our series, a macrophagic pattern of ALTR was seen in

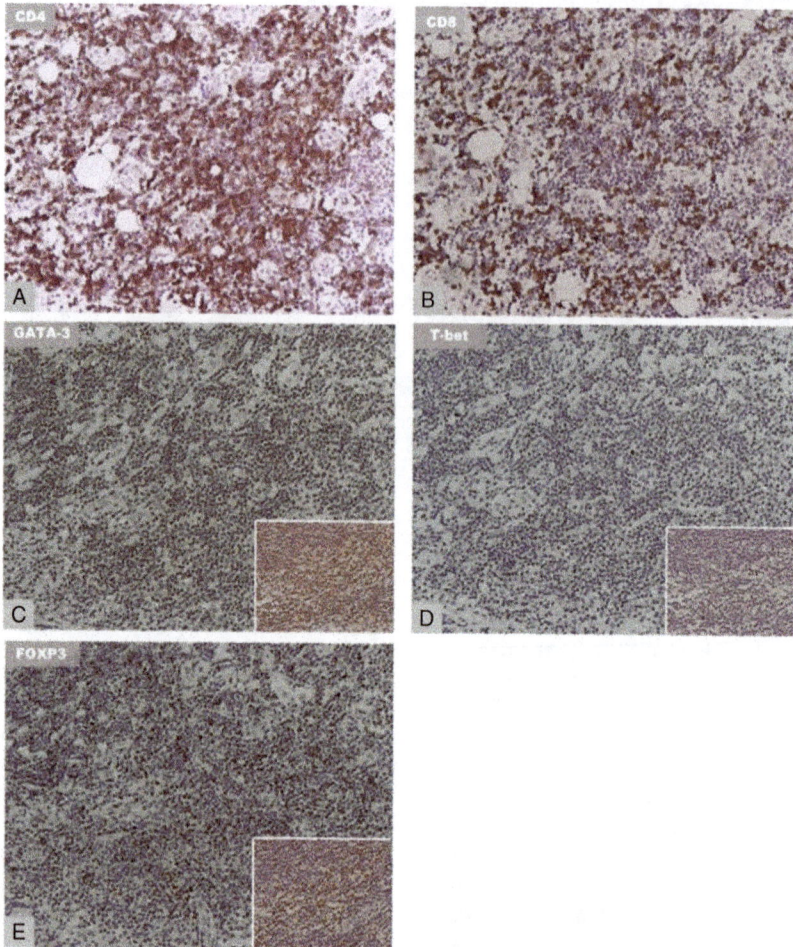

**Figure 5 Immunohistochemistry in the Dual-Modular Neck and MoM THA groups (all 200X magnification).** Perivascular lymphocytic infiltrate demostrates **A)** CD4 positivity and **B)** CD8 positivity. Further subclassification of perivascular lymphocytes shows **C)** T cell GATA-3 positivity, **D)** T cell T-bet positivity, and **E)** T cell FOXP3 positivity.

0% and 5.2% of cases of ALTR in the DMN and the MoM THA respectively with absent or minimal lymphocytic response (Table 6). The second, and most common, subtype was the mixed inflammatory pattern. An increased percentage of cases with germinal centers were seen in the DMN group (Table 6). Granulomatous pattern was seen more commonly in the DMN group (Table 6). In the inflammatory and granulomatous groups, ALVAL with necrosis was observed in certain cases.

## Discussion

Failure due to ALTR has previously been described for MoM bearing surfaces and modular junctions at the head-neck and neck-stem [4,9-14,21-23,35,38,39]. The purposes of this study were to compare implant-based differences in periprosthetic tissue structure, organization, corrosion product morphology, and cellular composition by conventional

histology and immunohistochemistry in ALTR resulting from two common implant configurations. Our results demonstrate that similarities between these two implants included spectrum of histologic patterns, composition of the inflammatory infiltrate, and presence of corrosion products. Differences between these implant types included macrophage and lymphocyte distributions, and corrosion product morphology. This is the first study to our knowledge to compare the histologic and immunohistochemical features of ALTR in two different classes of implants.

We have shown convincing histological evidence that similar common morphologic features exist in ALTR with an early phase of cellular activation and proliferation seen in neo-synovial reaction to other particulate implant materials (e.g. polyethylene) followed by a distinctive sequence of cellular and tissue reactions leading to formation of a variable amount of soft tissue necrosis/

**Table 6 Observed histologic subtypes in the Dual-Modular Neck and the Metal-on-Metal (MoM) total hip arthroplasty (THA) groups**

| Observed subtypes | Dual-Modular Neck THA (N = 54 hips) | MoM THA (N = 18 hips) |
|---|---|---|
| Macrophagic | 0 (0%) | 1 (5.2%) |
| Macrophagic with Mixed Lymphocytic Infiltrate | | |
| w/ Germinal Centers | 15 (27.2%) | 2 (11.1%) |
| w/o Germinal Centers | 30 (54.5%) | 14 (77.8%) |
| Granulomatous | 9 (16.4%) | 1 (5.2%) |

All values listed as number (percentage of cases) representing each histologic subtype.
Histologic Subtypes of Adverse Local Tissue Reaction.

infarction. Corroborating evidence is provided by the metachronous development of the reaction in various areas of the periprosthetic tissue, contiguous areas of superficial necrosis, preserved neo-synovial architecture, and absence of necrosis in the bursal tissue until dehiscence of the fluid contained within the pseudocapsule. The time to revision in the DMN group was significantly shorter than the MoM THA, and this suggests different progression rates of ALTR with different implant designs. Progression of ALTR may depend on length of device implantation, toxicity/immunogenicity of corrosion particles, implant design and alignment, patient comorbidities, and host immune reactivity. The modality of failure of the DMN and MoM THA implants analyzed in this study have been attributed in previous publications to the formation of corrosion products at the metallic interacting surfaces and not to technical mistakes or poor design resulting in mechanical failure of the implants [5,9,11]. Gill et al. also found that corrosion at the modular neck-stem junction resulted in early revision relative to the same monoblock stem and bearing components [9]. Additionally, Cooper et al. have shown a similar time to failure of the DMN implant used in our study, further corroborating our results were not due to technical error [11]. A possibility of bias in time to revision might exist because the DMN group had a publicized recall of the implant, however, all patients revised in both cohorts were indicated for revision due to elevated metal ion levels, symptomatic hip pain, MRI findings of moderate to severe adverse tissue reaction, and/or positive needle biopsies. Our observations are similar to previous studies that have illustrated the distinct histological aspects of the reaction, predominantly in MoM hip resurfacing implants or in mixed resurfacing and THA implants [10,13-19]. Previous publications examining ALTR have used the proposed ALVAL score by Campbell et al. as a grading system of the reaction [16,18,25]. If our interpretation of the natural history of the reaction is correct, the score would be an indication of developmental stage of the adverse reaction rather than a grading system of its biological severity, and therefore of limited clinical value in predicting the course or

the biological outcome of the reaction for each specific type of implant.

Different histologic subtypes were observed in ALTR in our study. A subset of patients in the MoM THA group had a macrophagic pattern of failure with minimal lymphocytic response and absent or minimal necrosis. These patients may have impingement related failure, suggested by black metallic particles in their soft tissue and/or an immunoprofile that is less responsive to wear debris. A second subgroup of patients had a mixed macrophagic and lymphocytic response with a variable number of plasma cells, eosinophils, and mast cells. This has been described frequently in ALTR from previous studies and represented the most common pattern we observed [13-18]. A third subgroup displayed a granulomatous pattern with or without inflammatory infiltrate or necrosis, and this patient subgroup may have unique immunologic responses to wear debris. We did not observe any cases with an exclusively lymphocytic pattern without presence of particle-laden macrophages, as described by Berstock et al. [37]. This difference may be due to the extensive sampling performed of periprosthetic tissue in our study. The association of these different histologic patterns and clinical outcomes needs to be investigated in future studies.

We demonstrated an association between the presence of extra-cellular and intra-cellular corrosion products in the periprosthetic tissue with the presence of interstitial and perivascular lymphocytic infiltrate. This association suggests that corrosion particle laden macrophages are instrumental in the formation of the lymphocytic infiltrate, although free particulate material can also significantly contribute to the response. Corroborative evidence of our interpretation was the presence of benign lymphocytic aggregates in the bone marrow associated with particle-laden macrophages as previously reported in hip resurfacing implants [15,40]. The appearance of corrosion materials was different between the two implant designs, which also were associated with differing levels of serum cobalt and chromium ions. The MoM THA has two possible sources of corrosion materials or metallic debris: the metal-on-metal articular surface and the head-neck taper junction. The dual modular neck implant also has two possible sources of corrosion: the head-neck taper junction and the neck-stem taper junction, although the predominant one appears to be the latter [11]. These different surface possibilities likely explain the variable corrosion material appearance and distribution. Xia et al. used electron microscopy and EDX to assess macrophage content in ALVAL due to failure of a MoM bearing surface and their results showed nanometer-sized inclusions within the phagosomes with significant chromium content by EDX [41]. We hypothesize that the numerous, predominantly globular small intracellular inclusions seen on light microscopy represent corrosion products generated at the bearing surface, which are not present in the dual-modular neck implant. This observation is confirmed by the presence of the same inclusions in resurfacing implants with the same bearing surface (data not shown). In contrast to intracellular corrosion material, both implant types had large extracellular corrosion aggregates of similar morphology. Our data indicate these materials represent corrosion products from the taper junctions at the head-neck and neck-stem, which is consistent with previous studies [5,11,35]. Analysis of material produced from head-neck taper corrosion suggested that chromium orthophosphate was the most common corrosion material produced at modular junctions, and this material could disseminate into the surrounding soft tissue [5,11,35]. These wear products differ in size and shape from the intracellular products that are seen from the bearing surface, possibly explaining biological or clinical differences between different implant types [42]. Moreover, the stratified appearance of the aggregates at light microscopy possibly suggests mixing of fluid proteins and secondary particles released from the exfoliated macrophages forming products of unknown and untested cytotoxicity. Early involvement of the hematopoietic bone marrow by macrophages and large aggregates of particles can also influence the adverse reaction, and this may have future biological significance.

The ALTR reaction seen in the DMN implant is unlikely to be influenced by polyethylene debris. There have been extensive publications in the literature about wear rates of highly cross-linked polyethylene in vivo, and for the X3, femoral head penetration rates remain low at two years (head penetration <0.06 mm) [43]. Moreover, between years 1 and 5, wear rates in vivo were less than 0.001 mm/year [44]. This data suggests that polyethylene wear is unlikely to contribute to the observed reaction to ALTR seen in our study in the DMN group. This is further corroborated by the fact that only 1 of 54 cases examined in our study had polyethylene debris in their periprosthetic tissue at light microscopy, suggesting that polyethylene debris is unlikely to play a major role in ALTR seen in our study.

Immunohistochemistry results showed a predominant T lymphocytic response with a variable B cell component with the formation in some cases of perivascular germinal centers and tall endothelial cell venules as previously reported [13-17,19]. The analysis of the T cell population pointed towards a mixed pattern with predominant GATA3 positivity (Th2 lymphocytes) but also substantial T-bet and FOXP3 expressing lymphocytes, representing Th1 and Treg subgroups respectively. These findings were associated with the presence of a population of macrophages strongly positive for CD163, a marker of M2 macrophages, a subset frequently correlated with Th2 cytokines [45]. The frequent finding of a variable number of CD117 positive mast cells is also a new important finding with implications in reaction initiation/progression due to their interactions between T and B cell lymphocytes and eosinophils, and their potential to produce M2 inducing cytokines such as IL-4 [46]. Reaction initiation and severity may be explained by the release of chemokines from macrophages under oxidative stress and/or direct lymphocyte cytotoxicity [47-50]. Similar lymphocyte distributions were observed in the cases of osteoarthritis at time zero, and the possibility of a non-specific common pathway in different inflammatory conditions of the synovial membrane not representative of the initial response of the adverse reaction must be considered and confirmatory studies with testing of other specific antibodies are needed. It is also possible that the lymphocyte distributions seen in our study reflect an innate immunologic profile of the synovium with subsequent adaptive modulation, and analysis of pathologic gene expression patterns could be helpful to elucidate the role of these lymphocytic subpopulations in initiation and progression of ALTR [51]. Collectively, the immunohistochemistry studies indicate a complex adaptive immune response potentially involving several cell types. Future molecular analysis will help define the signaling pathways that orchestrate the tissue necrosis and other pathologies underlying ALTR.

The main limitation of this study is the attempt to reconstruct the natural history of the reaction based on one cross sectional observation at the time of implant revision. We compensated for this limitation by extensive topographical sampling of the periprosthetic soft tissue, but we acknowledge that continued longitudinal observation would be needed to confirm our findings.

## Conclusion

In conclusion, a common spectrum of neo-synovial proliferation and subsequent necrosis are observed in both implant classes. These findings can represent temporal progression of the reaction, which could have implant-based and patient-based characteristics. The Campbell-ALVAL score would represent an index of the staging of this temporal progression and not of the grading of the severity of ALTR. Cellular composition showed subtle differences in macrophagic and lymphocytic distributions in the two implant classes, suggesting biological differences may exist between different implant classes. The prominence of corrosion products is a consistent feature of ALTR in both implant types; however, their morphologies differ based on implant design. Immunohistochemistry showed a complex adaptive immune response, and future studies on molecular signaling pathways in ALTR are needed. The immunogenicity and toxicity of the new particulate material formed at the implant interacting surfaces and their association with hematopoietic marrow cells are still unknown, especially in patients with pre-existing immunologic disease. Short- and long-term follow-up of all patients affected by ALTR is needed to monitor for local and systemic effects.

## Abbreviations
ALTR: Adverse local tissue reaction; DMN: Dual-modular neck implant; MoM: Metal-on-metal implant; THA: Total hip arthroplasty; ALVAL: Aseptic lymphocyte dominated vasculitis-associated lesions.

## Competing interests
There are no competing financial or non-financial interests in direct relation to this manuscript for any authors. Author S Jerabek is a consultant for Mako Surgical Corporation.

## Authors' contributions
GP conceived of the study, collected and analyzed synovial tissue, and drafted the manuscript. BR assisted with histologic and immunohistochemistry analysis and drafted the manuscript. SAJ analyzed the clinical data. GM performed immunohistochemistry and assisted with study design. GW and DM collected synovial tissue and assisted with manuscript preparation. SRG participated in study design and interpretation of data. PEP participated in study design and coordination. All authors read and approved the final manuscript.

## Acknowledgements
We would like to acknowledge the surgeons of the Adult Reconstruction and Joint Replacement Service at the Hospital for Special Surgery for providing periprosthetic tissue for this study; Irina Shuleshko and Yana Bronfman for technical assistance in histology preparation; Licia Montagna, Claudia Parolini, and Paola Piccoli at University of Verona for immunohistochemistry staining; and Philip Rusli for technical assistance for preparation of the manuscript.

## Author details
[1]Department of Pathology, Hospital for Special Surgery, 535 East 70th Street, New York, NY 10021, USA. [2]Department of Orthopedic Surgery, Hospital for Special Surgery, New York, NY, USA. [3]Department of Pathology and Diagnostics, University of Verona, Verona and Pederzoli Hospital, Peschiera, Italy. [4]Division of Research, Hospital for Special Surgery, New York, NY, USA.

## References
1. Amstutz HC, Grigoris P: Metal on metal bearings in hip arthroplasty. *Clin Orthop Relat Res* 1996, 329(Suppl):S11–S34.
2. Srinivasan A, Jung E, Levine BR: Modularity of the femoral component in total hip arthroplasty. *J Am Acad Orthop Surg* 2012, 20:214–222.
3. Cohen D: How safe are metal-on-metal hip implants? *BMJ* 2012, 344: e1410.
4. Kop AM, Swarts E: Corrosion of a hip stem with a modular neck taper junction: a retrieval study of 16 cases. *J Arthroplasty* 2009, 24:1019–1023.
5. Huber M, Reinisch G, Trettenhahn G, Zweymüller K, Lintner F: Presence of corrosion products and hypersensitivity-associated reactions in periprosthetic tissue after aseptic loosening of total hip replacements with metal bearing surfaces. *Acta Biomater* 2009, 5:172–180.
6. Bosker BH, Ettema HB, Boomsma MF, Kollen BJ, Maas M, Verheyen CC: **High incidence of pseudotumour formation after large-diameter metal-on-metal total hip replacement: a prospective cohort study.** *J Bone Joint Surg Br* 2012, 94:755–761.
7. Chana R, Esposito C, Campbell PA, Walter WK, Walter WL: **Mixing and matching causing taper wear: corrosion associated with pseudotumour formation.** *J Bone Joint Surg Br* 2012, 94:281–286.
8. Fabi D, Levine B, Paprosky W, Della Valle C, Sporer S, Klein G, Levine H, Hartzband M: **Metal-on-metal total hip arthroplasty: causes and high incidence of early failure.** *Orthopedics* 2012, 35:e1009–e1016.
9. Gill IP, Webb J, Sloan K, Beaver RJ: **Corrosion at the neck-stem junction as a cause of metal ion release and pseudotumour formation.** *J Bone Joint Surg Br* 2012, 94:895–900.
10. Meyer H, Mueller T, Goldau G, Chamaon K, Ruetschi M, Lohmann CH: **Corrosion at the cone/taper interface leads to failure of large-diameter metal-on-metal total hip arthroplasties.** *Clin Orthop Relat Res* 2012, 470:3101–3108.
11. Cooper HJ, Urban RM, Wixson RL, Meneghini RM, Jacobs JJ: **Adverse local tissue reaction arising from corrosion at the femoral neck-body junction in a dual-taper stem with a cobalt-chromium modular neck.** *J Bone Joint Surg Am* 2013, 95:865–872.
12. Werner SD, Bono JV, Nandi S, Ward DM, Talmo CT: **Adverse tissue reactions in modular exchangeable neck implants: a report of two cases.** *J Arthroplasty* 2013, 28:543.e13–5.
13. Davies AP, Willert HG, Campbell PA, Learmonth ID, Case CP: **An unusual lymphocytic perivascular infiltration in tissues around contemporary metal-on-metal joint replacements.** *J Bone Joint Surg Am* 2005, 87:18–27.
14. Willert HG, Buchhorn GH, Fayyazi A, Flury R, Windler M, Köster G, Lohmann CH: **Metal-on-metal bearings and hypersensitivity in patients with artificial hip joints. A clinical and histomorphological study.** *J Bone Joint Surg Am* 2005, 87:28–36.
15. Mahendra G, Pandit H, Kliskey K, Murray D, Gill HS, Athanasou N: **Necrotic and vinflammatory changes in metal-on-metal resurfacing hip arthroplasties.** *Acta Orthop* 2009, 80:653–659.
16. Campbell P, Ebramzadeh E, Nelson S, Takamura K, De Smet K, Amstutz HC: **Histological features of pseudotumor-like tissues from metal-on-metal hips.** *Clin Orthop Relat Res* 2010, 468:2321–2327.
17. Natu S, Sidaginamale RP, Gandhi J, Langton DJ, Nargol AV: **Adverse reactions to metal debris: histopathological features of periprosthetic soft tissue reactions seen in association with failed metal on metal hip arthroplasties.** *J Clin Pathol* 2012, 65:409–418.
18. Grammatopoulos G, Pandit H, Kamali A, Maggiani F, Glyn-Jones S, Gill HS, Murray DW, Athanasou N: **The correlation of wear with histological features after failed hip resurfacing arthroplasty.** *J Bone Joint Surg Am* 2013, 95:e81.
19. Mittal S, Revell M, Barone F, Hardie DL, Matharu GS, Davenport AJ, Martin RA, Grant M, Mosselmans F, Pynsent P, Sumathi VP, Addison O, Revell PA, Buckley CD: **Lymphoid aggregates that resemble tertiary lymphoid organs define a specific pathological subset in metal-on-metal hip replacements.** *PLoS One* 2013, 8:e63470.
20. Gallo J, Vaculova J, Goodman SB, Konttinen YT, Thyssen JP: **Contributions of human tissue analysis to understanding the mechanisms of loosening and osteolysis in total hip replacement.** *Acta Biomater* 2014, 10:2354–2366.
21. Cooper HJ, Della Valle CJ, Berger RA, Tetreault M, Paprosky WG, Sporer SM, Jacobs JJ: **Corrosion at the head-neck taper as a cause for adverse local tissue reactions after total hip arthroplasty.** *J Bone Joint Surg Am* 2012, 94:1655–1661.
22. Fricka KB, Ho H, Peace WJ, Engh CA Jr: **Metal-on-metal local tissue reaction is associated with corrosion of the head taper junction.** *J Arthroplasty* 2012, 27(8 Suppl):26–31.e1.
23. Dyrkacz RM, Brandt JM, Ojo OA, Turgeon TR, Wyss UP: **The influence of head size on corrosion and fretting behaviour at the head-neck interface of artificial hip joints.** *J Arthroplasty* 2013, 28:1036–1040.
24. Hayter CL, Gold SL, Koff MF, Perino G, Nawabi DH, Miller TT, Potter HG: **MRI findings in painful metal-on-metal hip arthroplasty.** *AJR Am J Roentgenol* 2012, 199:884–893.
25. Nawabi DH, Hayter CL, Su EP, Koff MF, Perino G, Gold SL, Koch KM, Potter HG: **Magnetic resonance imaging findings in symptomatic versus**

asymptomatic subjects following metal-on-metal hip resurfacing arthroplasty. *J Bone Joint Surg Am* 2013, **95**:895–902.

26. Nawabi DH, Gold S, Lyman S, Fields K, Padgett DE, Potter HG: **MRI Predicts ALVAL and tissue damage in metal-on-metal hip arthroplasty.** *Clin Orthop Relat Res* 2014, **472**:471–481.

27. Nawabi DH, Nassif NA, Do HT, Stoner K, Elpers M, Su EP, Wright T, Potter HG, Padgett DE: **What causes unexplained pain in patients with metal-on metal hip devices? A retrieval, histologic, and imaging analysis.** *Clin Orthop Relat Res* 2014, **472**:543–554.

28. Willert HG, Semlisch M: **Reactions of the articular capsule to wear products of artificial joint prostheses.** *J Biomed Mater Res* 1977, **11**:157–164.

29. Holness CL, Simmons DL: **Molecular cloning of CD68, a human macrophage marker related to lysosomal glycoproteins.** *Blood* 1993, **81**:1607–1613.

30. Wang FQ, Chen G, Zhu JY, Zhang W, Ren JG, Liu H, Sun ZJ, Jia J, Zhao YF: **M2-polarised macrophages in infantile haemangiomas: correlation with promoted angiogenesis.** *J Clin Pathol* 2013, **66**:1058–1064.

31. Zheng W, Flavell RA: **The transcription factor GATA-3 is necessary and sufficient for Th2 cytokine gene expression in CD4 T cells.** *Cell* 1997, **89**:587–596.

32. Szabo SJ, Kim ST, Costa GL, Zhang X, Fathman CG, Glimcher LH: **A novel transcription factor, T-bet, directs Th1 lineage commitment.** *Cell* 2000, **100**:655–669.

33. Hori S, Nomura T, Sakaguchi S: **Control of regulatory T cell development by the transcription factor Foxp3.** *Science* 2003, **299**:1057–1061.

34. Iemura A, Tsai M, Ando A, Wershil BK, Galli SJ: **The c-kit ligand, stem cell factor, promotes mast cell survival by suppressing apoptosis.** *Am J Pathol* 1994, **144**:321–328.

35. Jacobs JJ, Urban RM, Gilbert JL, Skipor AK, Black J, Jasty M, Galante JO: **Local and distant products from modularity.** *Clin Orthop Relat Res* 1995, **319**:94–105.

36. Jacobs JJ, Gilbert JL, Urban RM: **Corrosion of metal orthopaedic implants.** *J Bone Joint Surg Am* 1998, **80**:268–282.

37. Berstock JR, Baker RP, Bannister GC, Case CP: **Histology of failed metal-on metal hip arthroplasty; three distinct sub-types.** *Hip Int* 2014, **5**:0.

38. Langton DJ, Joyce TJ, Jameson SS, Lord J, Van Orsouw M, Holland JP, Nargol AV, De Smet KA: **Adverse reaction to metal debris following hip resurfacing: the influence of component type, orientation and volumetric wear.** *J Bone Joint Surg Br* 2011, **93**:164–171.

39. Lindgren JU, Brismar BH, Wikstrom AC: **Adverse reaction to metal release from a modular metal-on-polyethylene hip prosthesis.** *J Bone Joint Surg Br* 2011, **93**:1427–1430.

40. Hinsch A, Vettorazzi E, Morlock MM, Rüther W, Amling M, Zustin J: **Sex differences in the morphological failure patterns following hip resurfacing arthroplasty.** *BMC Med* 2011, **9**:113.

41. Xia Z, Kwon YM, Mehmood S, Downing C, Jurkschat K, Murray DW: **Characterization of metal-wear nanoparticles in pseudotumor following metal-on-metal hip resurfacing.** *Nanomedicine* 2011, **7**:674–681.

42. Caicedo MS, Samelko L, McAllister K, Jacobs JJ, Hallab NJ: **Increasing both CoCrMo-alloy particle size and surface irregularity induces increased macrophage inflammasome activation in vitro potentially through lysosomal destabilization mechanisms.** *J Orthop Res* 2013, **31**:1633–1642.

43. Campbell DG, Field JR, Callary SA: **Second-generation highly cross-linked X3™ polyethylene wear: a preliminary radiostereometric analysis study.** *Clin Orthop Relat Res* 2010, **468**:2704–2709.

44. Callary SA, Field JR, Campbell DG: **Low wear of a second-generation highly crosslinked polyethylene liner: a 5-year radiostereometric analysis study.** *Clin Orthop Relat Res* 2013, **471**:3596–3600.

45. Mills CD: **M1 and M2 macrophages: oracles of health and disease.** *Crit Rev Immunol* 2012, **32**:463–488.

46. Amin K: **The role of mast cells in allergic inflammation.** *Respir Med* 2012, **106**:9–14.

47. Caicedo MS, Desai R, McAllister K, Reddy A, Jacobs JJ, Hallab NJ: **Soluble and particulate Co Cr-Mo alloy implant metals activate the inflammasome danger signaling pathway in human macrophages: a novel mechanism for implant debris reactivity.** *J Orthop Res* 2009, **27**:847–854.

48. Cobelli N, Scharf B, Crisi GM, Hardin J, Santambrogio L: **Mediators of the inflammatory response to joint replacement devices.** *Nat Rev Rheumatol* 2011, **7**:600–608.

49. Vanlangenakker N, Vanden Berghe T, Vandenabeele P: **Many stimuli pull the necrotic trigger, an overview.** *Cell Death Differ* 2012, **19**:75–86.

50. Samelko L, Caicedo MS, Lim SJ, Della-Valle C, Jacobs J, Hallab NJ: **Cobalt-alloy implant debris induce HIF-1α hypoxia associated responses: a mechanism for metal-specific orthopedic implant failure.** *PLoS One* 2013, **8**:e67127.

51. Fujishiro T, Moojen DJ, Kobayashi N, Dhert WJ, Bauer TW: **Perivascular and diffuse lymphocytic inflammation are not specific for failed metal-on metal hip implants.** *Clin Orthop Relat Res* 2011, **469**:1127–1133.

# 2

# Histological findings in infants with Gastrointestinal food allergy are associated with specific gastrointestinal symptoms

Neil Shah[1,3*†], Ru-Xin Melanie Foong[1†], Osvaldo Borrelli[1], Eleni Volonaki[1], Robert Dziubak[1], Rosan Meyer[1], Mamoun Elawad[1] and Neil J. Sebire[2]

## Abstract

**Background:** Gastrointestinal food allergy (GIFA) occurs in 2 to 4 % of children, the majority of whom are infants (<1 year of age). Although endoscopy is considered the gold standard for diagnosing GIFA, it is invasive and requires general anaesthesia. Therefore, we aimed to investigate whether in infants with GIFA, gastrointestinal symptoms predict histological findings in order to help optimise the care pathway for such patients.

**Methods:** All infants <1 year of age over a 20 year period who underwent an endoscopic procedure gastroscopy or colonoscopy for GIFA were evaluated for the study. Symptoms at presentation were reviewed and compared with mucosal biopsy histological findings, which were initially broadly classified for study purposes as "Normal" or "Abnormal" (defined as the presence of any mucosal inflammation by the reporting pathologist at the time of biopsy).

**Results:** Of a total of 1319 cases, 544 fitted the inclusion criteria. 62 % of mucosal biopsy series in this group were reported as abnormal. Infants presenting with diarrhoea, rectal (PR) bleeding, irritability and urticaria in any combination had a probability >85 % (OR > 5.67) of having abnormal histological findings compared to those without. Those with isolated PR bleeding or diarrhoea were associated with 74 % and 68 % probability (OR: 2.85 and 2.13) of an abnormal biopsy, respectively. Conversely, children presenting with faltering growth or reflux/vomiting showed any abnormal mucosal histology in only 50.8 % and 45.3 % (OR: 1.04 and 0.82) respectively.

**Conclusions:** Food allergy may occur in very young children and is difficult to diagnose. Since endoscopy in infants has significant risks, stratification of decision-making may be aided by symptoms. At least one mucosal biopsy demonstrated an abnormal finding in around half of cases in this selected population. Infants presenting with diarrhoea, PR bleeding, urticaria and irritability are most likely to demonstrate abnormal histological findings.

**Keywords:** Endoscopy, Infant, Food allergy, Biopsy, Histopathology, Eosinophil

## Background

Gastrointestinal food allergy (GIFA) is increasing in prevalence and usually affects very young children [1]. Approximately 2-4 % of children between the ages of 0-3 years are diagnosed with food allergy [2, 3] and up to 60 % of these children display gastrointestinal symptoms

such as abdominal pain, poor appetite, vomiting and diarrhoea. Other children may present with symptoms affecting skin, such as eczema, catarrhal problems or even anaphylaxis. Clinically, symptoms are often very pronounced and warrant investigations to eliminate other diagnoses before food allergy is considered [2, 4, 5]. Normally, the mucosal barrier in the gastrointestinal (GI) tract develops an "oral tolerance" to food antigens ingested [6]. However, in children with food allergy, this mechanism is believed to fail, resulting in allergic sensitisation and elicitation of allergy-type responses [6, 7]. This reaction, which

* Correspondence: neil.shah@gosh.nhs.uk
†Equal contributors
[1]Paediatric Gastroenterology Department, Great Ormond Street Hospital, London WC1N 3JH, United Kingdom
[3]Institute of Child Health/UCL, London WC1N 1EH, UK
Full list of author information is available at the end of the article

can manifest as a wide range of different symptoms, can be classified as immunoglobulin E (IgE)-mediated allergy, non-IgE mediated allergy or mixed IgE and non-IgE allergy [8]. Gastrointestinal food allergies (GIFA) are generally considered as non-IgE mediated, but eosinophilic dominant gastrointestinal disorders may be mixed IgE and non-IgE allergies. The most common age of presentation of non-IgE mediated allergies affecting the gut is in children under the age of one year, with cow's milk, soy protein, hens' egg and wheat being the most frequent causative foods [2, 4, 5, 9, 10].

The immunopathology of non-IgE mediated GIFA is still not fully understood, which makes diagnosis and management difficult, often requiring an elimination diet followed by food challenge [8, 11]. Endoscopy and biopsy has become increasingly important, with some considering endoscopic biopsy as the gold standard since it is relatively objective and may provide information regarding possible mechanisms. [4, 7] For example, in eosinophilic oesophagitis, the histological appearance defines the diagnosis [12]. However, endoscopy for very young children is often limited to specialised centres and involves general anaesthesia, requiring administration by paediatric anaesthetists, and procedural risks such as intestinal perforation [13, 14]. There are no studies investigating gastrointestinal symptoms in relation to histological features in infant GIFA [15]. Hence, the aim of this study was to investigate whether specific symptoms are associated with abnormal histological findings in endoscopic biopsies obtained from children with GIFA in order to optimise care pathway decision making.

## Methods

Routinely collected data was reviewed from children under the age of one-year referred to a tertiary paediatric gastroenterology centre during the study period (June 1987 to August 2007), who had undergone endoscopic biopsy. Jejunal biopsies performed by the now historical procedure of Crosby capsule (common in the early years of our study) were excluded, and we also excluded children biopsied for other indications unrelated to GIFA. For all cases clinical symptoms were assessed in relation to histopathological findings based on contemporaneous biopsy reports. A single researcher extracted data according to predefined objective criteria.

All biopsies were reported by specialist paediatric histopathologists from the same tertiary centre. For the purposes of this study, histopathological findings were coded as either "Normal" or "Abnormal" (presence of any significant abnormal finding at any biopsy site including acute or chronic inflammation, with or without increased mucosal eosinophil density [16], or other pathologies such as partial villous atrophy or *Helicobacter pylori* see Fig. 1). Chronic inflammation with predominantly excess mucosal eosinophil density was considered most suggestive of food allergy in this cohort of young children [12, 17, 18].

Data were analysed using IBM SPSS Statistics for Windows, Version 22 (Armonk, NY). Continuous variables

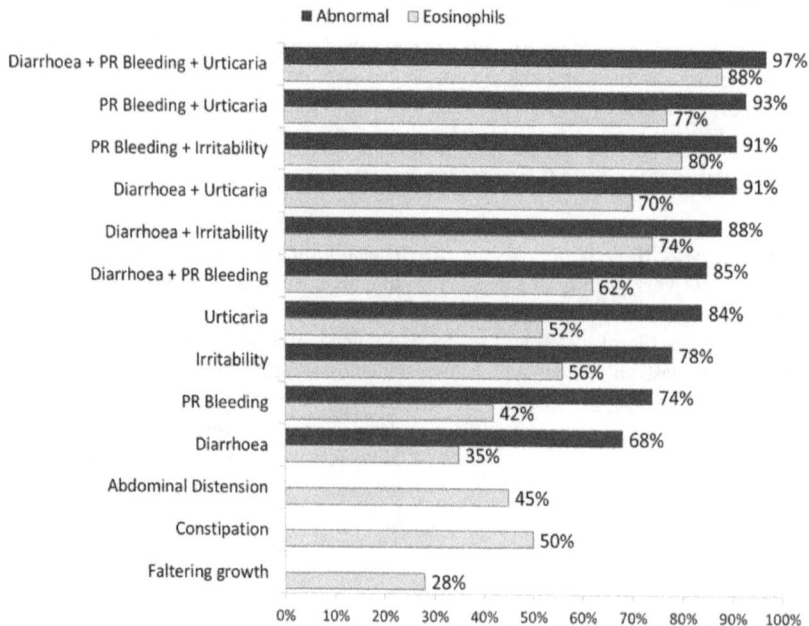

**Fig. 1** Frequencies of abnormal biopsy findings for single symptoms and combinations of symptoms common to two regression models

were presented as medians with interquartile ranges and categorical variables as frequencies and percentages. Mann-Whitney $U$ test and chi-square test were used to examine the differences between groups.

For all symptoms in isolation (in cases when the patient presented with only one symptom) Positive Predictive Values (PPV) of abnormal biopsy findings were calculated. Multiple logistic regression was used to investigate the relationship between biopsy findings and symptoms with adjustment for potential confounders of age and gender. Based on logistic regression models, probabilities of abnormal biopsy findings were calculated for combinations of symptoms using the median age. Goodness of fit of logistic regression models was based on Hosmer-Lemeshow test. All tests were two-tailed and significance level was set to 0.05. The study was approved by the local Research Ethics Committee (Bloomsbury REC). All data was retrospective and identified by study number only and individual patient consent was not required for data inclusion. The study conformed to the Helsinki declaration regarding research performance.

## Results

Of 1319 infants undergoing endoscopic biopsies, 318 were excluded due to insufficient clinical information, 265 due to being Crosby capsule biopsies and 60 due to specific non GIFA indications (congenital diarrhoea, autoimmune enteropathy, graft-versus-host disease, tufting enteropathy and disaccharidase deficiency), leaving 676 patients who met the inclusion criteria. Some patients had multiple endoscopies and repeat biopsies, 122 in total, which were also excluded and only the initial presentation biopsy included. 554 endoscopic biopsy series were therefore included. Fifty-one per cent (285/554) were male, median age 7 months (IQR = 0.2-12 months). Overall, 62 % (344/554) had abnormal mucosal biopsy findings. The median age of those with abnormal biopsy was significantly lower than those with normal findings (median 6.6 months versus median 7.5 months, $P < 0.001$).

The most common presenting symptoms as indications for endoscopy were reflux/vomiting (40 %), faltering growth (37 %), diarrhoea (35 %) and rectal (PR) bleeding (12 %). 309 (56 %) patients presented with one symptom, 190 (34 %) with two, 49 (9 %) with three and six patients (1 %) with four symptoms. Positive predictive values (PPV) for symptoms based on the patients who presented with one symptom ($n = 309$) are shown in Table 1.

Diarrhoea was associated with a significantly greater frequency of abnormal histological findings than faltering growth (70.8 % vs. 50.8 %, $p = 0.018$) or reflux (70.8 % vs. 45.3 %, $p = 0.001$). PR bleeding was associated with a significantly greater rate of abnormal histological

findings than faltering growth (74.2 % vs. 50.8 %, $p = 0.031$) or reflux (74.2 % vs. 45.3 %, $p = 0.004$). There were no significant differences between the frequency of abnormal biopsies between those presenting with diarrhoea and PR Bleeding, ($p = 0.728$) or those presenting with reflux and faltering growth, ($p = 0.484$).

Multiple logistic regression models were used to assess the frequency of any abnormal biopsy findings with combinations of symptoms (Hosmer-Lemeshow $p = 0.373$), as well as the probability of increased mucosal eosinophil density (Hosmer-Lemeshow $p = 0.413$), adjusted for differences in age and gender. Diarrhoea ($p < 0.001$), PR bleeding ($p < 0.01$), irritability ($p < 0.05$) and urticaria ($p < 0.05$) were significantly associated with both abnormal biopsy and excess eosinophils (Table 2). The site, Oesophagus, stomach, duodenum or colon, of the abnormal findings are shown in Table 3. Faltering growth, constipation and abdominal distension were also predictors of finding eosinophils in a biopsy ($p < 0.05$, $p < 0.01$, $p < 0.05$ respectively; Table 2). Age was an important confounding factor as we found a higher probability of an abnormal biopsy in younger children. Among others, reflux/vomiting was a poor predictor; therefore it was excluded from the models. Similarly, gender was not a significant confounding factor.

Specific symptom combinations were more likely to have biopsies with excess eosinophils present. For example, children who presented with a combination of diarrhoea, PR bleeding and urticaria had an 88 % frequency of excess eosinophils.

## Discussion

This is the first large study to examine whether specific symptoms at presentation in very young children are associated with abnormal endoscopic biopsy findings in children being assessed for GIFA. The findings demonstrate that younger infants are more likely to have abnormal mucosal histological findings, and those presenting with specific combinations of symptoms are associated with high frequency of abnormal mucosal biopsy findings, including increased mucosal eosinophil density. In the current patient population, first presentation of GI symptoms occurred at around five months of age. However, it is likely that this represents a highly selected group referred to a specialist centre who are likely to have been experiencing more severe symptoms and hence were evaluated earlier in life than the general population and were all deemed to have symptoms of sufficient severity to warrant endoscopic examination. The risks of undergoing a general anaesthetic procedure and associated potential complications involved in performing endoscopy in very young infants as well as the impact on families are important considerations when deciding on whether to perform an endoscopy [13, 14, 19].

**Table 1** Positive Predictive Values (PPV) of abnormal mucosal biopsies in infants being assessed for GIFA based on a single presenting gastrointestinal symptom based on 309/554 patients who presented with one symptom only

| | Number | Percent | Isolated increased mucosal eosinophil density | PPV | Any abnormal biopsy | PPV |
|---|---|---|---|---|---|---|
| | | | n | | n | |
| Reflux/vomiting | 117 | 37.9 % | 19 | 16.2 % | 53 | 45.3 % |
| Diarrhoea | 72 | 23.3 % | 30 | 41.7 % | 51 | 70.8 % |
| Faltering growth | 61 | 19.7 % | 19 | 31.1 % | 31 | 50.8 % |
| PR Bleeding | 31 | 10.0 % | 16 | 51.6 % | 23 | 74.2 % |
| Haematemesis | 7 | 2.3 % | 1 | 14.3 % | 4 | 57.1 % |
| Constipation | 6 | 1.9 % | 3 | 50.0 % | 3 | 50.0 % |
| Feeding difficulties | 4 | 1.3 % | 0 | 0.0 % | 0 | 0.0 % |
| Irritability | 4 | 1.3 % | 1 | 25.0 % | 2 | 50.0 % |
| Anaemia | 2 | 0.6 % | 0 | 0.0 % | 0 | 0.0 % |
| Hypoalbuminaemia | 2 | 0.6 % | 0 | 0.0 % | 2 | 100.0 % |
| Abdominal distension | 2 | 0.6 % | 1 | 50.0 % | 1 | 50.0 % |
| Recurrent Abdominal pain | 1 | 0.3 % | 0 | 0.0 % | 1 | 100.0 % |

The most common symptoms were diarrhoea, reflux/vomiting, PR bleeding and faltering growth. Of these, if isolated, infants presenting with diarrhoea or PR bleeding, had an approximate 70 % probability of a histologically abnormal biopsy. However, infants who presented with combinations of diarrhoea, PR bleeding, irritability and urticaria were both more likely to have abnormal biopsy findings and also more likely to demonstrate increased mucosal eosinophil density. For example, almost 90 % of those presenting with diarrhoea and irritability had an abnormal biopsy. There were few patients who presented with irritability in isolation (1.3 %). However, it is possible that parents and clinicians underreport this symptom especially in the presence of other more common and recognisable symptoms. [20, 21] The frequency of an abnormal biopsy was lower for infants presenting with reflux/vomiting (45 %) and faltering growth (51 %).

Food allergic diagnoses are classified according to the site and severity of inflammation, which influences the presenting symptoms. With gastrointestinal mucosal disease that is identified by endoscopic biopsy there is a close spatial relationship of inflammatory mediators known to be released by mucosal inflammatory cells and enteric nerves [2]. The exact mechanisms of the manifestations of gastrointestinal symptoms are slowly being unravelled with the concept of paracrine immune interaction on the enteric nervous system, being known as a neuro-immune interaction [22, 23] leading to the disturbed motility and symptoms seen in GIFA such as reflux, diarrhoea or constipation. Much workstill needs to be done to fully explain how these symptoms develop and respond to dietary or anti-inflammatory measures.

Limitations of the study are related to the retrospective nature of data collected over a long time period with possible associated variation in the clinical suspicion of GIFA and management of such infants by endoscopic examination and biopsy. In GIFA, despite adherence to the diagnosis only being made by clinicians in out unit

**Table 2** Multiple logistic regression models for association with abnormal mucosal biopsies in infants being assessed for GIFA

| | Regression model for excess eosinophils in biopsy | | Regression model for any Abnormal Biopsy | |
|---|---|---|---|---|
| Variables in the model | B | p-value | B | p-value |
| Constant | −0.96 | 0.001 | 0.49 | 0.05 |
| Age (months) | −0.07 | 0.033 | −0.06 | 0.041 |
| Urticaria | 1.50 | 0.007 | 1.59 | 0.038 |
| Irritability | 1.69 | <0.001 | 1.22 | 0.018 |
| PR Bleeding | 1.12 | < 0.001 | 1.00 | 0.002 |
| Diarrhoea | 0.79 | < 0.001 | 0.71 | < 0.001 |
| Constipation | 1.42 | 0.002 | n/a | n/a |
| Abdominal Distension | 1.24 | 0.045 | n/a | n/a |
| Faltering growth | 0.49 | 0.016 | n/a | n/a |

**Table 3** Symptoms related to the site of abnormal findings in cases with only a single site affected

|  | Oesophagus (n = 61) | Percent | Stomach (n = 16) | Percent | Duodenum (n = 50) | Percent | Colon (n = 44) | Percent |
|---|---|---|---|---|---|---|---|---|
| Reflux/Vomiting | 44 | 72 % | 5 | 31 % | 19 | 38 % | 15 | 34 % |
| FTT | 18 | 30 % | 5 | 31 % | 26 | 52 % | 18 | 41 % |
| Diarrhoea | 5 | 8 % | 6 | 38 % | 19 | 38 % | 18 | 41 % |
| PR Bleeding | 3 | 5 % | 0 | 0 % | 5 | 10 % | 10 | 23 % |
| Constipation | 0 | 0 % | 2 | 13 % | 3 | 6 % | 8 | 18 % |
| Anaemia | 0 | 0 % | 0 | 0 % | 0 | 0 % | 2 | 5 % |
| Feed Diff | 2 | 3 % | 2 | 13 % | 3 | 6 % | 2 | 5 % |
| Mouth Ulcers | 0 | 0 % | 0 | 0 % | 0 | 0 % | 0 | 0 % |
| Rash | 1 | 2 % | 0 | 0 % | 3 | 6 % | 2 | 5 % |
| Irritability | 2 | 3 % | 1 | 6 % | 4 | 8 % | 5 | 11 % |
| Haematemesis | 6 | 10 % | 3 | 19 % | 1 | 2 % | 0 | 0 % |
| Hypoalbuminaemia | 0 | 0 % | 1 | 6 % | 2 | 4 % | 1 | 2 % |
| Abd. Distension | 1 | 2 % | 0 | 0 % | 1 | 2 % | 5 | 11 % |
| RAP | 1 | 2 % | 0 | 0 % | 0 | 0 % | 3 | 7 % |

following elimination diet of major dietary antigens (Diary, egg, soya and wheat usually) with clinical improvement and subsequent reappearance of symptoms on rechallenge, the diagnosis remains subjective. The symptoms can be delayed and is unblended and subject to parental reporting. Furthermore, even with such a large dataset, for the purposes of this study we have classified mucosal biopsy findings broadly into normal versus abnormal, (with the only subcategory being those with apparently isolated increased mucosal eosinophil density at any site since this has been suggested as the most characteristic feature of GIFA) [12, 24]. More detailed sub-analysis of the relationship between other specific histological findings and their combinations with symptoms is not possible in this dataset and much larger numbers of cases, all of whom undergo multiple biopsies from small and large intestinal sites, would be required, but is unlikely to be available.

The clinical decision regarding whether an infant requires endoscopic examination and biopsy for diagnosis of food allergy can be difficult, since the procedure in this age group requires general anaesthesia with associated risks. The current data demonstrates that specific symptom patterns at presentation are associated with varying yield of abnormal mucosal histological findings, in particular, infants who experience diarrhoea, PR bleeding, irritability and urticaria having a high frequency of abnormal biopsies. This information may aid the decision making process for young children presenting with probable food allergy.

## Conclusions

Gastrointestinal food allergy (GIFA), may present with a wide variety of symptoms in the first year of life and specific symptom patterns at presentation are associated with varying yield of abnormal mucosal histological findings at endoscopic biopsy. Infants who experience diarrhoea, PR bleeding, irritability and urticaria have a high frequency of abnormal gastrointestinal mucosal biopsies, including prominent mucosal eosinophils.

**Competing interests**
Dr Shah has performed consultancy work for Mead Johnson Nutrition, unrelated to this project. The other authors declare that they have no competing interests and have not received reimbursements, fees, funding, or salary from an organization that may in any way gain or lose financially from the publication of this manuscript, either now or in the future.

**Authors' contributions**
NS, ME and NJS conceived and planned the study. RMF, EV, RD and RM performed the data extraction and analysis. All authors participated in drafting of the manuscript and read and approved the final manuscript.

**Acknowledgements**
NJS is part supported by an NIHR Senior Investigator award and the NIHR GOSH BRC. This report is independent research and the views expressed in this publication are those of the authors and not necessarily those of the NHS, the NIHR or the Department of Health.

**Author details**
[1]Paediatric Gastroenterology Department, Great Ormond Street Hospital, London WC1N 3JH, United Kingdom. [2]Histopathology Department, Great Ormond Street Hospital, London, United Kingdom. [3]Institute of Child Health/ UCL, London WC1N 1EH, UK.

**References**
1. Prescott SL, Pawankar R, Allen KJ, et al. A global survey of changing patterns of food allergy burden in children. World Allergy Organ J. 2013;6:21.
2. Meyer R, Schwarz C, Shah N. A Review of the Diagnosis and Management of Food-induced Gastrointestinal Allergies. Curr Allergy Clin Immunol. 2012;25:10–7.
3. Venter C, Pereira B, Voigt K, et al. Prevalence and cumulative incidence of food hypersensitivity in the first 3 years of life. Allergy. 2008;63:354–9.

4.   Maloney J, Nowak-Wegrzyn A. Educational clinical case series for pediatric allergy and immunology: Allergic proctocolitis, food protein-induced enterocolitis syndrome and allergic eosinophilic gastroenteritis with protein-losing gastroenteropathy as manifestations of non-IgE-mediated cow's milk allergy. Pediatr Allerg Immunol. 2007;18:360–7.

5.   Meyer R, Fleming C, Dominguez-Ortega G, et al. Manifestations of food protein induced gastrointestinal allergies presenting to a single tertiary paediatric gastroenterology unit. World Allergy Organ J. 2013;6:13–6.

6.   Dupont C. Food allergy: recent Advances in Pathophysiology and Diagnosis. Ann Nutr Metab. 2011;59:8–18.

7.   Vickery BP, Chin S, Burks AW. Pathophysiology of Food Allergy. Pediatr Clin North Am. 2011;58:363–76.

8.   Boyce JA, Assaad A, Burks AW, et al. Guidelines for the Diagnosis and Management of Food Allergy in the United States: Summary of the NIAID-Sponsored Expert Panel Report. Nutr Res. 2011;31:61–75.

9.   Husby S. Food Allergy as Seen by a Paediatric Gastroenterologist. J Ped Gast Nutr. 2008;47:S49–52.

10.  Fogg MI, Spergel JM. Management of food allergies. Expert Opin Pharmacother. 2003;4:1025–37.

11.  Sicherer SH, Sampson HA. Food Allergy. J Allergy Clin Immunol. 2010;125:S116–25.

12.  Liacouras CA, Furuta GT, Hirano I, et al. Eosinophilic esophagitis: Updated consensus recommendations for children and adults. J Allergy Clin Immunol. 2011;128:3–20.

13.  Jimenez SG, Catto-Smith AG. Impact of day-case gastroscopy on children and their families. J Gast Hepatol. 2008;23:379–84.

14.  Ammar MS, Pfefferkorn MD, Croffie JM, et al. Complications after outpatient upper GI endoscopy in children: 30-day follow-up. Am J Gastroenterol. 2003;98:1508–11.

15.  Volonaki E, Sebire NJ, Borrelli O, et al. Gastrointestinal Endoscopy and Mucosal Biopsy in the First Year of Life: Indications and Outcome. J Pediatr Gastro Nutr. 2012;55:62–5.

16.  Sebire NJ, Ramsay A, Smith W, Malone M, Risdon RA. Lamina propria eosinophil density in paediatric gastrointestinal mucosal biopsies. J Pathol. 2002;198:25a.

17.  Papadopoulou A, Koletzko S, Heuschkel R, et al. Management guidelines of Eosinophilic Esophagitis in Childhood. J Pediatr Gastrol Nutr. 2014;58:107–88.

18.  Atkins D, Furuta GT. Mucosal immunology, eosinophic esophagitis, and other intestinal inflammatory diseases. J Allergy Clin Immunol. 2010;125:S255–61.

19.  Melville D, da Silva MS, Young J, et al. Postprocedural effects of gastrointestinal endoscopy performed as a day case procedure in children: implications for patient and family education. Gastroenterology Nursing. 2007;30:426–34.

20.  National Institute for Health and Care Excellence (NICE). CG116 Food allergy in children and young people: NICE guideline 2012 http://guidance.nice.org.uk/CG116

21.  Venter C, Brown T, Shah N, et al. Diagnosis and management of non-IgE-mediated cow's milk allergy in infancy – a UK primary care practical guide. Clin Transl Allergy. 2013;3:23.

22.  Chandrasekharan B, Nezami BG, Srinivasan S. Emerging neuropeptide targets in inflammation: NPY and VIP. Am J Physiol Gastrointest Liver Physiol. 2013;304:G949–57.

23.  Wood JD. Enteric neuroimmunophysiology and Pathophysiology. Gastroenterol. 2004;127:635–57.

24.  Tunis MC, Marshall JS. Toll-Like Receptor 2 as a Regulator of Oral Tolerance in the Gastrointestinal Tract. Mediators Inflamm. 2014; 606383.

# 3

# Ultrastructural characterization of primary cilia in pathologically characterized human glioblastoma multiforme (GBM) tumors

Joanna J Moser, Marvin J Fritzler and Jerome B Rattner[*]

## Abstract

**Background:** Primary cilia are non-motile sensory cytoplasmic organelles that are involved in cell cycle progression. Ultrastructurally, the primary cilium region is complex, with normal ciliogenesis progressing through five distinct morphological stages in human astrocytes. Defects in early stages of ciliogenesis are key features of astrocytoma/glioblastoma cell lines and provided the impetus for the current study which describes the morphology of primary cilia in molecularly characterized human glioblastoma multiforme (GBM) tumors.

**Methods:** Seven surgically resected human GBM tissue samples were molecularly characterized according to IDH1/2 mutation status, EGFR amplification status and MGMT promoter methylation status and were examined for primary cilia expression and structure using indirect immunofluorescence and electron microscopy.

**Results:** We report for the first time that primary cilia are disrupted in the early stages of ciliogenesis in human GBM tumors. We confirm that immature primary cilia and basal bodies/centrioles have aberrant ciliogenesis characteristics including absent paired vesicles, misshaped/swollen vesicular hats, abnormal configuration of distal appendages, and discontinuity of centriole microtubular blades. Additionally, the transition zone plate is able to form in the absence of paired vesicles on the distal end of the basal body and when a cilium progresses beyond the early stages of ciliogenesis, it has electron dense material clumped along the transition zone and a darkening of the microtubules at the proximal end of the cilium.

**Conclusions:** Primary cilia play a role in a variety of human cancers. Previously primary cilia structure was perturbed in cultured cell lines derived from astrocytomas/glioblastomas; however there was always some question as to whether these findings were a cell culture phenomena. In this study we confirm that disruptions in ciliogenesis at early stages do occur in GBM tumors and that these ultrastructural findings bear resemblance to those previously observed in cell cultures. This is the first study to demonstrate that defects in cilia expression and function are a true hallmark of GBM tumors and correlate with their unrestrained growth. A review of the current ultrastructural profiles in the literature provides suggestions as to the best possible candidate protein that underlies defects in the early stages of ciliogenesis within GBM tumors.

**Keywords:** Primary cilia, Ciliogenesis, Cilium-pit, Centriole, Basal body, Distal appendages, Glioblastoma multiforme, EGFR amplification, IDH1/2 mutation, MGMT promoter methylation

* Correspondence: rattner@ucalgary.ca
Department of Biochemistry and Molecular Biology, Faculty of Medicine, University of Calgary, Calgary, AB, Canada

## Background

Primary cilia are non-motile sensory cytoplasmic organelles that have been implicated in signal transduction, cell to cell communication, left and right pattern embryonic development, sensation of fluid flow, regulation of calcium levels, mechanosensation, growth factor signaling and cell cycle progression [1,2]. They are present in the central nervous system and depletion of primary cilia in pro-opiomelanocortin hypothalamic neurons have induced hyperphagia [3,4]. Central nervous system primary cilia are key organelles required for Sonic hedgehog signalling (Shh) [5-8] where components Patched, Smoothened, Suppressor of fused and Gli transcription factors concentrate in the primary cilium [9-11]. It is currently thought that an intact primary cilium is required to enable proper Shh pathway function [12]. Subventricular zone astrocytes extend their primary cilium into the cerebral spinal fluid (CSF) suggesting they play a role in sensing ion concentration, pH, osmolarity, and changes in protein or glucose levels [13]. It is possible that astrocyte primary cilia can sense concentrations of neurotransmitters, growth factors, hormones, osmolarity, ions, pH and fluid flow in the extracellular space and relay homeostatic information (or lack thereof) to the centrosome.

Defects in the formation and/or function of primary cilia underlie a variety of human diseases that impact neurological development and are broadly referred to as ciliopathies and include diseases such as Alström, Bardet-Biedl, Joubert, Meckel-Gruber and oral-facial-digital type 1 syndromes. Common neurological phenotypes include obesity, ataxia and mental retardation [14]. The expression and function of primary cilia has become a focus of attention in a number of normal and malignant cells and tissues but have not been characterized in human glioblastoma tissue samples. Given that primary cilia are linked to cell cycle regulation and progression, several studies have suggested that primary cilia may play a role in tumor formation [15,16].

Previously our group undertook a comparative investigation of primary cilia in cultured primary human astrocytes and compared them to those found in five human astrocytoma/glioblastoma cell lines [17]. We demonstrated that the primary cilium region in cultured astrocyte cells is structurally complex, with ciliogenesis progressing through five distinct stages (Figure 1), and included foci for endocytosis-based signalling [17].

Further, we documented that in each of the five astrocytoma/glioblastoma cell lines studied (U-87 MG, T98G, U-251 MG, U-373 MG, U-138 MG), fully formed primary cilia are either expressed at a very low level, are completely absent or do not proceed through all the stages of ciliogenesis [17]. In addition, we noted several defects in the structure of astrocytoma/glioblastoma centrioles, including abnormal length and appendage architecture, that

were not observed in primary human astrocytes [17]. We concluded that aberrant ciliogenesis is common in cells derived from astrocytomas/glioblastomas and that this deficiency likely contributes to the phenotype of these malignant cells. These initial studies in astrocytoma/glioblastoma cell lines indicate that defects in primary cilium ciliogenesis do occur in glioblastoma cells and provided the impetus for this current study which characterizes the morphology of primary cilia and documents ciliogenesis defects in molecularly characterized human glioblastoma multiforme (GBM) tumors. Glioblastomas, although relatively uncommon with an annual incidence rate of 3–4 cases per 100,000 people, have disproportionately high morbidity and mortality rates with median survival pegged at 12–15 months [18,19]. Primary glioblastomas typically occur in patients older than 50 years of age and are characterized by epidermal growth factor receptor (EGFR) amplification and mutations, loss of heterozygosity of chromosome 10q and other abnormalities as reviewed in Wen and Kesari (2008) [20]. One of the most common defects in growth factor signalling involves EGFR [21] and amplification occurs almost exclusively in glioblastomas with 40-50% of patients containing EGFR amplification [20]. Isocitrate dehydrogenase (IDH) mutations are a strong predictor of a more favourable prognosis and a highly selective molecular marker for secondary glioblastomas [22]. Mutations of genes encoding *IDH1* and *IDH2*, as compared to no mutations, are associated with younger age and a better prognosis in adults with gliomas [23]. $O^6$-methylguanine-DNA methyltransferase (MGMT) promoter methylation silences the *MGMT* gene, decreasing DNA repair activity and increases the susceptibility of tumor cells to chemotherapeutic agents [20]. Recently it was shown that MGMT promoter methylation was associated with better overall survival in patients with GBM regardless of therapeutic intervention [24]. Given this burden of disease, it is important to determine the degree to which ciliogenesis is compromised in glioblastoma tumors as this information will inform the identity of altered mechanisms which may become targets for the development of future treatments.

Our hypothesis was that primary cilia in human GBM cells would be completely absent or show defects in the early stages of ciliogenesis. Our primary objective was to examine primary cilia expression and structure in human GBM tissue samples at both the light and ultrastructural level.

## Methods

### Ethics statement

Anonymized human brain tumor (GBM) tissue samples and basic clinico-pathologic data were obtained through the Clark Smith Brain Tumour and Tissue Bank at the

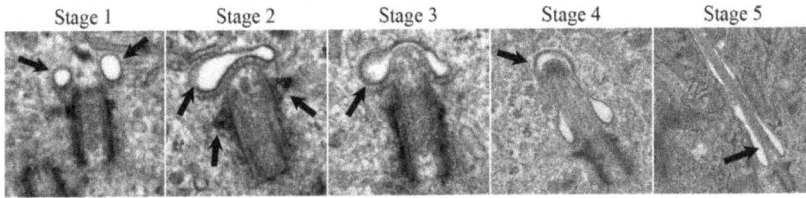

**Figure 1 Primary ciliogenesis progresses through five morphologically distinct stages in human astrocytes.** Key characteristics of each stage are indicated with arrows. Paired lateral vesicles are prominent at the distal end of the basal body in Stage 1. Distal appendages are triangular in appearance and reside at the distal end of the basal body (Stage 2). The paired lateral vesicles fuse to become a vesicular hat and become stretched by the outgrowth of the primary cilium and can be seen progressing through stages 2 through 4. Stage 5 shows a mature primary cilium with a surrounding cilium-pit. *Used with permission from Moser et al. BMC Cancer 2009, 9:448, Figure 2A © BioMed Central.*

University of Calgary and Calgary Laboratory Services, Calgary, AB (ethics approved for biobanking and previous patient consent granted at time of banking). Tissue was used according to the policies of the institutional review boards of Calgary Laboratory Services and the Calgary Health Region Ethics Board. Further ethics review and approval for this study (ID# E-23011) was provided by the Conjoint Health Research Ethics Board (University of Calgary, Calgary, AB).

### GBM tissue samples

All samples were part of routine clinical care for diagnostic and treatment purposes and were designated as excess material by the consulting and consenting neuropathologist. Hematoxylin and eosin stained formalin-fixed paraffin-embedded sections were reviewed by a neuropathologist for confirmation of a diagnosis of high-grade glioma (glioblastoma WHO grade IV) as per World Health Organization criteria [18].

### Molecular characterization of GBM tumors

Molecular characterization of IDH and EGFR was performed by the clinical Molecular Diagnostics Laboratory at Calgary Laboratory Services on formalin-fixed paraffin-embedded (FFPE) sections. Briefly, IDH1 and IDH2 mutational analyses were performed using a multiplexed SNaPshot® reaction and detection by capillary electrophoresis [25]. Analysis of EGFR amplification was performed by EGFR colorimetric *in situ* hybridization using standard methods with the EGFR probe #84-1300 (Zymed Laboratories), and scored by a neuropathologist as follows: 'amplified EGFR' indicates >10 signals/nucleus in >80% of tumor cells and 'not amplified' indicates 2 signals/nucleus in tumor cells.

### Antigen retrieval method (ARM)

Slides containing the FFPE tissue sections were deparaffinised in xylene and passed through a graded ethanol series, rinsed with cold tap water and transferred to a Coplin jar on a hot plate containing a 100°C Tris-EDTA-Tween (w/v)

solution (0.121% Tris HCl, 0.0379% EDTA, 0.05% Tween-20, pH adjusted to 9.0). The sections were boiled for 60 minutes and then allowed to reach room temperature while remaining in the same solution. The slides were washed in phosphate buffered saline (PBS) for 10 minutes and processed for IIF.

### Indirect immunofluorescence (IIF)

Formalin-fixed paraffin embedded tissue sections were treated with the above ARM (section 3.4.). Cells were blocked in 10% normal goat serum (NGS; Antibodies Incorporated, Davis, CA) and 2% bovine serum albumin (BSA; Sigma-Aldrich) for 30 minutes at room temperature (RT) and incubated with primary antibodies at appropriate working dilutions overnight at 4°C. Primary cilia were marked by mouse anti-acetylated tubulin at 1:100 dilution (Sigma, St. Louis, MO). After washing with PBS, cells were incubated for 2 hours in a dark chamber with Alexa Fluor (AF) 488 (green) secondary goat fluorochrome-conjugated antibodies at 1:100 dilution (Invitrogen). Slides were washed in several changes of PBS, cell nuclei counterstained with 4',6-diamidino-2-phenylindole (DAPI), mounted in Vectashield (Vector Laboratories, Burlingame, CA) and examined for IIF using a 100x objective on a Leica DMRE microscope equipped with epifluorescence and an Optronics camera. Appropriate IIF controls with no primary antibody revealed no detectable bleed-through between microscope filter sets.

### Electron microscopy (EM)

Fresh GBM samples were immersed in a fixative containing 3% glutaraldehyde in Millonig's phosphate buffer and stored at 4°C for 48 hours. Samples were immersed post-fixation in 2% $OsO_4$ for 20 minutes and then dehydrated in ethanol and infiltrated with Polybed 812 resin (Polysciences Inc., Warrington, PA). Polymerization was performed at 37°C for 24 hours. Silver-gray sections were cut with an ultramicrotome (Leica) equipped with a diamond knife, stained with uranyl acetate and lead citrate and then examined in a H-700 Hitachi electron microscope. For each sample, 10 grids were examined on standard sections. Approximately 500 cells were examined in each tissue sample.

## Results

We examined both formalin-fixed paraffin embedded (FFPE) and fresh-fixed tissue from seven cases of surgically resected brain tumors diagnosed by neuropathologists as grade IV glioblastoma/GBM using indirect immunofluorescence (IIF) and electron microscopy (EM), respectively.

The GBM tumors were molecularly characterized according to IDH 1/2 mutation status, EGFR amplification status and MGMT promoter status (Table 1). Our results showed that 71% of GBM patients had amplified levels of EGFR, 86% had no IDH1/2 mutations and 50% had methylated MGMT promoters (Table 1).

We examined the biopsy tissue from each of the 7 patients by light and electron microscopy. IIF examination of tissue from patient #1 showed typical primary cilia (Figure 2, top inset). Similarly, ultrastructural examination revealed a normal basal body with a fully formed mature primary cilium, consistent with normal morphology (Figure 2 compared to Figure 1). The cilium-pit was well defined (Figure 2) and the cilium contained well-formed microtubules with normal spacing between doublets (Figure 2, bottom inset). In addition, small vesicles were seen along the cilium microtubules and interfacing with the cilium-pit (Figure 2), which is consistent with previous findings that showed this is a site for endocytosis based signalling [17].

The GBM tissue from patient #2 failed to show abundant primary cilia by IIF. Ultrastructural examination revealed cells with basal bodies reminiscent of stage 1 ciliogenesis, however there were no paired vesicles present along the lateral sides of the distal end of the basal body/transition zone as observed in longitudinal and cross-sections (Figure 3A and inset compared to Figure 1). In addition to missing paired vesicles, patient #2 had basal bodies that presented with abnormal, vertically outstretched distal appendages (Figure 3B). Figure 3C shows another example of an abnormal basal body with

absent paired vesicles along the lateral sides of the distal end of the basal body/transition zone. Interestingly, the transition zone plate is present without the presence of the vesicles which suggests that the vesicles do not need to be present to allow the transition zone to form, but need to be present to allow ciliogenesis to progress beyond stage 1. In one rare example, a primary cilium which had progressed to stage 5 of ciliogenesis was found (Figure 3D). On close examination, this cilium displayed a disrupted ciliary membrane which was also the site of cytoplasmic extrusions into the surrounding environment (Figure 3D). These abnormal primary cilia also have a dark pericentriolar material (PCM)-like collection of material clumped along the transition zone of the primary cilium with darkening of the cilia microtubules at the proximal end of the cilium shaft (Figure 3D).

The tissue from patient #3 revealed an absence of mature primary cilia by IIF and ultrastructural examination showed that 70% of centrosome/basal body profiles were at stage 1 while the remaining 30% of profiles examined displayed stage 2/3 of ciliogenesis (Figure 4). Many of the immature cilia contained electron dense material along the cilium shaft (Figure 4 compared to Figure 1). The stretched vesicular hat that is so prominent in normal cells at stage 2/3 was irregular, thin and misshapen in patient #3 GBM cells (Figure 4). The microtubules of the cilium appear irregular, lack organization and do not display the normal architectural characteristics of the transition zone (Figure 4). There were no cilia in stages 4–5 observed for patient #3.

GBM tissue from patient #4 failed to display mature primary cilium by IIF. Ultrastructurally, patient #4 expressed basal bodies that were similar to stage 1 with a transition zone plate formed along the distal end (Figure 5A compared to Figure 1). It is important to note that in many of these electron microscope centrosome/basal body profiles there was only 1 vesicle present (as opposed to the normal 2 vesicles) at the distal end and the vesicle was positioned directly above the transition zone plate (as opposed to the normal lateral orientation beside the transition zone plate) (Figure 5A). The architecture of

**Table 1 Molecularly characterized grade IV glioblastoma GBM tumors**

| Patient no. | IDH 1/2 | EGFR amplification | MGMT promoter |
|---|---|---|---|
| 1 | No mutations detected | Amplified | Not assessed |
| 2 | No mutations detected | Amplified | Un-methylated |
| 3 | No mutations detected | Amplified | Un-methylated |
| 4 | IDH1 exon 4 R132H mutation detected; no mutation in exon 4 of IDH2 | Amplified | Methylated |
| 5 | No mutations detected | Not amplified | Methylated |
| 6 | No mutations detected | Amplified | Methylated |
| 7 | No mutations detected | Not amplified | Un-methylated |

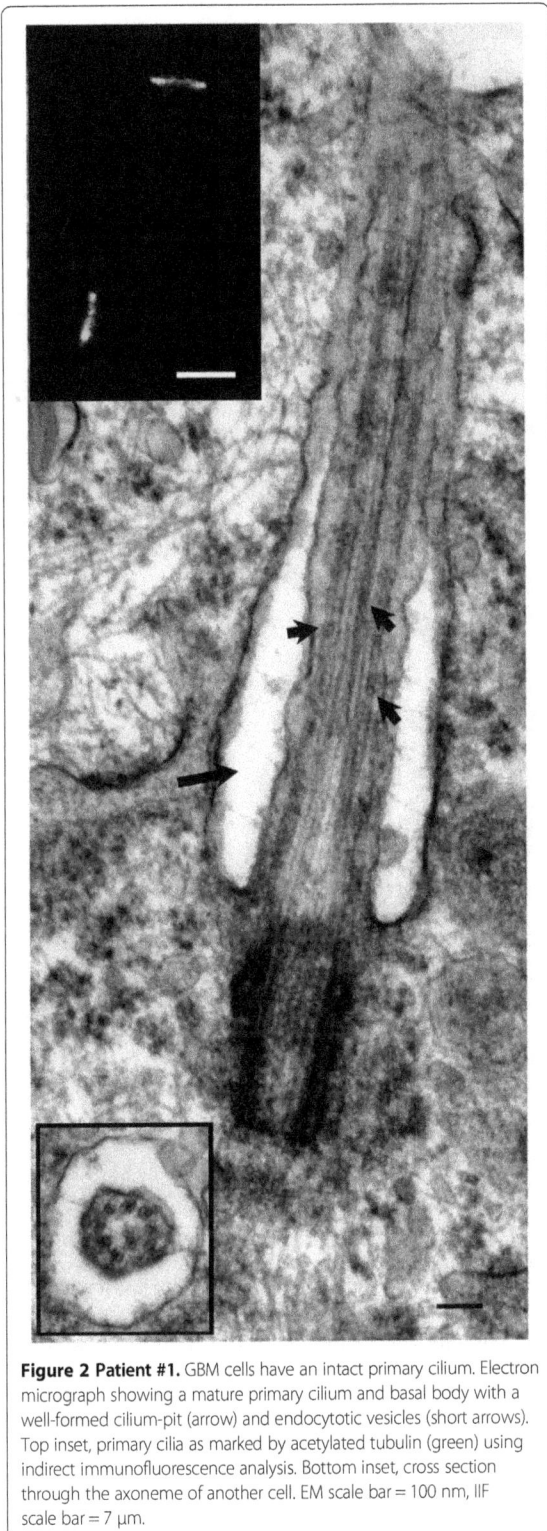

**Figure 2 Patient #1.** GBM cells have an intact primary cilium. Electron micrograph showing a mature primary cilium and basal body with a well-formed cilium-pit (arrow) and endocytotic vesicles (short arrows). Top inset, primary cilia as marked by acetylated tubulin (green) using indirect immunofluorescence analysis. Bottom inset, cross section through the axoneme of another cell. EM scale bar = 100 nm, IIF scale bar = 7 μm.

the distal appendages along the basal body was also abnormal given their outstretched vertical appearance (Figure 5A) as opposed to the normal horizontal appearance displayed in Figure 1. Figure 5B, illustrates a discontinuity present in one of the centriole microtubule blades, although this centriole was 357 nm in length (Figure 5B) which falls within normal parameters [17].

Samples from patient #5 did not show mature primary cilia by IIF. Ultrastructural examination revealed either basal bodies with an immature transition zone or profiles similar to stage 1 (Figure 6 compared to Figure 1). The transition zone was not visible in the electron micrograph centrosome/basal body profiles from this patient and we did not observe any paired vesicles similar to that seen in patient #2 (Figure 6). There also appears to be minimal PCM distributed in the cytoplasmic area surrounding the basal body and centriole (Figure 6).

There were no observable primary cilia staining by IIF in the GBM tissue from patient #6, although ultrastructural examination showed cilia at multiple stages (Figure 7). We observed profiles at stage 1 with a well-defined plate within the transition zone lacking paired laterally placed vesicles (Figure 7A). We observed many cilia at stage 1 with either multiple irregular abnormally shaped vesicles formed at the distal end of the basal body or 4 distinct vesicles above the plate within the transition zone (Figure 7B). In the latter case, distal appendages were absent. In rare cases, a cilium with a short axoneme was detected (Figure 7C). These cilia appeared to have a truncated cilium-pit so that the distal end of the cilium is continuous with the cytoplasm, a configuration reminiscent of a regressing cilium [26].

GBM tissue from patient #7 also did not show any primary cilia by IIF staining. Ultrastructurally, primary ciliogenesis occurred in profiles to a maximum of stage 2 (Figure 8 compared to Figure 1). These cells had vesicular hats that were misshaped and swollen (Figure 8A and B) and had outstretched, vertical distal basal body appendages (Figure 8B). These characteristics were similar to those observed in other astrocytoma/glioblastoma cell lines, particularly in U-373 MG and U-138 MG cells (Figure 2B in [17]).

## Discussion

The expression of a primary cilium relies on two main events: 1) activation of ciliogenesis and 2) orderly progression through a series of developmental stages so that a structurally and functionally competent mature cilium is formed [27-29]. Our study illustrates that ciliogenesis was activated in all the GBM samples examined but cilium morphogenesis beyond stage 1 was rare in the majority of tumors. These findings support our previous examination of several astrocytoma/glioblastoma cell lines [17]. Thus,

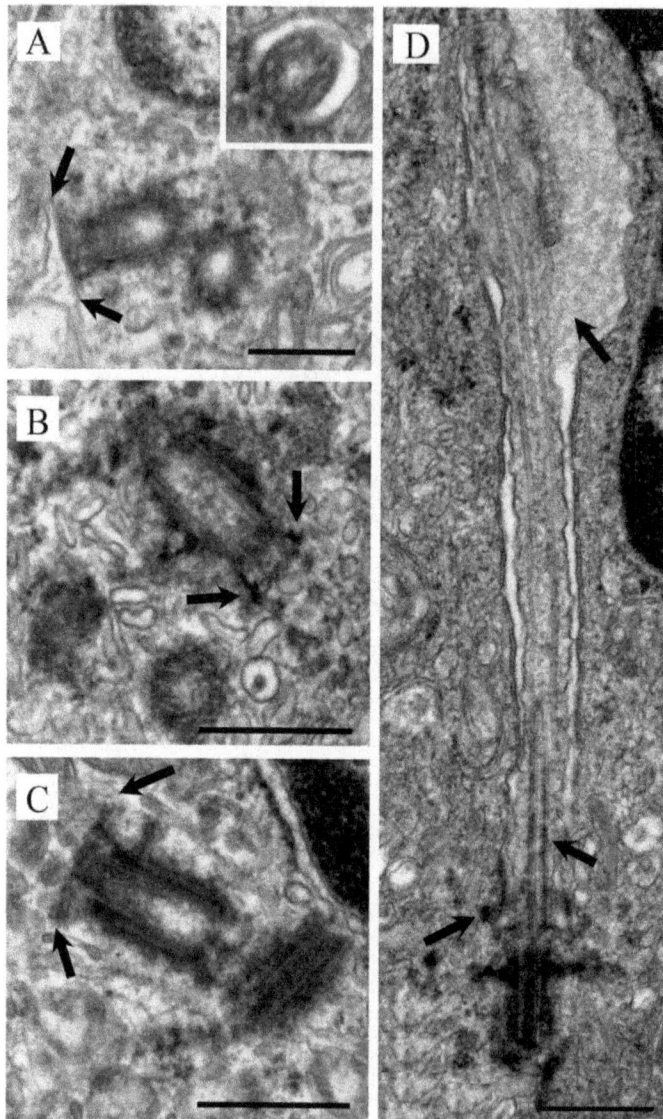

**Figure 3 Patient #2.** GBM cells are halted at stage 1 of ciliogenesis with rare cells progressing to stage 5. **(A)** Basal body and abnormal stage 1 cilium with absent paired lateral vesicles. Inset cross section through the transition zone from another cell. **(B)** Basal body and abnormal stage 1 cilium with vertically outstretched distal appendages and no vesicles. **(C)** Basal body with clear transition zone and abnormal stage 1 cilium with absent vesicles. **(D)** Rare occurrence of a primary cilium at stage 5 with abnormal destruction of the cilium-pit with cytoplasmic extrusion, darkened microtubules at proximal end of cilium and electron dense collection of material at the transition zone. EM scale bars = 500 nm.

cells from each of these sources (cell line or tumor tissue) express a similar defect or set of defects that targets the earliest stages of ciliogenesis and does not inhibit the cells ability to proliferate.

These findings are compatible with previous studies of melanoma, renal cell carcinoma and pancreatic cancer, which found that primary cilia loss was independent of Ki67 staining (cell proliferation marker) suggesting that cilia loss is not the result of altered cellular proliferation

rates but rather may be due to aberrations in another mechanism that is inherent to ciliogenesis [30-32]. Yang and colleagues (2013) recently showed that cell cycle-related kinase (CCRK) and its substrate intestinal cell kinase inhibited ciliogenesis in a glioblastoma cell line [33]. Specifically, they showed that dysregulated high levels of CCRK are present in U-251 MG glioblastoma cells whereby knockdown of CCRK led to the formation of primary cilia indicating that CCRK depletion restored

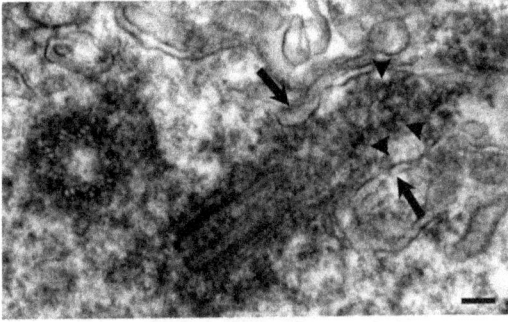

**Figure 4 Patient #3.** GBM cells are halted at stage 3 of ciliogenesis and display electron dense material clustered along the cilium shaft (arrow heads) and an irregular vesicular hat (arrows). EM scale bar = 100 nm.

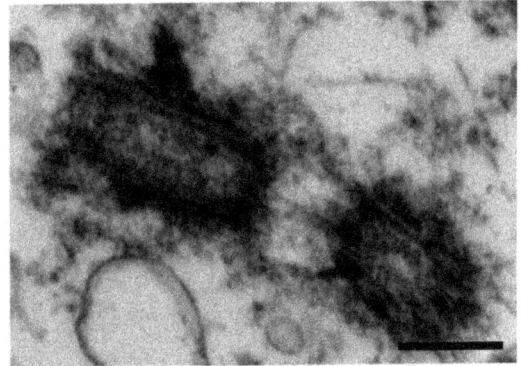

**Figure 6 Patient #5.** GBM cells were characterized by abnormal primary cilia that were halted at or before stage 1 of ciliogenesis with no evidence of paired vesicles or a transition zone plate. EM scale bar = 250 nm.

primary ciliogenesis [33]. Furthermore, it was demonstrated that the inhibition of ciliogenesis by over-expression of CCRK in U-251 MG glioblastoma cells promoted cell proliferation capacity [33].

From our ultrastructural studies in astrocytoma/glioblastoma cell lines and GBM tumor tissues it is interesting to note that profiles occasionally displayed centriole/basal bodies with structural abnormalities (i.e. altered length or microtubule integrity). This suggests that it is possible for such structural alterations to be tolerated by the cycling cell, perhaps by being repaired, or that these defects underlie further aberrant cancer cell behaviour.

It is important to note that in the majority of previously published studies, IIF alone was used to evaluate ciliogenesis status. This technique alone does not allow for the precise identification or characterization of the earliest stages of ciliogenesis. Thus, truncated cilia such as that seen in a few patients within our study may be more common that previously indicated. Our ultrastructural data not only reveals a defect in early ciliogenesis but also shows that this defect specifically

affects the initial elaboration of the distal surface of the basal body and its ability to associate with Golgi derived vesicles. There have been a number of proteins shown to act at the distal end of the basal body, particularly at the distal appendage region, and they include; Cep170 [34], ninein [8,35], ε-tubulin [36], cenexin/ODF2 [37] (likely cenexin1 [38]) and by association Rab8a [39], centriolin/Cep110 [8,40], Cep164 [41] and Cep123 [42] reviewed in [1]. For example, in neuronal primary cilia, B9-C2 containing proteins have been shown to collect at the base of the primary cilium in the transition zone [43-47] and physically interact and with ciliary protein localization [48] (and reviewed in [49]). One B9-C2 family gene in particular named Stumpy (or *B9d2*) is required for mammalian ciliogenesis where knockout mutants displayed near-complete loss of neuronal primary cilia with remaining cilia displaying dysmorphic stump-like ultrastructures [43].

Of particular interest, a distal appendage protein, Cep 123, has recently been shown to be required for initiation

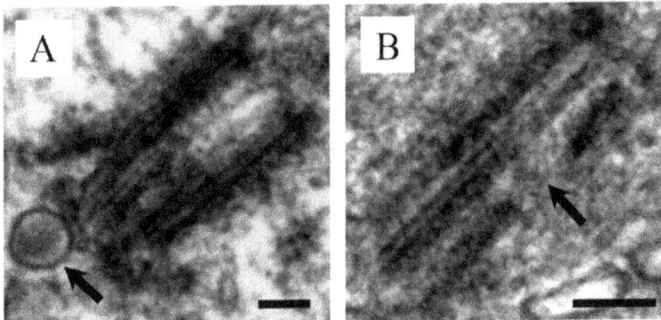

**Figure 5 Patient #4.** GBM cells were characterized by **(A)** primary cilia that were halted at stage 1 of ciliogenesis with a single vesicle present above the transition plate and abnormal distal appendages and **(B)** breakages in the basal body/centriole microtubules. EM scale bars = 100 nm.

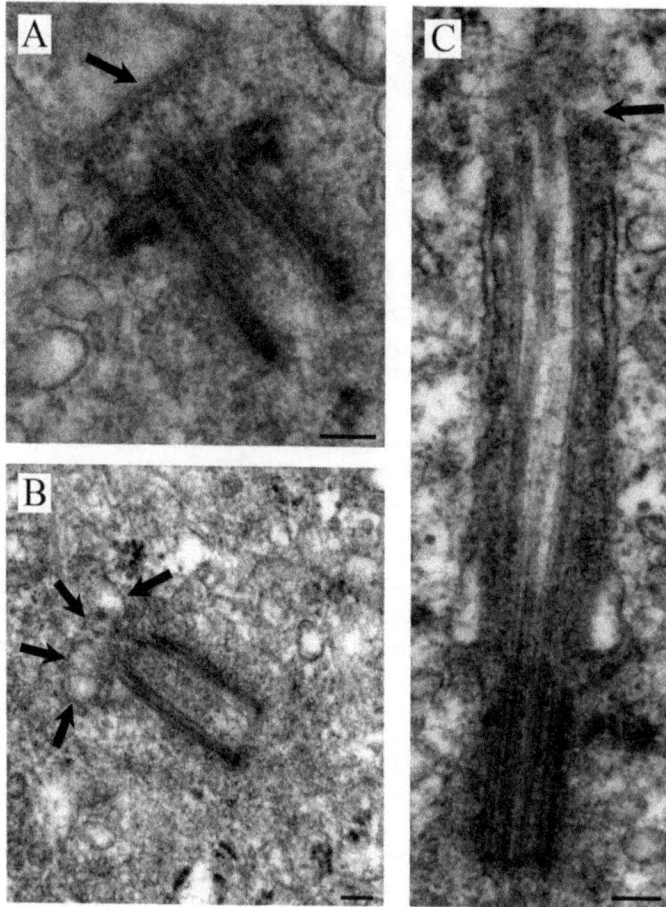

**Figure 7 Patient #6.** GBM cells were characterized by abnormal primary cilia at **(A, B)** stage 1/2 and **(C)** 4/5 of ciliogenesis with either absent lateral vesicles, aberrant supernumerary vesicles along the length of the transition zone plate or abrupt cessation of the cilium shaft. EM scale bars = 100 nm.

of ciliogenesis by modulation of capping the distal end of the mother centriole with a ciliary vesicle [42]. Sillibourne and colleagues (2013) showed that Cep123 is required for assembly of a primary cilium but not the maintenance of the axoneme in human retinal pigment epithelial (RPE1) cells [42]. Depletion of Cep123 using Cep 123 siRNA perturbed ciliary vesicle formation at the distal end of the basal body which suggests that distal appendage proteins are critical for progression of cilia beyond the early stages of ciliogenesis [42]. These knockdown studies are captured in Figure 6B by Sillibourne *et al.* (2013) [42] and are very similar in appearance to the abnormal early stages of ciliogenesis seen in our GBM tumors. Given this high degree of ultrastructural similarity, Cep123 may be the best candidate to explain the defects we observed in GBM tumors. Although a review of the glioblastoma literature does not highlight Cep123 as being defective in patients with GBM tumors, our study

suggests that it is a reasonable target for future expression studies and ultrastructural analysis in GBM tumors.

Limitations of the current study are small sample size and lack of normal brain tissue for comparison. Given the small incidence of malignant gliomas per year, we collected samples over a 5 year period and eliminated those samples that were not grade IV glioblastomas/ GBM. To respect the ethics of collection of normal human brain tissue from our patients, we compared the GBM patient results to those previously established in normal human astrocyte cells that were used between passages 3–5 in culture [17]. Although 10 grids were examined for each patient sample, there were noticeable differences between tumor samples in terms of cellularity and patient heterogeneity. It is important to emphasize that this is a complex mixture of cells and extracellular matrixof GBM brain tissue and that some cell types are ciliated whereas others are not ciliated. Because of the

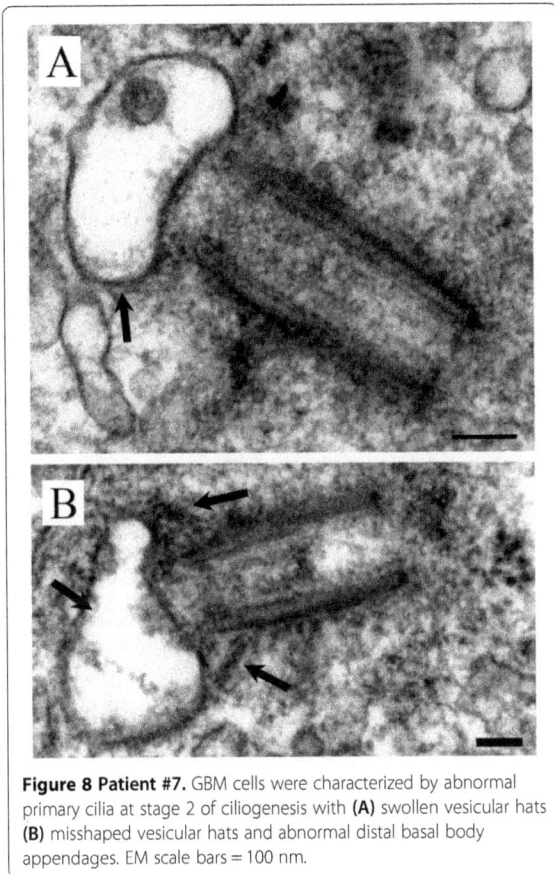

**Figure 8 Patient #7.** GBM cells were characterized by abnormal primary cilia at stage 2 of ciliogenesis with **(A)** swollen vesicular hats **(B)** misshaped vesicular hats and abnormal distal basal body appendages. EM scale bars = 100 nm.

tissue complexity and heterogeneity, it is impossible to identify all the cells which have the potential to undergo ciliogenesis. When we do see profiles, we can quantitate the number of cells undergoing abnormal ciliogenesis (including profiles at stages 3/4/5) which is summarized as follows. Patient #1: 20 cells with profiles, 2 cells with normal cilia, 0 cells with abnormal cilia. Patient #2: 9 cells with profiles, 0 cells with normal cilia, 2 cells with abnormal cilia. Patient #3: 20 cells with profiles, 0 cells with normal cilia, 2 cells with abnormal cilia. Patient #4: 22 cells with profiles, 0 cells with normal cilia, 0 cells with abnormal cilia. Patient #5: 20 cells with profiles, 0 cells with normal cilia, 0 cells with abnormal cilia. Patient #6: 30 cells with profiles, 0 cells with normal cilia, 3 cells with abnormal cilia. Patient #7: 15 cells with profiles, 0 cells with normal cilia, 0 cells with abnormal cilia. Taken together, only one patient expressed morphologically normal cilia. As a whole, we did see the same types of abnormalities in the early stages of ciliogenesis amongst tumor samples which suggests that early ciliogenesis defects are a generalized problem in GBM tumors. In summary, we can say that the large majority of grade 4 glioblastoma/astrocytomas (i.e. GBM tumors) are likely to express

abnormal immature primary cilia suggesting that this defect may be a hallmark of GBMs. We have not detected a clear correlation between abnormal ciliogenesis and the 3 main molecular characterizations examined in these patient samples. It must be kept in mind that our patient sample size may not be sufficient to reveal correlations with molecular markers and this might require a larger study.

In summary, we found that ciliogenesis is activated in GBM tumors but the normal development of a mature cilium is perturbed at early stages of ciliogenesis. The aberrant ultrastructural profiles observed in our survey of GBM tumors and a review of the current ultrastructural profiles present in the literature suggest the possibility that at present the best possible candidate protein underlying defects in the early stages of ciliogenesis within GBM tumors might involve Cep123.

## Conclusions

The major finding of this report is that primary ciliogenesis is disrupted at an early stage in the majority of human GBM tumors. This finding is important for several reasons. First, these results confirm astrocytoma/glioblastoma cell culture data. Second, it indicates that defects in ciliogenesis are a hallmark of GBM tumor pathology and provides impetus for further study of the relationship between primary cilium defects and other brain tumors such as astrocytoma, oligodendroglioma and medulloblastoma. Third, it provides further evidence that the early stages of ciliogenesis are a critical time in the process of ciliogenesis, thus narrowing the number of target proteins that may underlie these defects. Fourth, it catalogues and describes the key basal body/cilium-related ultrastructural abnormalities that are common between GBM tumors. The ultrastructural description of this study informs which proteins are involved in early ciliogenesis defects and identifies candidates that are currently in the literature. In future, it will be important to elucidate which specific proteins are involved in this critical time period and whether alterations in their expression can restore ciliogenesis and thus restore cell cycle control.

**Abbreviations**
ARM: Antigen retrieval method; CCRK: Cell cycle-related kinase; CSF: Cerebral spinal fluid; DAPI: 4',6-diamidino-2-phenylindole; EM: Electron microscopy; EGFR: Epidermal growth factor receptor; FFPE: Formalin-fixed paraffin embedded; GBM: Glioblastoma multiforme; IIF: Indirect immunofluorescence; IDH: Isocitrate dehydrogenase; MGMT: $O^6$-methylguanine-DNA methyltransferase; PBS: Phosphate buffered saline; PCM: Pericentriolar material; RPE1: Retinal pigment epithelial; Shh: Sonic hedgehog signalling; WHO: World Health Organization.

**Competing interests**
The authors declare that they have no competing interests.

**Authors' contributions**
JJM and JBR obtained the molecular characterization data, carried out the electron microscopy studies, performed indirect immunofluorescence experiments and wrote the first draft of the manuscript. JJM, MJF and JBR conceived of the study design, participated in obtaining ethics approval,

interpretation of the data, read, edited and approved the final manuscript. All authors read and approved the final manuscript.

## Acknowledgements

We thank neuropathologists, Drs. Jennifer Chan and Leslie Hamilton, University of Calgary for providing the samples, diagnoses and clinico-pathological information on the tissues obtained from Calgary Laboratory Services. This work was supported in part by the Canadian Institutes for Health Research Grant MOP-57674 (MJF) and the Natural Sciences and Engineering Research Council of Canada Grant 690481 (JBR).

## References

1. Moser JJ, Fritzler MJ, Ou Y, Rattner JB: The PCMbasal body/primary cilium coalition. *Semin Cell Dev Biol* 2010, 21:148–155.
2. Hassounah NB, Bunch TA, McDermott KM: Molecular pathways: the role of primary cilia in cancer progression and therapeutics with a focus on hedgehog signaling. *Clin Cancer Res* 2012, 18:2429–2435.
3. Davenport JR, Watts AJ, Roper VC, Croyle MJ, van Groen T, Wyss JM, Nagy TR, Kesterson RA, Yoder BK: Disruption of intraflagellar transport in adult mice leads to obesity and slow-onset cystic kidney disease. *Curr Biol* 2007, 17:1586–1594.
4. Satir P: Cilia biology: stop overeating now! *Curr Biol* 2007, 17:R963–R965.
5. Ingham PW: Transducing hedgehog: the story so far. *EMBO J* 1998, 17:3505–3511.
6. Dahmane N, Altaba A: Sonic hedgehog regulates the growth and patterning of the cerebellum. *Development* 1999, 126:3089–3100.
7. Wallace VA: Purkinje-cell-derived Sonic hedgehog regulates granule neuron precursor cell proliferation in the developing mouse cerebellum. *Curr Biol* 1999, 9:445–448.
8. Ou YY, Mack GJ, Zhang M, Rattner JB: CEP110 and ninein are located in a specific domain of the centrosome associated with centrosome maturation. *J Cell Sci* 2002, 115:1825–1835.
9. Corbit KC, Aanstad P, Singla V, Norman AR, Stainier DYR, Reiter JF: Vertebrate Smoothened functions at the primary cilium. *Nature* 2005, 437:1018–1021.
10. Haycraft C, Banizs B, Aydin-Son Y, Zhang Q, Michaud EJ, Yoder BK: Gli2 and Gli3 localize to cilia and require the intraflagellar transport protein polaris for processing and function. *PLoS Genet* 2005, 1:e53.
11. Rohatgi R, Milenkovic L, Scott MP: Patched1 regulates hedgehog signaling at the primary cilium. *Science* 2007, 317:372–376.
12. Breunig JJ, Sarkisian MR, Arellano JI, Morozov YM, Ayoub AE, Sojitra S, Wang B, Flavell RA, Rakic P, Town T: Primary cilia regulate hippocampal neurogenesis by mediating sonic hedgehog signaling. *Proc Natl Acad Sci* 2008, 105:13127–13132.
13. Danilov AI, Gomes-Leal W, Ahlenius H, Kokaia Z, Carlemalm E, Lindvall O: Ultrastructural and antigenic properties of neural stem cells and their progeny in adult rat subventricular zone. *Glia* 2009, 57:136–152.
14. Badano JL, Mitsuma N, Beales PL, Katsanis N: The ciliopathies: an emerging class of human genetic disorders. *Annu Rev Genomics Hum Genet* 2006, 7:125–148.
15. Wong SY, Seol AD, So PL, Ermilov AN, Bichakjian CK, Epstein EH, Dlugosz AA, Reiter JF: Primary cilia can both mediate and suppress Hedgehog pathway-dependent tumorigenesis. *Nat Med* 2009, 15:1055–1061.
16. Han YG, Kim HJ, Dlugosz AA, Ellison DW, Gilbertson RJ, Alvarez-Buylla A: Dual and opposing roles of primary cilia in medulloblastoma development. *Nat Med* 2009, 15:1062–1065.
17. Moser JJ, Fritzler MJ, Rattner JB: Primary ciliogenesis defects are associated with human astrocytoma/glioblastoma cells. *BMC Cancer* 2009, 9:448.
18. Louis D, Ohgaki H, Wiestler O, Cavenee W, Burger P, Jouvet A, Scheithauer B, Kleihues P: The 2007 WHO classification of tumours of the central nervous system. *Acta Neuropathol* 2007, 114:547.
19. Ostrom QT, Gittleman H, Farah P, Ondracek A, Chen Y, Wolinsky Y, Stroup NE, Kruchko C, Barnholtz-Sloan JS: CBTRUS Statistical Report: Primary Brain and Central Nervous System Tumors Diagnosed in the United States in 2006-2010. *Neuro Oncol* 2013, 15(suppl 2):ii1–ii56.
20. Wen PY, Kesari S: Malignant gliomas in adults. *N Engl J Med* 2008, 359:492–507.
21. Furnari FB, Fenton T, Bachoo RM, Mukasa A, Stommel JM, Stegh A, Hahn WC, Ligon KL, Louis DN, Brennan C, Chin L, DePinho RA, Cavanee WK: Malignant astrocytic glioma: genetics, biology, and paths to treatment. *Genes Dev* 2007, 21:2683–2710.
22. Nobusawa S, Watanabe T, Kleihues P, Ohgaki H: IDH1 mutations as molecular signature and predictive factor of secondary glioblastomas. *Clin Cancer Res* 2009, 15:6002–6007.
23. Yan H, Parsons DW, Jin G, McLendon R, Rasheed BA, Yuan W, Kos I, Batinic-Haberle I, Jones S, Riggins GJ, Friedman H, Friedman A, Reardon D, Herndon J, Kinzler KW, Velculescu VE, Vogelstein B, Bigner DD: IDH1 and IDH2 mutations in gliomas. *N Engl J Med* 2009, 360:765–773.
24. Zhang K, Wang XQ, Zhou B, Zhang L: The prognostic value of MGMT promoter methylation in Glioblastoma multiforme: a meta-analysis. *Fam Cancer* 2013, 12:449–458.
25. Perizzolo M, Winkfein B, Hui S, Krulicki W, Chan JA, Demetrick DJ: IDH mutation detection in formalin-fixed paraffin-embedded gliomas using multiplex PCR and single-base extension. *Brain Pathol* 2012, 22:619–624.
26. Williams NE, Frankel J: Regulation of microtubules in tetrahymena : I. electron microscopy of oral replacement. *J Cell Biol* 1973, 56:441–457.
27. Sorokin S: Centrioles and the formation of rudimentary cilia by fibroblasts and smooth muscle cells. *J Cell Biol* 1962, 15:363–377.
28. Hagiwara H, Ohwada N, Aoki T, Takata K: Ciliogenesis and ciliary abnormalities. *Med Electron Microsc* 2000, 33:109–114.
29. Hagiwara H, Ohwada N, Takata K: Cell Biology of normal and abnormal ciliogenesis in the ciliated epithelium. In *International Review of Cytology*, Volume 234. Academic Press: Kwang WJ; 2004:101–141. ISBN ISBN 9780123646385.
30. Tukachinsky H, Lopez LV, Salic A: A mechanism for vertebrate Hedgehog signaling: recruitment to cilia and dissociation of SuFuGli protein complexes. *J Cell Biol* 2010, 191:415–428.
31. Schraml P, Frew IJ, Thoma CR, Boysen G, Struckmann K, Krek W, Moch H: Sporadic clear cell renal cell carcinoma but not the papillary type is characterized by severely reduced frequency of primary cilia. *Mod Pathol* 2008, 22:31–36.
32. Seeley ES, Carrière C, Goetze T, Longnecker DS, Korc M: Pancreatic cancer and precursor pancreatic intraepithelial neoplasia lesions are devoid of primary cilia. *Cancer Res* 2009, 69:422–430.
33. Yang Y, Roine N, Makela TP: CCRK depletion inhibits glioblastoma cell proliferation in a cilium-dependent manner. *EMBO Rep* 2013, 14:741–747.
34. Guarguaglini G, Duncan PI, Stierhof YD, Holmstrom T, Duensing S, Nigg EA: The Forkhead-associated domain protein Cep170 Interacts with Polo-like Kinase 1 and serves as a marker for mature centrioles. *Mol Biol Cell* 2005, 16:1095–1107.
35. Mogensen MM, Malik A, Piel M, Bouckson-Castaing V, Bornens M: Microtubule minus-end anchorage at centrosomal and non-centrosomal sites: the role of ninein. *J Cell Sci* 2000, 113:3013–3023.
36. Chang P, Giddings TH, Winey M, Stearns T: epsilon-Tubulin is required for centriole duplication and microtubule organization. *Nat Cell Biol* 2003, 5:71–76.
37. Ishikawa H, Kubo A, Tsukita S, Tsukita S: Odf2-deficient mother centrioles lack distal/subdistal appendages and the ability to generate primary cilia. *Nat Cell Biol* 2005, 7:517–524.
38. Soung NK, Park JE, Yu LR, Lee KH, Lee JM, Bang JK, Veenstra TD, Rhee K, Lee KS: Plk1-dependent and -independent roles of an ODF2 splice variant, hCenexin1, at the centrosome of somatic cells. *Dev Cell* 2009, 16:539–550.
39. Si Y, Egerer J, Fuchs E, Haas AK, Barr FA: Functional dissection of Rab GTPases involved in primary cilium formation. *J Cell Biol* 2007, 178:363–369.
40. Gromley A, Jurczyk A, Sillibourne J, Halilovic E, Mogensen M, Groisman I, Blomberg M, Doxsey S: A novel human protein of the maternal centriole is required for the final stages of cytokinesis and entry into S phase. *J Cell Biol* 2003, 161:535–545.
41. Graser S, Stierhof YD, Lavoie SB, Gassner OS, Lamla S, Le Clech M, Nigg EA: Cep164, a novel centriole appendage protein required for primary cilium formation. *J Cell Biol* 2007, 179:321–330.
42. Sillibourne JE, Hurbain I, Grand-Perret T, Goud B, Tran P, Bornens M: Primary ciliogenesis requires the distal appendage component Cep123. *Biol Open* 2013.
43. Town T, Breunig JJ, Sarkisian MR, Spilianakis C, Ayoub AE, Liu X, Ferrandino AF, Gallagher AR, Li MO, Rakic P, Flavell RA: The stumpy gene is required for mammalian ciliogenesis. *Proc Natl Acad Sci* 2008, 105:2853–2858.

44. Garcia-Gonzalo FR, Corbit KC, Sirerol-Piquer MS, Ramaswami G, Otto EA, Noriega TR, Seol AD, Robinson JF, Bennett CL, Josifova DJ, García-Verdugo JM, Katsanis N, Hildebrandt F, Reiter JF: A transition zone complex regulates mammalian ciliogenesis and ciliary membrane composition. *Nat Genet* 2011, **43**:776–784.

45. Williams CL, Li C, Kida K, Inglis PN, Mohan S, Semenec L, Bialas NJ, Stupay RM, Chen N, Blacque OE, Yoder BK, Leroux MR: MKS and NPHP modules cooperate to establish basal body/transition zone membrane associations and ciliary gate function during ciliogenesis. *J Cell Biol* 2011, **192**:1023–1041.

46. Chih B, Liu P, Chinn Y, Chalouni C, Komuves LG, Hass PE, Sandoval W, Peterson AS: A ciliopathy complex at the transition zone protects the cilia as a privileged membrane domain. *Nat Cell Biol* 2012, **14**:61–72.

47. Zhang D, Aravind L: Identification of novel families and classification of the C2 domain superfamily elucidate the origin and evolution of membrane targeting activities in eukaryotes. *Gene* 2010, **469**:18–30.

48. Dowdle W, Robinson J, Kneist A, Sirerol-Piquer M, Frints S, Corbit K, Zaghloul N, van Lijnschoten G, Mulders L, Verver D, *et al*: Disruption of a Ciliary B9 protein complex causes Meckel syndrome. *Am J Hum Genet* 2011, **89**:94–110.

49. Gate D, Danielpour M, Levy R, Breunig J, Town T: Basic biology and mechanisms of neural ciliogenesis and the B9 family. *Mol Neurobiol* 2012, **45**:564–570.

# 4

# Primary gastric actinomycosis: report of a case diagnosed in a gastroscopic biopsy

Khaleel Al-Obaidy[1], Fatimah Alruwaii[1], Areej Al Nemer[1], Raed Alsulaiman[2], Zainab Alruwaii[3] and Mohamed A Shawarby[1*]

## Abstract

**Background:** Primary gastric actinomycosis is extremely rare, the appendix and ileocecal region being the most commonly involved sites in abdominopelvic actinomycosis. Herein, we report a case of primary gastric actinomycosis. The diagnosis was made on microscopic evaluation of gastroscopic biopsy specimens. To the best of our knowledge, this is the third case to be reported in the literature, in which the diagnosis was made in a gastroscopic biopsy rather than a resection specimen.

**Case presentation:** An 87-year-old Saudi male on medication for cardiomyopathy, premature ventricular contractions, renal impairment, hypertension, and dyslipidemia, presented to the emergency department with acute diffuse abdominal pain, abdominal distension, constipation and vomiting for two days, with no history of fever, abdominal surgery or trauma. The patient was admitted to the hospital with an impression of gastric outlet obstruction. Based on radiologic and gastroscopic findings, a non-infectious etiology was suspected, possibly adenocarcinoma or lymphoma. Gastroscopic biopsies showed an actively inflamed, focally ulcerated atrophic fundic mucosa along with fragments of a fibrinopurulent exudate containing brownish, iron negative pigment and abundant filamentous bacteria, morphologically consistent with *Actinomyces*.

**Conclusion:** Althuogh extremely rare, primary gastric actinomycosis should be considered in the differential diagnosis of radiologic and gastroscopic diffuse gastric wall thickening and submucosal tumor-like or infiltrative lesions, particularly in patients with history of abdominal surgery or trauma, or those receiving extensive medication. A high level of suspicion is required by the pathologist to achieve diagnosis in gastroscopic biopsies. Subtle changes such as the presence of a pigmented inflammatory exudate should alert the pathologist to perform appropriate special stains to reveal the causative organism.

**Keywords:** Actinomycosis, Gastric, Grocott's, Gram, PAS

## Background

Actinomycosis is a chronic suppurative granulomatous inflammation caused by anaerobic, filamentous, Gram-positive bacteria of *Actinomyces* species, most often *Actinomyces israelii*. There are three main forms of actinomycosis, namely, cervicofacial (31%-65%), abdominopelvic (20%-36%) and thoracic (15%-30%) [1-4]. In abdominopelvic actinomycosis, the appendix and ileocecal region are the most commonly involved sites (65%) [2,3,5-7]. Primary gastric actinomycosis is extremely rare, with only 23 cases reported to date [5,6,8-20]. Herein, we report a case of primary gastric

actinomycosis. The diagnosis was made on microscopic evaluation of gastroscopic biopsy specimens. To the best of our knowledge, this is the third case to be reported in the literature, in which the diagnosis was made in a gastroscopic biopsy rather than a resection specimen [6,8].

## Case presentation

### Clinical and laboratory findings

An 87-year-old Saudi male on medication for non-ischemic cardiomyopathy, frequent premature ventricular contractions, renal impairment, hypertension, and dyslipidemia, presented to the emergency department with acute diffuse abdominal pain, abdominal distension, constipation and vomiting of two days duration, with no history of fever, abdominal surgery or trauma. Medications received by the

\* Correspondence: melshawarby46@hotmail.com
[1]Pathology Department, College of Medicine, University of Dammam, P.O. Box 1982, Dammam 31441, Saudi Arabia
Full list of author information is available at the end of the article

patient for the last four years included, mainly, daily acetyl salicylic acid 81 mg, atorvastatin 40 mg, irbesartan 300 mg and hydrochlorothiazide 25 mg. Abdominal examination revealed stable vital signs along with positive findings of abdominal distension and mild epigastric tenderness. Laboratory investigations showed leucocytosis (16.6 k/µl with 89% segmented cells), mild normocytic normochromic anemia (Hgb 11.5 g/dl, MCV 93.7 fl, MCH 31.7 pg), elevated serum lipase (1123 U/L), amylase (269 U/L), and creatinine (1.4 mg/dl), and low potassium (3.1 mEq/L). Plain abdominal X-ray showed a markedly dilated stomach (Figure 1a). The patient was admitted to the hospital with an impression of gastric outlet obstruction. NGT was inserted & aspiration yielded a large amount of greenish fluid. The patient was then immediately put on empiric antibiotic coverage for 5 days with 2 doses of IV levofloxacin and 3 doses of IV metronidazole administered. Contrast CT-scan, performed to rule out an organic cause for the gastric outlet obstruction, showed a significantly distended stomach with thickened wall and abnormal configuration, and a single air-fluid level (Figure 1b). Two gastroscopies were then performed, 1 week apart, and revealed a deformed stomach with a hard mass infiltrating the greater curvature in the fundic area, covered by necrotic greenish brown material, along with absent peristaltic movement and no apparent organic obstruction to the gastric outlet (Figure 2). Based on the radiologic and gastroscopic findings, a non-infectious etiology was suspected, possibly adenocarcinoma or lymphoma. Biopsies obtained from the edge and the centre of the fundic mass during both gastroscopies were sent for pathological examination. Histologic examination showed an actively inflamed, focally ulcerated, atrophic fundic mucosa with variable, focal eosinophilic infiltration, edema, and variably dilated foveolae with focal regenerative epithelial atypia (Figure 3). There were also fragments of a fibrinopurulent exudate mixed with brownish, iron negative pigment (Perl's stain) and abundant PAS, Grocott's, and Gram positive rod-

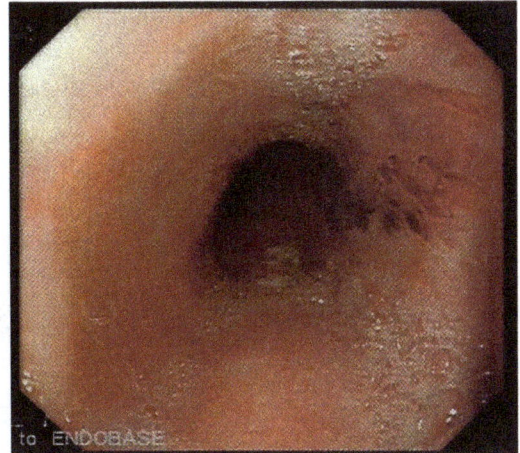

**Figure 2 Gastroscopy.** Deformed stomach, with rotation like appearance. There are inflamed areas with greenish brown material over the surface.

like and filamentous bacteria, morphologically consistent with *Actinomyces* (Figure 4). The organisms were overlooked in the first biopsy. The second biopsy was performed because a diagnosis of malignancy was still in suspicion, despite the negative result of the first biopsy. A revisit to the first biopsy confirmed negativity for malignancy but revealed the presence of organisms identical to those noted in the second biopsy. Culturing of gastric contents following the second gastroscopy, yielded only *Streptococcus viridans* with no *Actinomyces* identified. However, anaerobic culture was not specifically ordered by the clinician. Consequently *Actinomyces*, known to be strictly anaerobic, were not detected. Despite the negative culture, the typical morphology of the organisms in tissue sections confirmed by positive Grocott, PAS and Gram staining was considerd sufficient

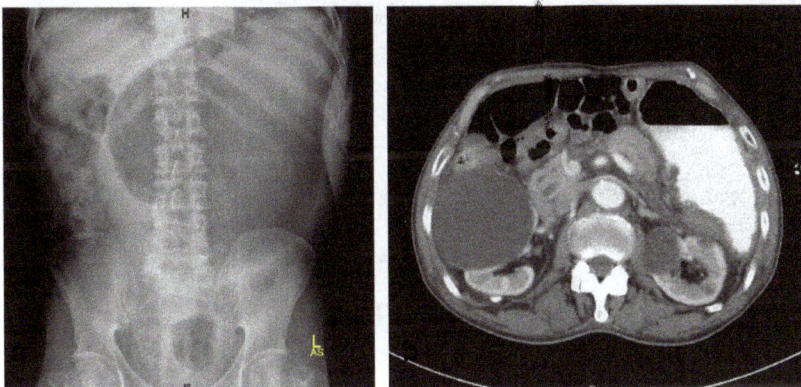

**Figure 1 Radiologic findings. a**. Plain abdominal X-ray showing a markedly dilated stomach  **b**. Contrast CT-scan showing a significantly distended stomach with thickened wall and abnormal configuration. Note also air-fluid level.

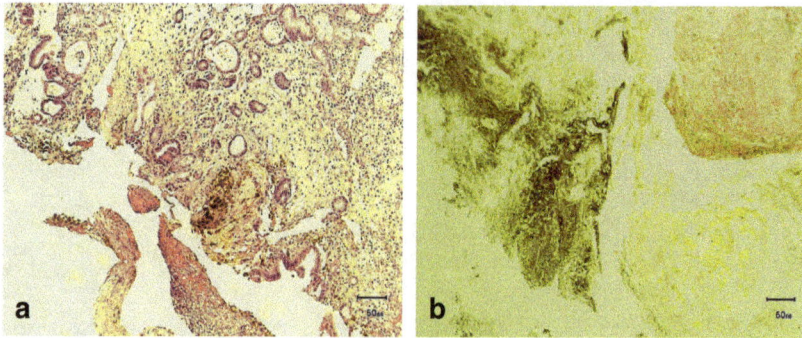

**Figure 3 Gastroscopic biopsies. a**. Inflamed atrophic mucosa with dilated foveolae and pigmented fibrinopurulent inflammatory exudate. H & E x 100 **b**. Perl's stain showing iron negative brownish pigment. x 400.

for diagnosis with no necessity for confirmation by repeat culturing under anaerobic conditions.

The patient was then managed conservatively in the hospital. A third gastroscopic biopsy two weeks later revealed chronic atrophic gastritis with no *Actinomyces* detected, and the patient appeared in a good health status. A plan was set up to start him on the appropriate antibiotic therapy for actinomycosis with follow up gastroscopy after one month. However, the patient chose to continue treatment somewhere else. So he was discharged on his request and never showed up again in our institution.

## Discussion

Actinomycosis in human is most commonly caused by *Actinomyces israelii* [1,3,21-26] which is an endogenous commensal present in the oral and GI-tract flora [9,10,12,22,27]. Actinomycetes typically invade injured mucosa with opportunistic infection occuring if there is a break in the mucosal barrier. Factors that precipitate intra-abdominal actinomycosis include GI surgery, inflammation, and visceral perforation [28,29]. However, in most cases of gastric actinomycosis, it has been impossible to trace the mechanism by which *Actinomyces* had reached the gastric wall [30]. Our patient had no past

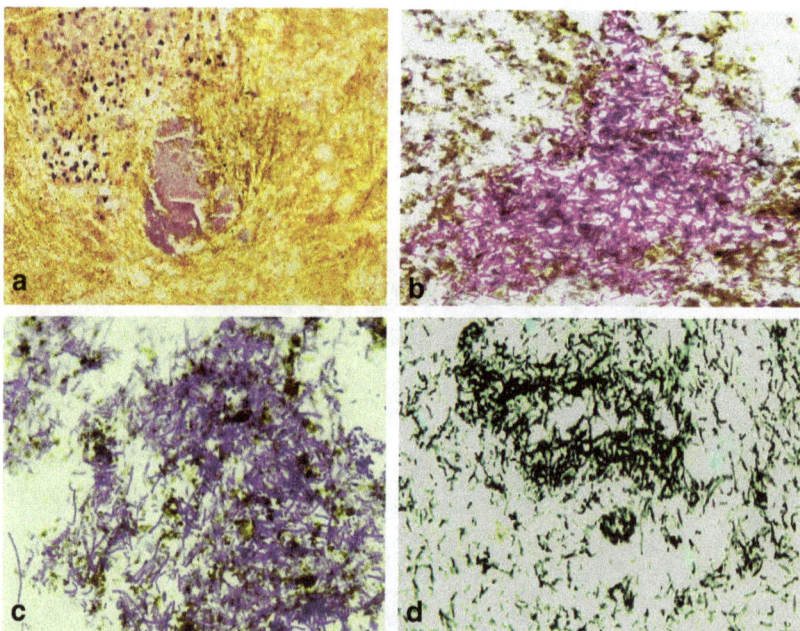

**Figure 4 Filamentous and rod-like bacteria consistent with *Actinomyces* in gastroscopic biopsies. a**. H & E x 400 **b**. PAS x 1000 **c**. Gram x 1000 **d**. Grocott's x 1000.

history of abdominal surgery or trauma. However, he was on prolonged medication for non-ischemic cardiomyopathy, premature ventricular contractions, renal impairment, hypertension, and dyslipidemia. Such extensive medication may have caused physical or functional gastric mucosal damage that facilitated entry of the organisms into the gastric wall. Numerous drugs, acting through various mechanisms, have been associated with gastric mucosal damage [31]. Age related mucosal atrophy may have also contributed to diminished mucosal resistance.

The rarity of gastric involvement by actinomycosis has been attributed to the high lumenal acidity of the stomach. As a result of the low gastric pH, the organisms may be killed or growth is inhibited [9].

The usual presenting clinical manifestations of gastric actinomycosis are low-grade fever, epigastric pain, weight loss, and upper GI bleeding [1,3,10,12,20]. One patient developed symptoms of gastric outlet obstruction [19]. The duration of symptoms ranged from two weeks to several years [3,8,9,11,19]. Our patient presented with acute diffuse abdominal pain, abdominal distension, constipation and vomiting for two days duration, with no history of fever. The clinical impression was that of gastric outlet obstruction.

There is no specific radiological or endoscopic appearance for gastric actinomycosis. CT findings have mostly demonstrated an infiltrative lesion with diffuse gastric wall thickening. The appearance suggested adenocarcinoma or lymphoma of the stomach [2,20,32]. In our case, contrast CT-scan showed a significantly distended stomach with thickened wall and abnormal configuration. Similar to radiologic studies, the endoscopic findings of the disease may simulate a gastric neoplasm and include submucosal tumor-like or infiltrative lesions and, occasionally, mucosal ulceration [13]. A non-infectious etiology was initially suspected in our patient based on radiologic and endoscopic findings, possibly adenocarcinoma or lymphoma, and the gastric outlet obstruction subsequently interpreted as functional due to absence of peristaltic movement consequent to infiltration of the gastric wall by actinomycosis. An associated paralytic ileus due to acute pancreatitis may be an alternative explanation for the obstruction as suggested by elevated serum lipase and amylase levels. Such obstruction may have also contributed to the gastric localization of the actinomycosis, so that the clinical manifestations may be a consequence of acute pancreatitis with secondary gastric overinfection by *Actinomyces*, facilitated by the mucosal damage.

Because of the submucosal localization of the inflammatory process, gastroscopic biopsy specimens usually reveal nonspecific inflammatory changes [3,14,18,19]. In most cases, the diagnosis was made after surgery and histopathological examination of the resected specimen [9,12,19,20,22]. Only two cases have been reported in which the diagnosis

of gastric actinomycosis was made on microscopic evaluation of a gastroscopic biopsy specimen [6,8]. In our case, the diagnosis was, likewise, established through histologic examination of gastroscopic biopsies in which abundant PAS, Grocott's, and Gram positive rod-like and filamentous bacteria, morphologically consistent with *Actinomyces* were identified. The presence of a brownish, iron negative pigment in the fibrinopurulent inflammatory exudate (that was also visible endoscopically) alerted us to the possibility of actinomycosis which was established by appropriate special staining that revealed the microorganisms. It is well known that the main sources of natural pigments are plants and microorganisms, including *Actinomycets* [33].

Culturing is negative in most cases of gastric actinomycosis (>76%) [19,24,25]. In our case, culturing yielded only *Streptococcus viridans*, another endogenous aerobic/anaerobic facultative commensal present in the oral and GI-tract flora [34]. Despite the negative culture, the typical morphology of the organisms in tissue sections confirmed by positive Grocott, PAS and Gram staining was considered sufficient for the diagnosis of *Actinomyces* infection with no necessity for culture confirmation.

Most anaerobic bacteria recovered from clinical infections are found mixed with other anaerobic organisms [35]. Polymicrobial infections are known to be more pathogenic for experimental animals than are those involving single organisms [35]. Whether *Streptococcus viridans*, known to be an organism of low virulence, had contributed to the gastritis in our case remains unclear.

Primary gastric actinomycosis is an indolent infection. If the disease is recognized, the prognosis is good because antibiotic treatment, particularly penecillin is very effective [4,19]. Our patient received 2 doses of IV levofloxacin and 3 doses of IV metronidazole and appeared in a good health status, two weeks after diagnosis.

## Conclusions

Althuogh extremely rare, primary gastric actinomycosis should be considered in the differential diagnosis of radiologic and gastroscopic diffuse gastric wall thickening and submucosal tumor-like or infiltrative lesions, particularly in patients with history of abdominal surgery or trauma or those receiving extensive medication. A high level of suspicion is required by the pathologist to achieve diagnosis in gastroscopic biopsies. Subtle changes such as the presence of a pigmented inflammatory exudate should alert the pathologist to perform appropriate special stains to reveal the causative organism.

## Consent

Written informed consent was obtained from the patient for publication of this case report and any accompanying images. A copy of the written consent is available for review by the Editor of this journal.

**Competing interests**
The authors declare that they have no competing interests.

**Authors' contributions**
KA-O shared in analysis of histologic, clinical and radiologic findings and significantly contributed to drafting of the article. FA shared in analysis of histologic findings and contributed to drafting of the article. AAN shared in interpretation of histologic findings and performed critical review of the article. RA provided and interpreted clinical, endoscopic and radiological findings. ZA shared in analysis of histologic findings and performed critical review of the article. MAS performed interpretation and analysis of histologic findings, closely supervised progress of the study and completed drafting and editing of the article. All authors have read and approved the final manuscript.

**Acknowledgements**
The authors acknowledge Dr Amani Al Nemer, Assistant Professor, Microbiology Department, University of Dammam for reviewing the results of H & E and special staining of micro-organisms in tissue sections. The authors also acknowledge the services of Mr Shakir Ahmed and Mrs Maria Rosario Lazaro from the histopathology laboratory of the University of Dammam, Saudi Arabia for conducting the histology technical work.

**Author details**
[1]Pathology Department, College of Medicine, University of Dammam, P.O. Box 1982, Dammam 31441, Saudi Arabia. [2]Department of Internal Medicine, College of Medicine, University of Dammam, P.O. Box 1982, Dammam 31441, Saudi Arabia. [3]King Fahd Hospital of the University, University of Dammam, P.O. Box 2208, Al-Khobar 31952, Saudi Arabia.

**References**
1.  Choi MM, Beak JH, Lee JN, Park S, Lee WS. Clinical features of abdominopelvic actinomycosis: report of twenty cases and literature review. Yonsei Med J. 2009;50:555–9.
2.  Isik B, Aydin E, Sogutlu G, Ara C, Yilmaz S, Kirimlioglu V. Abdominal actinomycosis simulating malignancy of the right colon. Dig Dis Sci. 2005;50:1312–4.
3.  Lee YM, Law WL, Chu KW. Abdominal actinomycosis. Aust N Z J Surg. 2001;71:261–3.
4.  Wang YH, Tsai HC, Lee SS, Mai MH, Wann SR, Chen YS, et al. Clinical manifestations of actinomycosis in Southern Taiwan. J Microbiol Immunol Infect. 2007;40:487–92.
5.  Oksüz M, Sandikçi S, Culhaci A, Egesel T, Tuncer I. Primary gastric actinomycosis: a case report. Turk J Gastroenterol. 2007;18:44–6.
6.  Lee SH, Kim HJ, Kim HJ, Chung IK, Kim HS, Park SH, et al. Primary gastric actinomycosis diagnosed by endoscopic biopsy: case report. Gastrointest Endosc. 2004;59:586–9.
7.  Evans J, Chan C, Gluch L, Fielding I, Eckstein R. Inflammatory pseudotumour secondary to actinomyces infection. Aust N Z J Surg. 1999;69:467–9.
8.  Minamino H, Machida H, Tominaga K, Kameda N, Okazaki H, Tanigawa T, et al. A case report on primary gastric actinomycosis. Gastroenterol Endosc. 2011;53(2):262–9.
9.  Skoutelis A, Panagopoulos C, Kalfarentzos F, Bassaris H. Intramural gastric actinomycosis. South Med J. 1995;88:647–50.
10. Lee CM, Ng SH, Wan YL, Tsai CH. Gastric actinomycosis. J Formos Med Assoc. 1996;95:66–8.
11. Fernández-Aceñero MJ, Silvestre V, Fernández-Roldán R, Cortes L, Garcia-Blanch G. Gastric actinomycosis: a rare complication after gastric bypass for morbid obesity. Obes Surg. 2004;14:1012–5.
12. Van Olmen G, Larmuseau MF, Geboes K, Rutgeerts P, Penninckx F, Vantrappen G. Primary gastric actinomycosis: a case report and review of the literature. Am J Gastroenterol. 1984;79(7):512–6.
13. Mazuji MK, Henry JS. Gastric actinomycosis: case report. Arch Surg. 1967;94:292–3.
14. Urdaneta LF, Belin RP, Cueto J, Doberneck RC. Intramural gastric actinomycosis. Surgery. 1967;62:431–5.
15. Figueras Felip J, Martín Rague J, Madesvall N, Norquera C, Casias AL. Intramural gastric abscess. Rev Esp Enfer Apar Dig. 1979;56:267–70.
16. Dellagi K, Kchir N, Mezni F, Boubaker S, el Quertani L, Zitouni MM, et al. Abdominal actinomycosis: a rare complication of gastric surgery? A propos of a case. Ann Gastroenterol Hepatol. 1986;22:391–3.
17. Eastridge CE, Prather JR, Hughes FA. Actinomycosis: a 24-year experience. South Med J. 1972;65:839–43.
18. Wilson E. Abdominal actinomycosis with special reference to the stomach. Br J Surg. 1961;49:266–70.
19. Lee DL, Kang JY, Kim H, Lee KH, Choi GY, Jeon WJ, et al. A case of primary gastric actinomycosis. Korean J Med. 2009;77:S27–30.
20. Euanorasetr C, Sornmayura P. Gastric Outlet Obstruction Secondary to Gastric Actinomycosis: A Case Report and Literature Review. The THAI Journal of SURGERY. 2010;31:63–8.
21. Kaszuba M, Tomaszewska R, Pityński K, Grzanka P, Bazan-Socha S, Musail J. Actinomycosis mimicking advanced cancer. Pol Arch Med Wewn. 2008;118:581–4.
22. Berardi RS. Abdominal actinomycosis. Surg Gynecol Obstet. 1979;149:257–66.
23. Sumer Y, Yilmaz B, Emre B, Ugur C. Abdominal mass secondary to actinomyces infection: an unusual presentation and its treatment. J Postgrad Med. 2004;50:115–7.
24. Huang CJ, Huang TJ, Hsieh JS. Pseudo-colonic carcinoma caused by abdominal actinomycosis: report of two cases. Int J Colorectal Dis. 2004;19:283–6.
25. Wagenlehner FM, Mohren B, Naber KG, Mannl HF. Abdominal actinomycosis. Clin Microbiol Infect. 2003;9:881–5.
26. Alam MK, Khayat FA, Al-Kayali A, Al-Suhaibani YA. Abdominal actinomycosis: case reports. Saudi J Gastroenterol. 2001;7:37–9.
27. Russo TA. Agents of actinomycosis. In: Mandell GL, Bennett JE, Dolin R, editors. Principles and practice of infectious diseases. 4th ed. New York: Churchill Livingstone; 1995. p. 2280–4.
28. Weese WC, Smith IM. A study of 57 cases of actinomycosis over a 36-year period. Arch Intern Med. 1975;135:1562–8.
29. Yang SH, Li AF, Lin JK. Colonoscopy in abdominal actinomycosis. Gastrointest Endosc. 2000;51:236–8.
30. Brown JR. Human actinomycosis: a study of 181 subjects. Hum Pathol. 1973;4:319–30.
31. Srivastava A, Lauwers GY. Pathology of non-infective gastritis. Histopathology. 2007;50:15–29.
32. Das N, Lee J, Madden M, Elliot CS, Bateson P, Gilliland R. A rare case of abdominal actinomycosis presenting as an inflammatory pseudotumor. Int J Colorectal Dis. 2006;21:483–4.
33. Chattopadhyay P, Chatterjee S, Sen SK. Biotechnological potential of natural food grade biocolorants. Afr J Biotech. 2008;17:2972–85.
34. Tunkel AR, Sepkowitz KA. Infections Caused by Viridans Streptococci in Patients with Neutropenia. Clin Infect Dis. 2002;34(11):1524–9.
35. Brook I, Hunter V, Walker RI. Synergistic effects of anaerobic ccocci, Bacteroides, Clostridia, Fusobacteria, and anaerobic bacteria on mouse and induction of substances abscess. J Infect Dis. 1984;149:924–8.

# 5

# Tumor-specific expression of HMG-CoA reductase in a population-based cohort of breast cancer patients

Emma Gustbée[1], Helga Tryggvadottir[1,2], Andrea Markkula[1], Maria Simonsson[1], Björn Nodin[1], Karin Jirström[1], Carsten Rose[3], Christian Ingvar[4], Signe Borgquist[1,2] and Helena Jernström[1*]

## Abstract

**Background:** The mevalonate pathway synthetizes cholesterol, steroid hormones, and non-steriod isoprenoids necessary for cell survival. 3-Hydroxy-3-methylglutaryl-coenzyme A reductase (HMGCR) is the rate-limiting enzyme of the mevalonate pathway and the target for statin treatment. HMGCR expression in breast tumors has recently been proposed to hold prognostic and treatment-predictive information. This study aimed to investigate whether HMGCR expression in breast cancer patients was associated with patient and tumor characteristics and disease-free survival (DFS).

**Methods:** A population-based cohort of primary breast cancer patients in Lund, Sweden was assembled between October 2002 and June 2012 enrolling 1,116 patients. Tumor tissue microarrays were constructed and stained with a polyclonal HMGCR antibody (Cat. No HPA008338, Atlas Antibodies AB, Stockholm, Sweden, diluted 1:100) to assess the HMGCR expression in tumor tissue from 885 patients. HMGCR expression was analyzed in relation to patient- and tumor characteristics and disease-free survival (DFS) with last follow-up June 30th 2014.

**Results:** Moderate/strong HMGCR expression was associated with less axillary lymph node involvement, lower histological grade, estrogen and progesterone receptor positivity, HER2 negativity, and older patient age at diagnosis compared to weak or no HMGCR expression. Patients were followed for up to 11 years. The median follow-up time was 5.0 years for the 739 patients who were alive and still at risk at the last follow-up. HMGCR expression was not associated with DFS.

**Conclusion:** In this study, HMGCR expression was associated with less aggressive tumor characteristics. However, no association between HMGCR expression and DFS was observed. Longer follow-up may be needed to evaluate HMGCR as prognostic or predictive marker in breast cancer.

**Keywords:** Breast cancer, HMG-CoA reductase, Tumor characteristics, Treatment, Early breast cancer events, Prognosis

## Introduction

New prognostic and treatment-predictive markers are needed to improve treatment decisions and consequently prognosis and treatment response in breast cancer patients. Recent data suggest that the enzyme 3-hydroxy-3-methylglutaryl-coenzyme A reductase (HMGCR), which is inhibited by statins that are commonly used as a cholesterol-lowering treatment, may be associated with breast tumor characteristics, prognosis and treatment response [1–3]. HMGCR is the rate-limiting enzyme in the mevalonate pathway [4]. The mevalonate pathway produces cholesterol, steroid hormones, and non-steroid isoprenoids, which are necessary for cell survival [5]. Previous studies demonstrated that HMGCR inhibitors (e.g., statins) exert anti-carcinogenic effects by inducing apoptosis and inhibiting inflammation [6], proliferation and migration [7–9]. HMGCR inhibitors can also inhibit angiogenesis [10]. Whether statins also reduce the risk of

* Correspondence: helena.jernstrom@med.lu.se
[1]Division of Oncology and Pathology, Department of Clinical Sciences, Lund, Lund University, Barngatan 2B, SE 22185 Lund, Sweden
Full list of author information is available at the end of the article

cancer remains debated [11–17]. HMGCR is differentially expressed among breast cancers, as well as between normal epithelial cells and tumor cells, with higher expression in the tumor cells. This difference is presumably caused by resistance against the feedback system of the mevalonate pathway [18]. Several studies examined the relationship between tumor-specific HMGCR expression and other tumor characteristics [1, 2]. In previous studies, stronger expression of HMGCR was associated with a less aggressive tumor profile, such as a low histological grade, a small tumor size, estrogen receptor (ER) positivity, and low proliferation [1, 2]. One study reported that patients with HMGCR-positive tumors exhibited longer recurrence-free survival, which was more pronounced in patients with ER-positive tumors [2]. Another study observed longer recurrence-free survival in patients treated with tamoxifen who had HMGCR-positive and ER-positive tumors compared to patients who had ER-positive and HMGCR-negative tumors, indicating that HMGCR may predict tamoxifen response [3].

### Hypothesis and aim

We hypothesized that stronger HMGCR expression was associated with markers of good prognosis and prolonged disease-free survival (DFS), as well as a better response to tamoxifen, in this population-based unselected cohort of primary breast cancer patients. The aims of the study were to investigate whether HMGCR expression in breast cancer was associated with patient and tumor characteristics, prognosis and treatment response.

## Materials and methods

### Patients

Women diagnosed with a primary breast cancer at Skåne University Hospital in Lund, Sweden between October 2002 and June 2012 were invited to take part in an ongoing prospective cohort study: the Breast Cancer (BC) Blood study. During the inclusion period, 1,116 patients were included in the study and followed-up until June 30th, 2014. Patients with a previous breast cancer diagnosis or another cancer diagnosis during the previous ten years were not included. The aim was to study factors that could affect prognosis or treatment response and to identify new markers that may help better tailor adjuvant therapy to individual breast cancer patients. The study was approved by Lund University Ethics Committee (Dnr LU75-02, LU37-08, LU658-09, LU58-12, and LU379-12). All patients signed a written informed consent. The study adhered to the REMARK criteria [19].

All patients completed questionnaires preoperatively. Post-operative questionnaires were completed after 3–6 months, 7–9 months, and 1, 2, 3, 5, 7, 9 and 11 years. The questionnaires included questions concerning medication intake during the last week, lifestyle, and reproductive factors. Medications were coded according to the Anatomic Therapeutic Chemical (ATC) classification system codes [20]. Patients who reported smoking during the last week or smoking at parties were considered current smokers. Coffee consumption was categorized as 0–1 or 2+ cups/day, as previously described [21]. A research nurse obtained body measurements, including, height, weight, waist and hip circumferences, and breast volumes, at the pre-operative visit. Breast volume was measured as previously described [22, 23].

Tumor characteristics were acquired from the patients' pathology reports. The estrogen receptor (ER) and progesterone receptor (PgR) expression were analyzed in the Department of Pathology at Skåne University Hospital in Lund, Sweden. Until December 2009, immunohistochemistry was performed using the Dako LSAB kit system (Dako, Glostrup, Denmark) and the M7047 (ER) and M3569 (PgR) antibodies (DAKO) [24, 25]. From 2010 onwards, the ER (SP1) and PgR (1E2) antibodies from Ventana Medical Systems (Ventana, AZ, USA) were used in combination with a Ventana Benchmark Ultra instrument (Ventana Medical Systems) [26]. Tumors with more than 10 % positive nuclear staining were considered ER-positive or PgR-positive according to current Swedish clinical guidelines. Histological type was classified into ductal, lobular and 'other' types. Ten tumors had a mixed ductal and lobular histology and were classified as 'other'. Since the tumors were not routinely analyzed for HER2 amplification until November 2005, patients included in the study prior to that time were excluded from analyses that included HER2 status.

Information on type of surgery, treatment, and breast cancer related events was obtained from patient charts and the regional tumor registry. The date of death was collected from the Swedish Population Registry. Patients who had received preoperative treatment (n = 51) and patients with cancer in situ (n = 39) were excluded from the analyses, leaving 1,026 preoperatively untreated patients with invasive breast cancer as the study population (Fig. 1).

### Tissue microarray construction

Tumor tissue was available from 992 of the 1,026 patients. Tissue microarrays (TMAs) for the tumors were constructed by sampling 1 mm duplicate cores from representative, non-necrotic tumor regions from the donating formalin-fixed paraffin-embedded tumor tissue block from surgical resection, using a semi-automated tissue array device (Beecher Instruments, Sun Prairie, WI, USA).

### Immunohistochemistry

An automatic PT-link system (DAKO, Glostrup, Denmark) was used to deparaffinize and pretreat 4 μm TMA-sections for HMGCR staining. HMGCR staining was performed

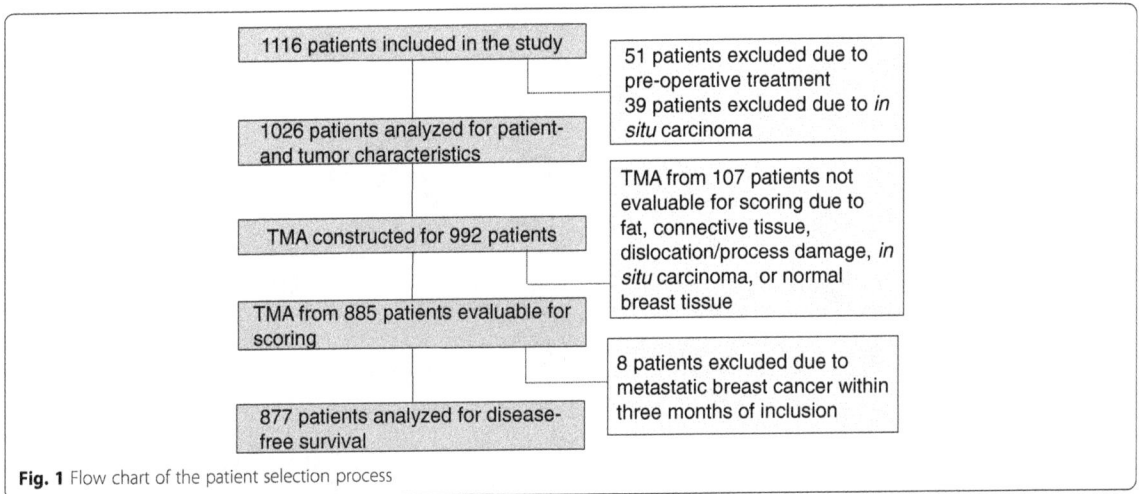

**Fig. 1** Flow chart of the patient selection process

using an Autostainer Plus, according to the manufacturer's instructions (DAKO). The staining procedure employed an HMGCR antibody (Cat. No HPA008338, Atlas Antibodies AB, Stockholm, Sweden) (diluted 1:100) and an EnVision FLEX high-pH kit. HMGCR expression could be evaluated in tumors from 885/992 patients. In 57 cases, the TMA-cores contained non-representative tissue, in 27 cases, the cores were damaged or lost during processing, and in 23 cases, the cores could not be evaluated due to a combination of the reasons mentioned above. HMGCR expression was evaluated based on the staining intensity in the cytoplasm (i.e., negative = 0, weak = 1, moderate = 2, and strong = 3), as shown in Fig. 2, and based on the fraction of HMGCR-positive cells (0 % = 0, 1-10 % = 1, 11-50 % = 2, 51-100 % = 3). Two investigators, who were blinded to the patient data and clinical outcome, evaluated all samples simultaneously (EG, HT). When the two investigators could not reach a consensus, a senior investigator (SB) was consulted and a consensus was reached. The HMGCR expression differed between the duplicate cores for 109 patients. In all cases but one, the intensity only differed by one step. Discordant cores were reevaluated jointly to obtain a pooled score based on the intensity represented in the majority of cancer cells. When one core was classified as negative and the other core was classified as positive, the pooled score was classified as positive. Only 22 tumors showed strong intensity of HMGCR expression, and this group was combined with tumors expressing HMGCR with a moderate intensity (n = 195). A total of 28 of the 1,026 patients had bilateral tumors; tissue from both tumors was available for 15 patients. Scoring of both bilateral tumors was possible for 10 of these patients. For the three cases where the intensity differed, the highest intensity was used. In most cases (94.9 %) for which the staining was positive in any cell, HMGCR

was expressed in the majority of the cells (51-100 %). Therefore, the fraction of HMGCR-positive cells was excluded from further analyses.

**Statistics**

The statistical analyses were performed using SPSS Statistics 19 (IBM, Chicago, IL, USA). Patient and tumor characteristics were analyzed in relation to HMGCR expression. The Chi-square and Linear-by-Linear tests were used for categorical variables. The Kruskal-Wallis and Jonckheere-Terpstra tests were used for continuous variables because some of these variables were not normally distributed. Tumor characteristics in relation to HMGCR tumor expression were also analyzed with linear regression and adjusted for age as a continuous variable. The DFS was calculated from the date of inclusion until the first breast cancer related event (i.e., local or regional recurrence, contralateral breast cancer, or distant metastasis); in cases with no breast cancer related events, DFS was calculated using the last study follow-up or death before July 1st, 2014. Non-breast cancer-related death was censored at the time of death. Patients with distant metastases detected earlier than three months after inclusion were excluded from the survival analyses (n = 8). Univariable survival analyses were calculated using Log-Rank tests. Cox proportional hazard regression was used for multivariable testing, with adjustments for invasive tumor size (>20 mm or muscular or skin involvement), axillary lymph node involvement, histological grade (III), ER and PgR status (positive/negative), age <50 years (yes/no), current preoperative smoking (yes/no), and body mass index (BMI) <25 kg/m$^2$ (yes/no) [27]. All statistical tests were two-tailed. $P$-values < 0.05 were regarded as statistically significant. Nominal $P$-values were presented without adjustment for multiple testing.

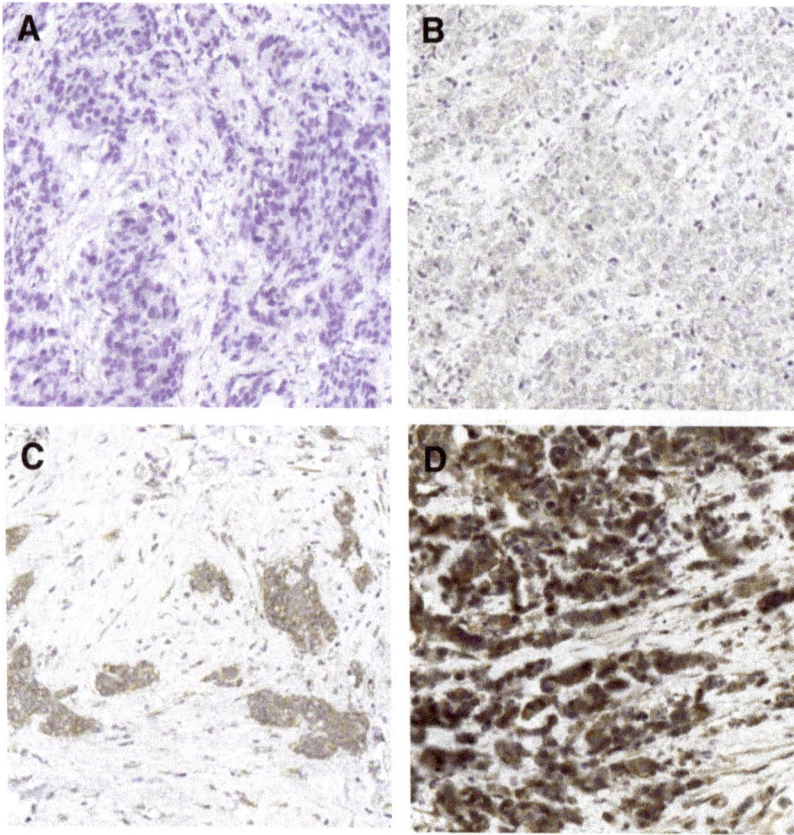

**Fig. 2** Examples of HMGCR expression, representing no staining (**a**), and weak (**b**), moderate (**c**), and strong (**d**) expression. The original magnification before scale-down was 20x for each example

## Results

### Patient characteristics and HMGCR expression

The patient characteristics are presented in relation to the HMGCR expression (Table 1). Of the 885 cases evaluable for scoring, the intensity of HMGCR expression was negative in 113 cases (12.8 %), weak in 555 cases (62.7 %), and moderate/strong in 217 (24.5 %) cases. Patients of all ages were included (range 24–99 years). The median age at inclusion in the study was 61.1 years (interquartile range 52.1 to 68.1). Patients younger than 50 years at inclusion were significantly taller, had a lower BMI, and had smaller waist and hip circumferences, waist-to-hip ratios, and breast volumes than older patients ($P \leq 0.001$ for all comparisons); however, these patients had a weight similar to that of older patients. The final surgery performed included partial mastectomy in 531 cases (60 %) and modified radical mastectomy in 354 cases (40 %). Postoperative radiotherapy was given to 559 patients (63.2 %) and 226 patients (25.5 %) received adjuvant chemotherapy. As adjuvant endocrine therapy, tamoxifen treatment was prescribed to 466 patients (52.7 %) and 302 patients (34.1 %) were

treated with aromatase inhibitors. As of November 2005, 55 patients (8.6 %) had received adjuvant treatment with trastuzumab (n = 640). Patients often received more than one type of treatment.

Patients with tumors that expressed moderate/strong HMGCR were significantly older than patients in the other HMGCR intensity groups at inclusion. Patients with tumors that expressed weak HMGCR were significantly taller than patients in the other HMGCR intensity groups. No other significant associations were observed between patient characteristics and HMGCR expression. The results remained essentially the same when excluding patients who reported statin usage preoperatively (n = 99).

### HMGCR expression and established tumor characteristics

Table 2 displays the tumor characteristics in relation to HMGCR expression. Tumor size was not associated with HMGCR expression. Tumors that expressed moderate/strong HMGCR were of significantly lower histological grade, were more frequently ER-positive, PgR-positive, and HER2-negative, and were less likely to show axillary lymph

**Table 1** Association of HMGCR expression with patient characteristics

| | All patients median (IQR) or % | Missing | Patients with evaluable TMA | HMGCR expression-Intensity median (IQR) or % | | | |
| --- | --- | --- | --- | --- | --- | --- | --- |
| | | | | No staining = 0 | Weak = 1 | Moderate/Strong = 2/3 | P-value |
| n= | 1026 | | 885 | 113 | 555 | 217 | |
| Age at inclusion, yrs | 61.1 (52.1-68.1) | 0 | 60.9 (52.2-67.9) | 61.2 (53.7-69.2) | 60.1 (51.6-67.4) | 64.3 (53.9-69.4) | 0.004[c] |
| Body mass index (BMI), (kg/m-2) | 25.1 (22.5-28.3) | 28 | 25.2 (22.5-28.4) | 25.7 (23.2-28.7) | 25.0 (22.4-28.3) | 25.3 (22.5-29.0) | 0.39[c] |
| Height (cm) | 165 (162–170) | 26 | 165 (162–170) | 164 (160–169) | 166 (162–170) | 165 (161–169) | 0.03[c] |
| Weight (kg) | 69 (62–78) | 26 | 69 (62–78) | 70 (62–79) | 69 (62–78) | 69 (61–80) | 0.91[c] |
| Waist-Hip-Ratio | 0.86 (0.81-0.9) | 38 | 0.86 (0.81-0.90) | 0.86 (0.81-0.92) | 0.85 (0.80-0.90) | 0.86 (0.81-0.90) | 0.32[c] |
| Waist (cm) | 87 (79–97) | 38 | 87 (80–97) | 89 (82–97) | 87 (79–97) | 89 (80–98) | 0.24[c] |
| Hip (cm) | 102 (97–109) | 38 | 102 (97–109) | 104 (99–109) | 102 (97–109) | 102 (96–111) | 0.57[c] |
| Breast volume (ml) | 1000 (650–1500) | 161 | 1000 (650–1550) | 1000 (700–1550) | 950 (640–1500) | 1000 (656–1600) | 0.28[c] |
| Age at menarche, yrs | 13 (12–14) | 7 | 13 (12–14) | 13 (13–14) | 13 (12–14) | 13 (12–14) | 0.68[c] |
| Nulliparous | 124 (12.1 %) | 1 | 109 (12.3 %) | 17 (15.0 %) | 67 (12.1 %) | 25 (11.5 %) | 0.41[d] |
| Parity | 2 (1–3) | 1 | 2 (1–3) | 2 (1–3) | 2 (1–3) | 2 (1–2) | 0.46[c] |
| Age at first child, years* | 25 (22–28) | 6 | 24 (22–28) | 24 (21–27) | 25 (21–28) | 25 (22–29) | 0.09[b] |
| Ever use of HRT | 449 (43.9 %) | 3 | 386 (43.8 %) | 55 (48.7 %) | 231 (41.8 %) | 100 (43.8 %) | 0.28[a] |
| Ever oral contraceptives | 726 (70.8 %) | 1 | 625 (70.7 %) | 82 (72.6 %) | 394 (71.1 %) | 149 (68.7 %) | 0.42[d] |
| Current smoker | 210 (20.5 %) | 2 | 177 (20.0 %) | 26 (23.0 %) | 111 (20.1 %) | 40 (18.4 %) | 0.34[d] |
| Coffee, 2+ cups per day | 832 (81.4 %) | 4 | 708 (80.4 %) | 89 (78.8 %) | 448 (81.3 %) | 171 (78.8 %) | 0.66[a] |
| Alcohol abstainer | 107 (10.5 %) | 7 | 96 (10.9 %) | 15 (13.3 %) | 56 (10.1 %) | 25 (11.6 %) | 0.58[a] |

*Among Parous women, IQR = Inter quartile range [a]Chi-Square, [b]Jonckheere-Terpstra, [c]Kruskal-Wallis, [d]Linear-by-linear

node involvement compared to patients whose tumors had weak or no HMGCR expression. Histological type was not associated with HMGCR expression. HER2 amplification was more common among patients with HMGCR-negative tumors. These associations remained significant after adjustment for age. The results remained essentially the same after exclusion of patients with preoperative statin usage. Ki67 was only available for 365 patients (41.2 %) and was not further analyzed.

### Risk of early breast cancer related events

Patients were followed for up to 11 years. The median follow-up time was 5.0 years (interquartile range 3.0-7.2 years) for the 739 patients who were alive and still at risk at the last follow-up. The total number of patients with a breast cancer related event during follow-up was 104, of whom 68 patients were diagnosed with distant metastases. Of these 104 patients with a breast cancer related event, 53 patients subsequently died during follow-up. An additional 34 patients died without a prior recorded breast cancer related event. No significant association was observed between HMGCR expression and DFS either in univariable (Log-Rank $P_{trend} = 0.42$) (Fig. 3) or or multivariable models (Table 3). Likewise, no difference in DFS was observed between patients with any HMGCR expression and patients with HMGCR-negative tumors (Log-Rank $P_{trend} = 0.90$). In

addition, no significant association was observed between HMGCR expression and distant metastasis-free survival (Log-Rank $P_{trend} = 0.44$), or overall survival (Log-Rank $P_{trend} = 0.87$). The results remained essentially the same in analyses restricted to patients with ER-positive tumors. Further stratification according to ER status, treatment (e.g., tamoxifen, aromatase inhibitors, radiotherapy, or chemotherapy), age or BMI failed to yield any significant associations between HMGCR expression and DFS in either univariable or multivariable models. The results remained essentially the same when excluding preoperative statin users. Similarly, the results did not differ when three patients with *in situ* breast cancer related events were excluded.

### Discussion

The main finding of this study was that moderate/strong HMGCR expression was significantly associated with several indolent tumor characteristics, including lower histological grade, ER and PgR positivity, HER2 negativity, and less axillary lymph node involvement. These findings are largely consistent with a previous study that reported an association between stronger HMGCR expression and small tumor size, low histological grade, low Ki67, and ER expression [1]. However, in the present study, no association was observed between tumor size and HMGCR expression, and Ki67 was not included in

**Table 2** Association of HMGCR expression with tumor characteristics

| | All patients median (IQR) or % | Missing | Patients with evaluable TMA | HMGCR expression-Intensity median (IQR) or % | | | |
| --- | --- | --- | --- | --- | --- | --- | --- |
| | | | | No staining = 0 | Weak = 1 | Moderate/Strong = 2/3 | P-value |
| n= | 1026 | | 885 | 113 | 555 | 217 | |
| pT | | 0 | | | | | 0.77[a] |
| 1 | 740 (72.1 %) | | 631 (71.3 %) | 77 (68.1 %) | 404 (72.8 %) | 150 (69.1 %) | |
| 2 | 269 (26.2 %) | | 238 (26.9 %) | 34 (30.1 %) | 140 (25.2 %) | 64 (29.5 %) | |
| 3 | 15 (1.5 %) | | 14 (1.6 %) | 2 (1.8 %) | 9 (1.6 %) | 31 (1.4 %) | |
| 4 | 2 (0.2 %) | | 2 (0.2 %) | 0 (0 %) | 2 (0.4 %) | 0 (0 %) | |
| Axillary node involvement | | 2 | | | | | 0.020[b] |
| 0 | 627 (61.2 %) | | 532 (60.2 %) | 60 (53.1 %) | 330 (59.6 %) | 142 (65.7 %) | |
| 1-3 | 306 (29.9 %) | | 270 (30.6 %) | 37 (32.7 %) | 177 (31.9 %) | 56 (25.9 %) | |
| 4+ | 91 (8.9 %) | | 81 (9.2 %) | 16 (14.2 %) | 47 (8.5 %) | 18 (8.3 %) | |
| Histological grade | | 1 | | | | | 0.013[b] |
| I | 252 (24.6 %) | | 203 (22.9 %) | 20 (17.7 %) | 126 (22.7 %) | 57 (26.3 %) | |
| II | 511 (49.9 %) | | 443 (50.1 %) | 54 (47.8 %) | 278 (50.1 %) | 111 (51.2 %) | |
| III | 262 (25.6 %) | | 239 (27.0 %) | 39 (34.5 %) | 151 (27.2 %) | 49 (22.6 %) | |
| Histological type | | 1 | | | | | 0.512[a] |
| Mainly ductal | 836 (81.6 %) | | 737 (83.4 %) | 96 (85.0 %) | 467 (84.3 %) | 174 (80.2 %) | |
| Mainly lobular | 121 (11.8 %) | | 97 (11.0 %) | 11 (9.7 %) | 55 (9.9 %) | 31 (14.3 %) | |
| Other or mixed | 66 (6.4 %) | | 50 (5.7 %) | 6 (5.3 %) | 32 (5.8 %) | 12 (5.5 %) | |
| Hormone receptor status | | 2 | | | | | |
| ER+ | 896 (87.5 %) | | 771 (87.2 %) | 84 (74.3 %) | 484 (87.4 %) | 203 (93.5 %) | <0.0001[b] |
| PgR+ | 726 (70.9 %) | | 627 (70.9 %) | 70 (61.9 %) | 389 (70.2 %) | 168 (77.4 %) | 0.003[b] |
| HER 2 amplification* | | 59 | | | | | 0.009[b] |
| HER 2 positive | 86 (11.7 %) | | 71 (11.1 %) | 13 (21.0 %) | 46 (11.2 %) | 12 (7.2 %) | |
| HER 2 negative | 601 (81.4 %) | | 527 (82.3 %) | 47 (75.8 %) | 340 (82.7 %) | 140 (83.8 %) | |

*Patients younger than 70 years of age and included as of November 2005 [a]Chi-Square, [b]Linear-by-linear

the analyses as this marker was not routinely analyzed until March 2009 [28].

Patients with tumors that expressed moderate/strong HMGCR were significantly older at the time of inclusion in the present study, and only one of the patients with strong HMGCR staining was less than 50 years of age. This finding is consistent with another study that studied premenopausal patients and reported no tumors with strong expression of this marker [3]. ER-positive tumors are more common in postmenopausal patients than in premenopausal patients [29]. In the present study, moderate/strong HMGCR expression was associated with ER positivity, indicating that there might be an association between age, HMGCR expression and ER-positive tumors. This association may be linked to 27-hydroxycholesterol (27HC), which is a primary cholesterol metabolite and a selective estrogen receptor modulator (SERM) exerting ER agonistic effects, as recently shown in a study of murine models [30, 31]. The study demonstrated how conversion of cholesterol to 27HC was necessary for effects on ER-positive breast cancer cells and how the actions of 27HC

on tumor growth were dependent on ER. Those findings shed light on how 27HC may promote cancer growth and serve as the link between hypercholesterolemia and ER-positive breast cancer in postmenopausal women.

Normal cells can obtain cellular cholesterol in two ways; either via receptor-mediated uptake (low-density-lipoprotein receptor) or by synthesizing cholesterol through the mevalonate pathway and the activity of HMGCR. The normal cellular response to low intracellular cholesterol levels is to increase HMGCR activity to maintain an intact mevalonate pathway. However, tumor cells that fail to respond to this feed-back loop might have lost the checkpoint controls that maintain an intact pathway or may have a deregulated pathway [1, 32]. This dysregulation of the mevalonate pathway and HMGCR activity can contribute to the transformation involved in oncogenesis and may be essential for the metabolic transformation of tumor cells, at least in some cancers [32]. Therefore, potential biomarkers within the mevalonate pathway that could predict the response to statin treatment are of interest.

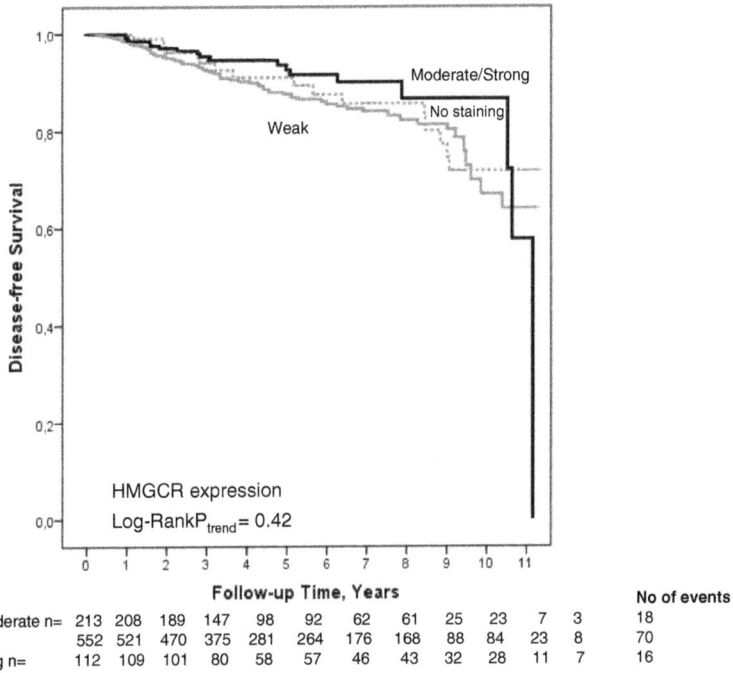

**Fig. 3** Kaplan-Meier estimate of DFS in relation to HMGCR expression. The number of patients at each follow-up is indicated. Since this study is an on-going study, the number of patients decreases with each follow-up

A previous study has reported that ER-negative breast cancer is less likely to arise among statin users and that ER-negative cell lines are more sensitive to statin inhibition than ER-positive cell lines [33]. In the present study, tumors that were negative for both ER and HMGCR had a higher histological grade significantly more often than tumors that were positive for these markers (data not shown). This association may reflect an inability of less differentiated cancer cells to maintain an intact mevalonate pathway. It was previously proposed that

some cancer cells could be statin-sensitive and unable to maintain adequate levels of mevalonate end products when exposed to statins, resulting in apoptosis [32]. In contrast, statin-insensitive tumor cells demonstrate a feedback response similar to that of normal cells, in which HMGCR is up-regulated; this response may protect these cells from the anticancer effects of statins [32]. It is possible that well-differentiated cancer cells but not less differentiated cancer cells are capable of initiating this response. Further studies are needed to explain the role of HMGCR in breast cancer.

**Table 3** Multivariable analysis of risk for breast cancer related events in relation to HMGCR status in all patients

| | HR | 95 % CI Lower | Upper |
|---|---|---|---|
| HMGCR no staining | 1.000 | | |
| HMGCR weak expression | 1.389 | 0.792 | 2.436 |
| HMGCR moderate/strong expression | 1.103 | 0.548 | 2.218 |
| Invasive tumor size ≥ 21 mm or muscular/skin involvement | 2.041 | 1.329 | 3.133 |
| Axillary nodal involvement | 1.427 | 0.946 | 2.153 |
| Histological grade III | 1.292 | 0.789 | 2.115 |
| ER status | 0.596 | 0.316 | 1.125 |
| PgR status | 0.740 | 0.448 | 1.223 |
| Age ≥ 50 years | 0.647 | 0.416 | 1.005 |
| BMI ≥ 25 kg/m$^2$ | 1.305 | 0.867 | 1.966 |
| Preoperative smoker | 1.289 | 0.811 | 2.050 |

No significant association was observed between HMGCR expression and DFS in the present study. Two previous studies reported associations between recurrence-free survival and HMGCR expression [2, 3]. However, the median follow-up time of the present study was only 5.0 years, compared to median follow-up times of 10.7 years [2] and 13.9 years [3] in the previous studies. Moderate/strong HMGCR expression was strongly associated with ER-positive tumors. ER-positive tumors are known to relapse later than ER-negative tumors; because 87.5 % of the patients in the present study had ER-positive tumors, a longer follow-up time may be needed [34].

HMGCR expression was negative in 12.8 % of the cases in this study. The percentage of tumors with negative staining varied between 18 % and 52.7 % of cases in previous studies [1–3, 35]. However, these studies had fewer tumors that stained for HMGCR. In addition, one study included only premenopausal patients [3], which may have affected the results because HMGCR was significantly associated with age in the present study. Although the intensity varied between studies, the finding in the current study that HMGCR is expressed in the majority of the cells when present is consistent with other studies [2, 3].

HMGCR is differentially expressed and often overexpressed in tumor cells [18] and high expression appears to be associated with less aggressive tumor characteristics [1, 2]. Previous studies reported that HMGCR expression was a good prognostic marker [2, 3]. A previous window-of-opportunity study demonstrated that patients who were treated with statins for two weeks pre-operatively exhibited increased expression of HMGCR in the tumor and a reduced proliferation rate of Ki67 [35]. The increase of HMGCR expression that occurs after statin treatment indicate that statins affected the tumor either directly through inhibition of HMGCR and the mevalonate pathway within the tumor or indirectly through lowered circulating levels of cholesterol and in both cases, a negative feed-back loop resulting in elevated intratumoral HMGCR levels [32]. Associations of HMGCR expression with more favorable tumor characteristics and a prolonged survival have also been demonstrated in patients with other types of cancer such as colorectal cancer [36].

Some limitations of this study should be considered. One weakness of the present study may be that HMGCR expression was evaluated on TMAs rather than in whole slide tumor tissue sections. However, a previous study stained five whole slide tumor tissue sections for HMGCR and this marker was homogeneously expressed in all of the sections [1]. Therefore, we believe that the HMGCR results obtained from TMAs are representative. The BC-blood study is an ongoing, population-based prospective study, which limits the risk for recall bias. The most common reason that patients did not participate in the present study was the lack of available research nurses. A previous study demonstrated that the patients who did not participate had patient and tumor characteristics similar to those who did participate [28]. This similarity makes the findings generalizable for breast cancer patients at Skåne University Hospital in Lund, Sweden. The patients were never asked about ethnicity. However, the majority of the patients were ethnic Swedes. To the authors' knowledge, the variation of HMGCR expression in cancer cells among different ethnic groups has not been investigated previously.

In conclusion, high HMGCR expression appears to be associated with less aggressive tumor characteristics in this population-based cohort of unselected primary breast cancer patients. Despite this finding, no association between HMGCR expression and short-term DFS was observed. Since previous studies had longer follow-up times, their findings can be neither confirmed nor rejected. Further studies and a prolonged follow-up time are needed to evaluate HMGCR as a prognostic and treatment-predictive marker.

**Abbreviations**
ATC: Anatomic Therapeutic Chemical; BMI: Body mass index; DFS: Disease-free survival; ER: Estrogen receptor; HER2: Human epidermal growth factor 2; HMGCR: 3-hydroxy-3-methylglutaryl-coenzyme A reductase; 27-OHC: 27-hydroxycholesterol; PgR: Progesterone receptor; REMARK: Recommendations for tumour MARKer prognostic studies; TMA: Tissue micro array.

**Competing interests**
The authors declare that they have no competing interests.

**Authors' contributions**
EG and HT performed the immunohistochemical evaluation. EG performed the statistical analyses and drafted the manuscript. HT has been involved in analysis and interpretation of data, and in revising the manuscript critically. AM and MS have been involved in acquisition of data and have revised the manuscript. BN constructed TMAs, carried out the IHC staining, and assisted with the immunohistochemical evaluation. KJ evaluated all tumors prior to TMA construction and revised the manuscript critically for important intellectual content. CI and CR have been involved in conception and design of the study and have revised the manuscript. SB was involved in conception and design of the study, performed immunohistochemical re-evaluation of selected cases, analysis and interpretation of data and revising the manuscript critically for important intellectual content. HJ has been involved in acquisition of data, in conception and design of the study, analysis and interpretation of data, in drafting the manuscript, and has revised the manuscript critically for important intellectual content. All authors have read and approved the final version of the manuscript.

**Acknowledgments**
This work was supported by grants from The Swedish Cancer Society (CAN 2011/497), the Swedish Research Council (K2012-54X-22027-01-3) (PI H Jernström), the Medical Faculty at Lund University, the Mrs. Berta Kamprad Foundation, the Gunnar Nilsson Foundation, the Swedish Breast Cancer Group (BRO), the South Swedish Health Care Region (Region Skåne ALF), Konung Gustaf V:s Jubileumsfond, the Lund Hospital Fund, the RATHER consortium (http://www.ratherproject.com/) and the Seventh Framework programme. The funding sources had no involvement in the collection, analysis and interpretation of data; in the writing of the report; or in the decision to submit the article for publication.
We thank our research nurses Maj-Britt Hedenblad, Karin Henriksson, Anette Möller, Monika Meszaros, Anette Ahlin Gullers, Anita Schmidt Casslén, Helén Thell, Linda Ågren, and Jessica Åkesson. We thank Erika Bågeman, Maria Hietala, and Maria Henningson for data entry, Elise Nilsson for TMA construction, and Kristina Lövgren and Catarina Blennow for sectioning.

**Author details**
[1]Division of Oncology and Pathology, Department of Clinical Sciences, Lund, Lund University, Barngatan 2B, SE 22185 Lund, Sweden. [2]Department of Oncology, Skåne University Hospital, Lund, Sweden. [3]CREATE Health and Department of Immunotechnology, Lund University, Medicon Village, Building 406, Lund, Sweden. [4]Department of Clinical Sciences, Division of Surgery, Lund, Lund University, Lund, Sweden and Skåne University Hospital, Lund, Sweden.

**References**
1. Borgquist S, Djerbi S, Ponten F, Anagnostaki L, Goldman M, Gaber A, et al. HMG-CoA reductase expression in breast cancer is associated with a less aggressive phenotype and influenced by anthropometric factors. Int J Cancer. 2008;123:1146–53.
2. Borgquist S, Jögi A, Ponten F, Rydén L, Brennan DJ, Jirström K. Prognostic impact of tumour-specific HMG-CoA reductase expression in primary breast cancer. Breast Cancer Res. 2008;10:R79.
3. Brennan DJ, Laursen H, O'Connor DP, Borgquist S, Uhlen M, Gallagher WM, et al. Tumor-specific HMG-CoA reductase expression in primary premenopausal breast cancer predicts response to tamoxifen. Breast Cancer Res. 2011;13:R12.
4. Goldstein JL, Brown MS. Regulation of the mevalonate pathway. Nature. 1990;343:425–30.
5. Mo H, Elson CE. Studies of the isoprenoid-mediated inhibition of mevalonate synthesis applied to cancer chemotherapy and chemoprevention. Exp Biol Med. 2004;229:567–85.
6. Jain MK, Ridker PM. Anti-inflammatory effects of statins: clinical evidence and basic mechanisms. Nat Rev Drug Discov. 2005;4:977–87.
7. Campbell MJ, Esserman LJ, Zhou Y, Shoemaker M, Lobo M, Borman E, et al. Breast cancer growth prevention by statins. Cancer Res. 2006;66:8707–14.
8. Wejde J, Blegen H, Larsson O. Requirement for mevalonate in the control of proliferation of human breast cancer cells. Anticancer Res. 1992;12:317–24.
9. Wong WW, Dimitroulakos J, Minden MD, Penn LZ. HMG-CoA reductase inhibitors and the malignant cell: the statin family of drugs as triggers of tumor-specific apoptosis. Leukemia. 2002;16:508–19.
10. Dulak J, Jozkowicz A. Anti-angiogenic and anti-inflammatory effects of statins: relevance to anti-cancer therapy. Curr Cancer Drug Targets. 2005;5:579–94.
11. Friis S, Poulsen AH, Johnsen SP, McLaughlin JK, Fryzek JP, Dalton SO, et al. Cancer risk among statin users: a population-based cohort study. Int J Cancer. 2005;114:643–7.
12. Strandberg TE, Pyorala K, Cook TJ, Wilhelmsen L, Faergeman O, Thorgeirsson G, et al. Mortality and incidence of cancer during 10-year follow-up of the Scandinavian Simvastatin Survival Study (4S). Lancet. 2004;364:771–7.
13. Beck P, Wysowski DK, Downey W, Butler-Jones D. Statin use and the risk of breast cancer. J Clin Epidemiol. 2003;56:280–5.
14. Boudreau DM, Yu O, Miglioretti DL, Buist DS, Heckbert SR, Daling JR. Statin use and breast cancer risk in a large population-based setting. Cancer Epidemiol Biomarkers Prev. 2007;16:416–21.
15. Desai P, Chlebowski R, Cauley JA, Manson JE, Wu C, Martin LW, et al. Prospective analysis of association between statin use and breast cancer risk in the women's health initiative. Cancer Epidemiol Biomarkers Prev. 2013;22:1868–76.
16. Kaye JA, Jick H. Statin use and cancer risk in the General Practice Research Database. Br J Cancer. 2004;90:635–7.
17. Nielsen SF, Nordestgaard BG, Bojesen SE. Statin use and reduced cancer-related mortality. N Engl J Med. 2012;367:1792–802.
18. Elson CE, Peffley DM, Hentosh P, Mo H. Isoprenoid-mediated inhibition of mevalonate synthesis: potential application to cancer. Exp Biol Med. 1999;221:294–311.
19. McShane LM, Altman DG, Sauerbrei W, Taube SE, Gion M, Clark GM. REporting recommendations for tumor MARKer prognostic studies (REMARK). Breast Cancer Res Treat. 2006;100:229–35.
20. Markkula A, Hietala M, Henningson M, Ingvar C, Rose C, Jernstrom H. Clinical profiles predict early nonadherence to adjuvant endocrine treatment in a prospective breast cancer cohort. Cancer Prev Res. 2012;5:735–45.
21. Simonsson M, Söderlind V, Henningson M, Hjertberg M, Rose C, Ingvar C, et al. Coffee prevents early events in tamoxifen-treated breast cancer patients and modulates hormone receptor status. Cancer Causes Control. 2013;24:929–40.
22. Ringberg A, Bågeman E, Rose C, Ingvar C, Jernström H. Of cup and bra size: reply to a prospective study of breast size and premenopausal breast cancer incidence. Int J Cancer. 2006;119:2242–3. author reply 2244.
23. Markkula A, Bromee A, Henningson M, Hietala M, Ringberg A, Ingvar C, et al. Given breast cancer, does breast size matter? Data from a prospective breast cancer cohort. Cancer Causes Control. 2012;23:1307–16.
24. Bågeman E, Ingvar C, Rose C, Jernström H. Coffee consumption and CYP1A2*1 F genotype modify age at breast cancer diagnosis and estrogen receptor status. Cancer Epidemiol Biomarkers Prev. 2008;17:895–901.
25. Jernström H, Bågeman E, Rose C, Jönsson PE, Ingvar C. CYP2C8 and CYP2C9 polymorphisms in relation to tumour characteristics and early breast cancer related events among 652 breast cancer patients. Br J Cancer. 2009;101:1817–23.
26. Simonsson M, Markkula A, Bendahl PO, Rose C, Ingvar C, Jernström H. Pre- and postoperative alcohol consumption in breast cancer patients: impact on early events. SpringerPlus. 2014;3:261.
27. World Health Organization. BMI Classification. 2006. http://apps.who.int/bmi/index.jsp?introPage = intro_3.html Access date March 24, 2014
28. Lundin KB, Henningson M, Hietala M, Ingvar C, Rose C, Jernström H. Androgen receptor genotypes predict response to endocrine treatment in breast cancer patients. Br J Cancer. 2011;105:1676–83.
29. Rose DP, Vona-Davis L. Interaction between menopausal status and obesity in affecting breast cancer risk. Maturitas. 2010;66:33–8.
30. Nelson ER, Wardell SE, Jasper JS, Park S, Suchindran S, Howe MK, et al. 27-Hydroxycholesterol links hypercholesterolemia and breast cancer pathophysiology. Science. 2013;342:1094–8.
31. Warner M, Gustafsson JA. On estrogen, cholesterol metabolism, and breast cancer. N Engl J Med. 2014;370:572–3.
32. Clendening JW, Penn LZ. Targeting tumor cell metabolism with statins. Oncogene. 2012;31:4967–78.
33. Kumar AS, Benz CC, Shim V, Minami CA, Moore DH, Esserman LJ. Estrogen receptor-negative breast cancer is less likely to arise among lipophilic statin users. Cancer Epidemiol Biomarkers Prev. 2008;17:1028–33.
34. Osborne CK, Yochmowitz MG, Knight 3rd WA, McGuire WL. The value of estrogen and progesterone receptors in the treatment of breast cancer. Cancer. 1980;46:2884–8.
35. Bjarnadottir O, Romero Q, Bendahl PO, Jirström K, Rydén L, Loman N, et al. Targeting HMG-CoA reductase with statins in a window-of-opportunity breast cancer trial. Breast Cancer Res Treat. 2013;138:499–508.
36. Bengtsson E, Nerjovaj P, Wangefjord S, Nodin B, Eberhard J, Uhlen M, et al. HMG-CoA reductase expression in primary colorectal cancer correlates with favourable clinicopathological characteristics and an improved clinical outcome. Diagn Pathol. 2014;9:78.

# 6

# Comparison of time-motion analysis of conventional stool culture and the BD MAX™ Enteric Bacterial Panel (EBP)

Joel E. Mortensen[1*], Cindi Ventrola[1], Sarah Hanna[1] and Adam Walter[2]

## Abstract

**Background:** Conventional bacterial stool culture is one of the more time-consuming tests in a routine clinical microbiology laboratory. In addition, less than 5 % of stool cultures yield positive results. A molecular platform, the BD MAX™ System (BD Diagnostics, Sparks, MD) offers the potential for significantly more rapid results and less hands-on time. Time-motion analysis of the BD MAX Enteric Bacterial Panel (EBP) (BD Diagnostics, Quebec, Canada) on the BD MAX System was compared to conventional stool culture in the microbiology laboratory of a tertiary care pediatric hospital.

**Methods:** The process impact analysis of time-motion studies of conventional cultures were compared to those of EBP with 86 stool specimens. Sample flow, hands-on time, processing steps, and overall turnaround time were determined and analyzed. Data were obtained and analyzed from both standard operating procedures and direct observation. A regression analysis was performed to ensure consistency of measurements. Time and process measurements started when the specimens were logged into the accessioning area of the microbiology laboratory and were completed when actionable results were generated.

**Results:** With conventional culture, negative culture results were available from 41:14:27 (hours:minutes:seconds) to 54:17:19; with EBP, positive and negative results were available from 2:28:40 to 3:33:39.

**Conclusions:** This study supports the suggestion that use of the EBP to detect commonly encountered stool pathogens can result in significant time savings and a shorter time-to-result for patients with acute bacterial diarrhea.

**Keywords:** Time-motion analysis, BD MAX™, Diarrhea, Bacterial stool pathogens

## Background

The World Health Organization has reported that, worldwide, there are nearly 1.7 billion cases of diarrheal disease every year and that diarrheal disease is the second leading cause of death in children under five years old [1, 2]. Each year, diarrhea results in approximately 760,000 preventable deaths of children under the age of five years. Diarrhea in this age group is also a leading cause of malnutrition. Most cases of this disease are related to unsafe drinking-water, inadequate sanitation, and poor hygiene [1, 2].

Detection and identification of the etiological agents of acute bacterial diarrhea are important for both the treatment of individual patients and for the management of diarrheal diseases of public health importance. Conventional bacterial culture remains the gold standard for the aforementioned detection, even though stool culture has relatively low sensitivity and requires a significant amount of labor. The use of nucleic acid amplification methods to detect and identify the etiological agents of acute bacterial diarrhea could have a significant impact on the laboratory diagnostic process, clinical approach, and epidemiology of this disease [3–5].

The objective of this study was to examine the laboratory impact of a new molecular platform (use of the BD MAX Enteric Bacterial Panel on the BD MAX System) on turnaround time, associated laboratory processes, and the cost of providing results with this system compared to conventional culture methods. Results of both

* Correspondence: joel.mortensen@cchmc.org
[1]Department of Laboratory Medicine, Cincinnati Children's Hospital, MLC1010, 3333 Burnet Ave, 45229 Cincinnati, OH, USA
Full list of author information is available at the end of the article

conventional culture (including a commercial immuno-assay for shiga-toxin) and the EBP, which include tests for the detection of *Salmonella* spp., *Shigella* spp./ Enteroinvasive *Escherichia coli* (EIEC), *Campylobacter* spp. (*jejuni* and *coli*), and Shiga toxin 1 and 2 genes in stool specimens were evaluated. Lean and Six Sigma processes were used to analyze the time from sample receipt to actionable result for conventional stool culture and the EBP. The following "events or decisions per specimen" were determined: any action or thought process that must occur to process and issue a result, the overall distance traveled per sample as a measure of efficiency, and the operating costs of the two systems [6].

(The results of this study were presented, in part, at the 24th European Congress of Clinical Microbiology and Infectious Diseases, Barcelona, Spain, May 10–13, 2014 and at the 114th General Meeting of the American Society for Microbiology, Boston MA, May 17–20, 2014.)

## Methods

Lean and Six Sigma processing analysis were performed to evaluate time-to-results for both culture and EBP testing. By design, this study did not involve human subjects or any patient information. Observations were performed without patient identifiers and additional testing was carried out on discarded, anonymous samples. Any sample ordered for routine stool culture was eligible for inclusion in the study.

## Culture

Clinical stool samples were immediately accessioned and plated upon arrival in the laboratory following standard laboratory practices. They were not stored prior to culture. Sample flow, hands-on time, processing steps, overall turnaround time, and specimen travel distance were measured by two independent observers over the course of three separate observation periods; each observation period was five days. To eliminate any potential of operator-to-operator bias during the study, 11 different laboratory technologists were observed performing all pre-analytical, analytical, and post-analytical culture procedures which occurred at five different laboratory stations: specimen receipt, specimen plating and incubation, culture reading, automated identification (Vitek 2 System, bioMérieux, Marcy l'Etoile, France) and shiga-toxin testing (Immunocard STAT! EHEC, Meridian Bioscience, Cincinnati, Ohio, USA).

In brief, for this study, stool samples that were submitted for routine culture were transported in Cary Blair Transport Medium (Meridian Bioscience, Inc.). Specimens were processed within 2 h of receipt. Initially, samples were inoculated onto the following agar media: 5 % sheep blood, MacConkey, Sorbitol MacConkey, Hektoen, Campy CVA (BD Diagnostics, Sparks, MD, USA).

Cultures were incubated under standard conditions. Suspected bacterial pathogens were identified using the Vitek 2 System (bioMerieux) and standard conventional methodologies as needed. Additional testing may have included the following: Salmonella serotyping and Shigella serotyping Becton, Dickinson and Company, Sparks, MD, USA) and Remel RIM E. coli O157:H7 Latex Test (Remel, Lenexa, KS, USA).

Additional data were obtained and analyzed from laboratory Standard Operating Procedures (SOP) used routinely in this particular laboratory. In order to ensure consistency during the study, a regression analysis of measurements, processing, and adherence to the SOP was performed. Correlation studies were performed on independent data sets to ensure no bias was falsely introduced by operator-to-operator performance [7]. The following elements were analyzed: elapsed time, distance traveled, processing steps performed, and clinical decisions, from the time the specimens were logged into the accessioning area until the time actionable results were generated. Processing was observed and data were collected during each of the following notable events: specimen arrival, specimen accessioning, specimen plating and preparation, specimen incubation, first-day plate reading and workup, subsequent day(s) reading, including *Campylobacter* spp. cultures reading, automated identification and additional workup, shiga-toxin broth inoculation, shiga-toxin rapid testing, and verification of results, and entering results into the laboratory/hospital information system.

### EBP testing

Methods similar to those used to evaluate culture processes were measured and analyzed: elapsed time, distance traveled, processing steps, and clinical decisions (also from the time specimens were logged into the accessioning area to the time actionable results were generated). Processing was observed and data were collected during each of the following notable events: specimen arrival, specimen accessioning, control preparation, specimen preparation, instrument preparation, worklist preparation, instrument processing, and result verification. For BD MAX testing, the samples were batched and tested in different batch sizes. Batch sizes ranged from 4 to 24 samples in increments of 4 to mimic routine clinical testing.

### Cost analysis

Standard institutional cost analysis was used to determine the costs for conventional culture and for EBP. The main cost components of the analysis were labor, direct materials and supplies, and general shared costs (Test Site Burden). Hands-on time (minutes) for each step of the cultures and the EBP was multiplied by the average hourly technologist salary/min of labor to determine labor costs. The quantity of each item and the cost of each item used in culture and EBP testing were derived from institutional inventory data. Institutional overhead or Test Site Burden is the cost for basic services such as lights and heat and the cost of common shared laboratory equipment such as incubators, repeat pipettes, etc.

## Institutional review board

It was determined that this study did not meet regulatory criteria for research involving human subjects because the research did not obtain data through intervention or interaction with the individual or identifiable private information. All observations of process were made without any patient identifiers available to the observer. All specimens tested on the BD MAX were anonymous, discarded samples that were only used after clinical testing was completed and for which no patient identifiers were used.

## Results

86 patient specimens were examined. No pathogens under consideration in this study (i.e., *Salmonella, Campylobacter, Shigella* and shiga toxin producing organisms) were detected by culture or BD MAX EBP.

To enable a comparison, simultaneously, 84 alternate specimens tested by EBP were processed across six batches of differing size (4 to 24 samples each) on the BD MAX platform. Processing and turnaround times of routine cultures were compared to the process and turnaround times of EBP testing. The mean time to reportable result for 86 routine cultures was 44:37:00 (hours:minutes:seconds) (+/− 8 h, 10 min) (Fig. 1). If potential pathogens

were detected that required additional testing, the time to final result ranged from 97:18:17 to 145:27:11.

Although the time to perform EBP testing is approximately two hours, EBP is designed and best used to batch specimen testing at reasonable intervals as determined by each laboratory. If a reasonable operational model is two EBP runs per day (one in the morning, one in the afternoon), the time to reportable EBP results would be, at most, 07:06:00 (no standard deviation; all variability dependent upon batch size and timing of run). Hands-on time per specimen was 0:01:30 (+/− 19 s). With an assumption of two EBP runs per day and 90 s hands-on time/specimen, there was an 85 % reduction of time to reportable results compared to culture.

## Process Steps for Culture and EBP

Technologists made an average of 141 and 25 decisions per culture and EBP test, respectively. Thus, EBP testing required 82 % fewer decisions than did culture (Table 1). The number of steps and processes in each unique laboratory can be represented by a spaghetti diagram of process flow for culture and for EBP testing (Fig. 2).

## Cost analysis

Detailed costs are listed in Table 2. The basic labor to process and handle a stool culture was 0:15:00 − 0:17:00. Approximately 20 % of the cultures required additional process steps to rule out potential pathogens; these additional steps resulted in additional labor (0:35:00 − 0:40:00) and supplies. The EBP required 0:01:28 hands on time.

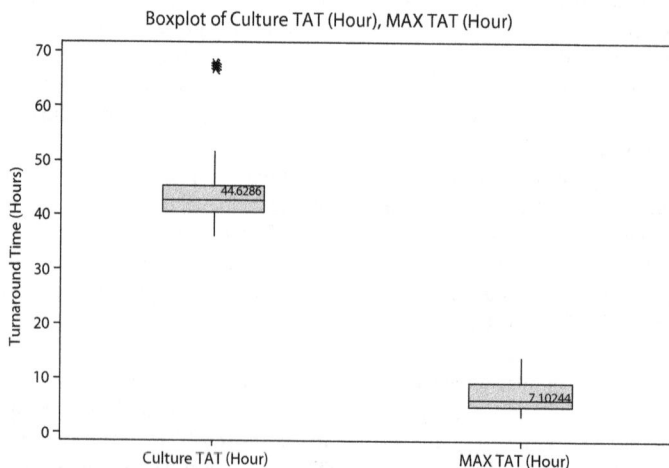

**Fig. 1** The mean turnaround time (TAT) to reportable results for 86 routine stool cultures and 84 samples tested with BD MAX EBP. Legend. *Represents 4 outlying culture results that required additional testing for confirmation of the results. All final culture results were negative for pathogens

**Table 1** Average Number of Process Steps (Decisions/Manipulations) Involved in Routine Culture and BD MAX EBP Testing

| Process Steps | Routine Culture | EBP |
|---|---|---|
| Receipt | 3 | 3 |
| Accession | 7 | 1 |
| Routine culture | | |
| Blood agar | 43 | - |
| MacConkey agar | 26 | - |
| Hektoen | 26 | - |
| Sorbitol MacConkey | 14 | - |
| Shiga toxin testing | 4 | - |
| Sample Preparation | - | 8 |
| System operation | - | 13 |
| Total activities | 141 | 25 |

## Discussion

A number of molecular platforms have been evaluated for specific specimen types, including stool, and potential pathogens in clinical laboratory settings and have been shown to be highly sensitive and specific when compared to conventional methods [3–5]. The BD MAX platform has been evaluated for the detection of MRSA and more recently stool pathogens [8, 9]. Recently, several investigators have recognized that beyond scientific validation, these platforms need to be evaluated for their impact on the operations and the time to reportable results in clinical laboratories [7, 10–12].

One of the more challenging parts of this study was accounting for all of the costs. The lack of positive samples with target stool pathogens did not allow a complete determination of the costs and labor associated with routine stool cultures. A community outbreak of acute bacterial diarrhea might significantly impact both labor and supplies for both of the methods in this study. In addition, it was difficult to account for the individual variability between technologists in the workup of stool cultures. Differences in individual technologists and their experience could have affected the extent of work and supplies needed for a culture. Nonetheless, including multiple technologists in the performance of this study more accurately represents real-world performance of the two methods than, for example, performing the study with specified research technologists. The use of a significant amount of shared equipment for routine cultures makes complete accounting for the portion of the cost of equipment such as water baths, incubators, storage rack, microscopes, etc. assigned to each culture difficult. At our institution, we use the somewhat arbitrary "Test Site Burden" as one mechanism of sharing these

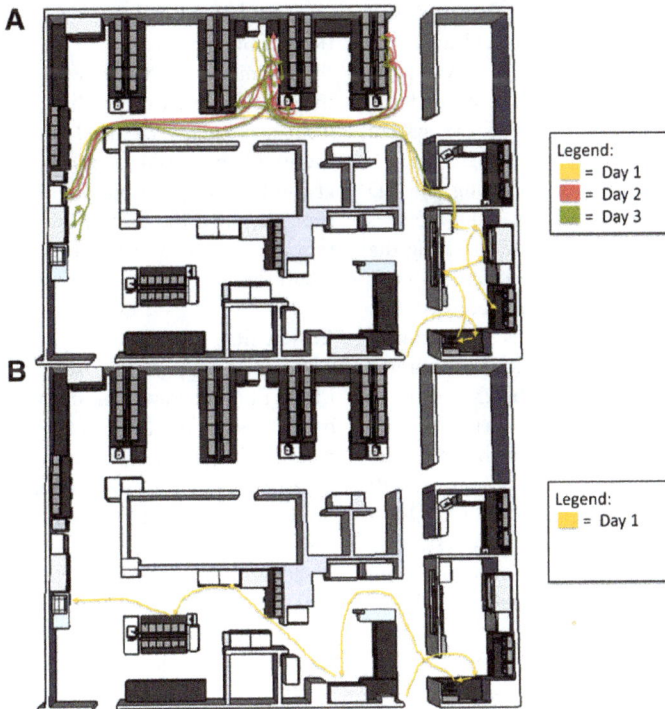

**Fig. 2** Spaghetti Diagram of Process Flow for Routine Stool Culture (**a**) and BD MAX EBP Testing (**b**)

**Table 2** Cost Analysis of Routine Stool Cultures and BD MAX EBP Testing

| | Stool Culture | | | EBP | | |
|---|---|---|---|---|---|---|
| | Cost/Unit | #Units | Cost | Cost/Unit | #Units | Cost |
| **Basic test** | | | | | | |
| Labor -Technologist time (minutes) | 0.45 | 15 - 17 | 6.75 – 7.65 | 0.45 | 1.48 | 0.67 |
| Information System labels | 0.05 | 3 | 0.15 | 0.05 | 2 | 0.1 |
| 5 % Sheep Blood agar plate | 0.25 | 1 | 0.25 | | | |
| MacConkey agar plate | 0.25 | 1 | 0.25 | | | |
| Campy agar plate and BioBag | 2.39 | 1 | 2.39 | | | |
| Hektoen Enteric agar plate | 0.31 | 1 | 0.31 | | | |
| MacConkey Sorbitol agar plate | 0.44 | 1 | 0.44 | | | |
| Shiga toxin test kit and MacConkey Broth | 13.52 | 1 | 13.52 | | | |
| Disposable 10 µl loop | | | | 0.02 | 1 | 0.02 |
| Enteric Panel Kit | | | | 30 – 35.00 | 1 | 30 – 25.00 |
| MAX test cartridge | | | | 0.40 – 0.65 | 1 | 0.40 – 0.65 |
| Test site burden | 1.00 | 2 | 2.00 | 1.00 | 1 | 1.00 |
| **Additional workup*** | | | | | | |
| Labor -Technologist time (minutes) | 0.45 | 35-40 | 15.75 – 18.00 | | | |
| 5 % Sheep Blood agar plate | 0.25 | 1-3 | 0.25 – 0.75 | | | |
| Vitek-Gram negative ID card | 6.00 | 1-3 | 6.00 – 18.00 | | | |
| RIM EC O157:H7 test | 0.59 | 1 | 0.59 | | | |
| **Total Cost (in $)** | | | $26.06 – 64.30 | | | $32.19–37.44 |

*20 % of cultures required additional labor and supplies to rule out potential pathogens

costs. An additional impact within the laboratory is the shift in supplies storage. A significant number of different media and tests are need for routine cultures and most of these require refrigerated storage. A move to the EBP assay would reduce the number of tests and the amount of media. In addition, adoption of the system would shift much of that storage to room temperature.

In contrast to culture, the cost of operating the BD MAX was more easily captured. However, there are several additional issues that affect the cost of operating the EBP assay that a clinical laboratory would need to consider. Because of how the disposables are constructed, samples can be run in various size batches. To optimize and reduce cost, the ideal batch size is 24. To optimize and reduce turnaround time, the ideal batch size is as small as possible. Use of fewer stools samples per batch would have a minor effect on the cost of the test. The cost of the EBP would not change with a positive result; however, a positive EBP would require a follow-up culture to allow serotyping, antimicrobial susceptibility testing as appropriate, and epidemiological studies, including time and supplies to send isolates to the State Public Health Laboratory. Depreciation of instruments is an important consideration if the instrumentation is purchased outright. Our analysis did not include the cost of the analyzer as that cost per assay is directly related to the volume of assays performed on the instrument. Finally, the cost of

service contracts is often not considered as part of the cost of a test, but can represent a significant cost to the operations of the laboratory.

As clinical microbiology laboratories move from traditional culture based methods to instrument based molecular methods, we need to look carefully at scientific merits of the various options, but we need also to look at the turnaround time of results, associated laboratory processes, and the cost of providing results with this system compared to conventional culture methods in our laboratories.

**Conclusion**

This study supports the suggestion that use of the BD MAX EBP can save significant time (over that required by culture) in the laboratory diagnosis of acute bacterial diarrhea caused by *Salmonella* spp., *Shigella* spp./(EIEC), *Campylobacter* spp. (*jejuni* and *coli*), and Shiga toxin producing *E. coli* which are responsible for 95 % of acute bacterial gastroenteritis. The use of a flexible and focused approach to identifying enteric pathogens (bacteria, viruses & parasites) based on patient history or risk, clinical presentation or clinician's preference is aligned with widely recommended clinical algorithms which not only potentially streamline laboratory testing and workflow in a cost effective manner, but also provide physicians with timely results which improve the standard of care for common causes of gastroenteritis. As additional nucleic amplification assays become available, the impact of the use of focused versus comprehensive panels will continue to be evaluated for their respective clinical relevance, cost and work flow implications.

## Abbreviations
EBP: Enteric bacterial panel; EIEC: Enteroinvasive *Escherichia coli*; SOP: Standard operating procedures; MRSA: Methicillin resistant *Staphylococcus aureus*.

## Competing interests
AW is an employee of BD Diagnostics. JEM has received honoraria from BD Diagnostics. Other authors have no competing interests.

## Authors' contributions
JEM conceived the study, analyzed the data and authored the manuscript. CV performed data collection, participated in the process measurements and performed the cost analysis. SH performed the BD MAX testing and data collection, and participated in the process measurements. AW contributed to the study design and performed the process measurements. All authors have reviewed the manuscript and accept responsibility for its content.

## Acknowledgements
BD Diagnostics (Sparks, MD) provided financial support and supplies for this project. BD Diagnostics did not design the study, interpret the data, write the manuscript or control submission of the manuscript for publication.

## Author details
[1]Department of Laboratory Medicine, Cincinnati Children's Hospital, MLC1010, 3333 Burnet Ave, 45229 Cincinnati, OH, USA. [2]BD Diagnostics, Sparks, MD, USA.

## References
1. WHO/UNICEF. Ending preventable child deaths from pneumonia and diarrhoea by 2025:The integrated Global Action Plan for Pneumonia and Diarrhoea (GAPPD). New York, N.Y: The United Nations CHildren's Fund(UNICEF)/World Health Organization (WHO); 2013.
2. Johansson EW, Wardlaw T, Binkin N, Brocklehurst C, Dooley T. Diarrhoea: why children are still dying and what can be done, (UNICEF). New York, N.Y: The United Nations CHildren's Fund(UNICEF)/World Health Organization (WHO); 2009.
3. Navidad JF, Griswold DJ, Gradus MS, Bhattacharyya S. Evaluation of Luminex xTAG gastrointestinal pathogen analyte-specific reagents for high-throughput, simultaneous detection of bacteria, viruses, and parasites of clinical and public health importance. J Clin Microbiol. 2013;51:3018–24.
4. Buchan BW, Olson WJ, Pezewski M, Marcon MJ, Novicki T, Uphoff TS, et al. Clinical evaluation of a real-time PCR assay for identification of Salmonella, Shigella, Campylobacter (Campylobacter jejuni and C. coli), and shiga toxin-producing Escherichia coli isolates in stool specimens. J Clin Microbiol. 2013;51(12):4001–7.
5. Patel A, Navidad J, Bhattacharyya S. Site-specific Clinical Evaluation of the Luminex xTAG Gastrointestinal Pathogen Panel for the Detection of Infectious Gastroenteritis in Fecal Specimens. J Clin Microbiol. 2013;52(8):3068–71.
6. Schweikhart SA, Dembe AE. The application of Lean and Six Sigma techniques to clinical and translational research. J Invest Med. 2009;57(7):748–55.
7. Felder RA, Foster ML, Lizzi MJ, Pohl BR, Diemert DM, Towns BG. Process evaluation of a fully automated molecular diagnostics system. J Assoc Lab Autom. 2009;14:262–8.
8. Widen R, Healer V, Silber S. Laboratory Evaluation of the BD MAX MRSA assay. J Clin Microbiol. 2014;52(7):2686–8.
9. Harrington SM, Buchan B, Doern C, Fader R, Ferraro MJ, Pillai D, et al. Multi-center evaluation of the BD MAX™ Enteric Bacterial Panel PCR assay for the rapid detection of Salmonella spp., Shigella spp., Campylobacter spp. (C. jejuni and C. coli), and Shiga toxin 1 and 2 genes. ASM General Meeting, 2014.
10. Hassell LA, Glass CF, Yip C, Eneff PA. The combined postive impact of Lean methology and Ventana Symphony autostainer on histology lab workflow. BMC Clin Path. 2010;10:2–10.
11. Felder RA, Jackson KD, Walter AM. Process Evaluation of an Open Architecture Real-Time Molecular Laboratory Platform. J Lab Autom. 2014;19(5):468–73.
12. Williams JA, Eddleman L, Pantone A, Martinez R, Young S, Van Der Pol B. Time-Motion Analysis of Four Automated Systems for the Detection of Chlamydia trachomatis and Neisseria gonorrhoeae by Nucleic Acid Amplification Testing. J Lab Autom. 2013;19(4):423–6.

# 7

# The use of dried blood spot sampling for the measurement of HbA1c

Claudio A. Mastronardi[1†], Belinda Whittle[2†], Robert Tunningley[2], Teresa Neeman[3] and Gilberto Paz-Filho[1*]

**Abstract**

**Background:** The use of dried blood spot (DBS) sampling is an alternative to traditional venous blood collection, and particularly useful for people living in rural and remote areas, and for those who are infirm, house-bound or time-poor. The objective of this study was to assess whether the measurement of glycated haemoglobin A1c (HbA1c) in DBS samples provided comparative and acceptably precise results.

**Methods:** Venous and capillary blood samples were collected from 115 adult participants. After proper instruction, each participant punctured his/her own finger and collected capillary blood samples on pieces of a proprietary cellulose filter paper. Each filter paper was subsequently placed inside a breathable envelope, stored at room temperature, and processed on the same day (D0), four (D4), seven (D7) and fourteen (D14) days after collection. HbA1c was measured in duplicates/triplicates in whole venous blood (WB), capillary blood (capDBS) and venous blood placed on the matrix paper (venDBS), by turbidimetric inhibition immunoassay. Intra-assay coefficients of variation (CV) were calculated. DBS values were compared to WB results using linear regression, Bland-Altman plots and cross-validation models.

**Results:** Eleven and 56 patients had type 1 and type 2 diabetes mellitus, respectively. Mean HbA1c levels were $6.22 \pm 1.11$ % for WB samples (n = 115). The median intra-assay CV was lower than 3 % for WB and capDBS on all days. Results from capDBS and venDBS showed high correlation and agreement to WB results, with narrow 95 % limits of agreement (except for results from D14 samples), as observed in Bland-Altman plots. When capDBS values were applied to equations derived from regression analyses, results approached those of WB values. A cross-validation model showed that capDBS results on D0, D4 and D7 were close to the WB results, with prediction intervals that were narrow enough to be clinically acceptable.

**Conclusions:** The measurement of HbA1c from DBS samples provided results that were comparable to results from WB samples, if measured up to seven days after collection. Intra-assay coefficients of variation were low, results were in agreement with the gold-standard, and prediction intervals were clinically acceptable. The measurement of HbA1c through DBS sampling may be considered in situations where traditional venipuncture is not available.

**Trial registration:** Australian New Zealand Clinical Trials Registry ID ACTRN12613000769785.

**Keywords:** Diabetes, Dried blood spot testing, HbA1c, Hemoglobin A1c, Turbidimetry

* Correspondence: Gilberto.Pazfilho@anu.edu.au
†Equal contributors
[1]Department of Genome Sciences, The John Curtin School of Medical Research, The Australian National University, 131 Garran Rd, Canberra, Acton ACT 2601, Australia
Full list of author information is available at the end of the article

## Background

Glycated haemoglobin (HbA1c) is a biomarker that is fundamental for the diagnosis of diabetes and for monitoring glycaemic control [1]. Traditionally, its measurement depends on venipuncture, and on processing, transportation and storage of whole blood (WB) samples, which can be logistically challenging [2]. These challenges can sometimes compromise proper diagnosis and treatment of patients with diabetes mellitus.

An alternative blood sampling method, based on the use of a dry matrix, was first described in the literature over a century ago [3], and subsequently applied in the clinics to detect metabolic defects through the collection of heel capillary blood samples from newborns [4]. This method is centred on collecting blood samples obtained from finger or heel puncturing on a matrix paper, which is subsequently dried. These dried blood spots (DBS) can then be used for the measurement of diverse substances, including HbA1c, and requires minimal training of staff, is cheaper and safer, eliminates the need for special transportation logistics, and is more acceptable to study participants [5–7].

DBS sampling has been routinely and successfully used for the screening of congenital metabolic and endocrine diseases, such as phenylketonuria and hypothyroidism [8]. More recently, studies have shown that measurements of inflammatory markers, cytokines, serum antibodies, human immunodeficiency virus (HIV) loads and blood hormone levels provide results that are comparable to those obtained from standard venous samples [5, 9–11].

Dried blood spot sampling is also useful for the measurement of HbA1c in individuals with and without diabetes. A recent meta-analysis of seventeen heterogeneous studies demonstrated that HbA1c results from DBS were correlated to those obtained through venipuncture [12]. However, there is still a need for standardisation of sample collection, transportation, storage and analysis. In this study, we evaluated HbA1c levels collected on a novel matrix paper and measured through immunoturbidity, up to 14 days after DBS collection. Subsequently, to demonstrate whether DBS provide results comparable to WB samples, DBS results were compared against those obtained from standard methods.

## Methods

This study was approved by the Australian National University Human Research Ethics Committee, and all participants provided informed consent. We recruited participants from the general population living within the Australian Capital Territory region, Australia. Inclusion criteria allowed all adults over 18 years-old from all genders and ethnicities that had no restrictions to having their blood drawn (*i.e.* due to religious matters, or blood donation in the previous 4 weeks, or

difficulty in providing venous blood samples). Participants were advised not to consume food, alcohol or caffeine for 12 h prior to the collection.

Venous blood was collected from an arm vein following standard sterile techniques, into EDTA-coated plastic tubes, providing WB samples. For the collection of capillary DBS (capDBS) samples, we used a 2 x 3 inch dry matrix cellulose paper with nine 10-mm outer diameter circles printed on the surface (ITL Healthcare Pty Ltd). Each printed circle has the capacity to hold 30 to 40 microlitres of blood. Participants were instructed to collect their capillary blood through finger pricking and placing one drop of blood onto each of the pre-defined circles of the dry matrix paper, at room temperature (23 ° C). The matrix paper was then placed into a breathable envelope (ITL Healthcare Pty Ltd) for transportation to the testing laboratory, and blood spots were allowed to dry at room temperature for >2 h before transportation. Forty-microlitre drops of venous blood were also pipetted from collection tubes with no anticoagulant and immediately placed on another dry matrix card, providing venous DBS (venDBS) samples.

All blood samples were transported to the pathology laboratory for analysis. HbA1c levels were determined by a direct turbidimetric inhibition immunoassay that determines HbA1c as a percentage of total haemoglobin (%HbA1c) (Thermo Fisher Scientific). Assays were performed on an Indiko Plus (Thermo Fisher Scientific) automated biochemistry analyser, and results were reported as %HbA1c NGSP values.

Processing of DBS samples (capDBS and venDBS): For each participant sample, two punches were taken from one DBS near the outer edge of the spot. Each punch had 3.2 mm in diameter and contains approximately 1.4 µL of serum. Punches were placed in haemolysing reagent (Thermo Fisher Scientific), in duplicate or triplicate, and incubated at room temperature with shaking. For each duplicate, one milliliter of haemolysate was processed in the Indiko analyser as per the standard protocol for whole blood. capDBS and venDBS samples were processed and analysed on the same day (D0), and on D4, D7 and D14, in duplicates or triplicates for the calculation of intra-assay coefficients of variation (CV).

Processing of WB samples: WB samples were prepared and processed as per standard protocol (Thermo Fisher Scientific). WB samples were processed and analysed on the same day (D0), in duplicates.

Results were presented as mean ± SD or median and range. Linear regression models for predicting WB from DBS were fit and goodness-of-fit measures [mean standard error (MSE) and R-squared] were estimated using cross-validation (R program developed for the cross-validation available upon request). From these models, we predicted WB from DBS values of 4 %, 7 %, 7.5 %

**Table 1** Characteristics of the studied population

|  | All | No diabetes | Type 1 diabetes | Type 2 diabetes |
|---|---|---|---|---|
| Gender (Males:Females) | 51 M:64 F | 20 M:28 F | 2 M:9 F | 28 M:28 F |
| Age (years; mean ± SD) | 55.9 ± 15.3 | 46.2 ± 14.4 | 45.0 ± 12.8 | 64.8 ± 10.0 |
| WB HbA1c (%; mean ± SD) | 6.22 ± 1.11 % | 5.41 ± 0.35 % | 7.80 ± 0.81 % | 6.61 ± 1.11 % |

Note: WB = whole blood; SD = standard deviation

and 10 % and in addition, obtained 95 % prediction intervals for all days. DBS values were applied to equations derived from linear regression analyses from D0, D4, D7 and D14 data, in order to obtain corrected DBS values (*i.e.*, to bring uncorrected DBS values closer to the line of equality). Bland-Altman plots were constructed with corrected D0, D4, D7 and D14 results.

## Results

A total of 115 participants (n = 51 males, n = 64 females) were recruited. Mean age was 55.9 ± 15.3 years-old; 11 participants (9.6 %) had been previously diagnosed with type 1 diabetes, and 56 individuals (48.7 %) had type 2 diabetes. Overall mean whole blood HbA1c levels were 6.22 ± 1.11 % (5.41 ± 0.35 % for participants without diabetes, 7.80 ± 0.81 % for volunteers with type 1 diabetes, and 6.61 ± 1.11 % among individuals with type 2 diabetes). Characteristics of the studied participants are summarised in Table 1.

Whole blood and dried blood spot samples (capillary and venous) were measured in duplicates or triplicates, allowing the determination of intra-assay CV. The median intra-assay CVs were 1.19 % for WB (range 0–4.1 %), and lower than 3 % for all other samples (Table 2).

Mean ± SD capillary DBS (capDBS) levels of HbA1c were 6.62 ± 1.16 % when measured on D0 (n = 77), 6.92 ± 1.32 % on D4 (n = 96), 6.85 ± 1.29 % on D7 (n = 81), and 6.62 ± 1.44 % on D14 (n = 79). Venous DBS (venDBS) samples ranged from 6.72 ± 1.20 % on D0 to 7.36 ± 1.47 % on D7. Mean capDBS and venDBS values were applied to correction formulas obtained from linear regression analyses for each day. Corrected DBS values were closer to WB results (except for D14). Table 2 summarizes the results from WB and DBS samples (corrected and uncorrected).

Bland-Altman plots of difference in HbA1c values in WB and corrected capDBS (Fig. 1), and in WB and corrected venDBS (Fig. 2) showed good correlation and agreement between the two methods, with few samples falling outside the 95 % limits of agreement for each comparison (average difference ± 1.96 standard deviation of the difference). However, limits of agreement were broader on D14 (Table 3).

From any given capDBS result, the linear regression models predicted WB values that were generally lower than the measured capDBS values. For example, for capDBS HbA1c results of 4 %, the predicted WB values were 3.84 % on Day 0, 3.86 % on Day 4, 3.97 % on Day 7, and 4.48 % on Day 14. For capDBS HbA1c results of 7 %, the predicted WB values were 6.76 % on Day 0, 6.33 % on Day 4, 6.37 % on Day 7, and 6.33 % on Day 14. For capDBS HbA1c results of 7.5 %, the predicted WB values were 7.25 % on Day 0, 6.73 % on Day 4, 6.77 % on Day 7, and 6.64 % on Day 14. For capDBS HbA1c results of 10 %, the predicted WB values were 9.69 % on Day 0, 8.79 % on Day 4, 8.78 % on Day 7, and 8.19 % on Day 14. The width of the 95 % prediction intervals (a measure of how precisely WB can be estimated) varied more broadly on D14. The estimated mean squared error (MSE) was lower on Days 0 and 4 when using the linear regression model, which also determined further decreases in $R^2$ values on D7 and D14 (Table 4).

**Table 2** Summary of HbA1c results from WB, capillary DBS and venous DBS samples

| Day | Sample | HbA1c (%, Mean ± SD) | Intra-assay CV % (median, range) |
|---|---|---|---|
| D0 | WB | 6.22 ± 1.11 (N = 115) | 1.19, 0–4.10 |
|  | Uncorrected capDBS | 6.62 ± 1.16 (N = 77) | 2.28, 0–10.10 |
|  | Corrected capDBS | 6.39 ± 1.17 (N = 77) | N/A |
|  | Uncorrected venDBS | 6.72 ± 1.20 (N = 81) | 1.68, 0–6.86 |
|  | Corrected venDBS | 6.42 ± 1.18 (N = 81) | N/A |
| D4 | Uncorrected capDBS | 6.92 ± 1.32 (N = 96) | 2.28, 0–9.87 |
|  | Corrected capDBS | 6.26 ± 1.18 (N = 96) | N/A |
|  | Uncorrected venDBS | 7.15 ± 1.39 (N = 81) | 2.14, 0–11.79 |
|  | Corrected venDBS | 6.42 ± 1.21 (N = 81) | N/A |
| D7 | Uncorrected capDBS | 6.85 ± 1.29 (N = 81) | 1.98, 0–16.04 |
|  | Corrected capDBS | 6.25 ± 1.15 (N = 81) | N/A |
|  | Uncorrected venDBS | 7.36 ± 1.47 (N = 75) | 2.81, 0–26.42 |
|  | Corrected venDBS | 6.51 ± 1.23 (N = 75) | N/A |
| D14 | Uncorrected capDBS | 6.62 ± 1.44 (N = 79) | 2.62, 0–17.68 |
|  | Corrected capDBS | 6.10 ± 1.33 (N = 79) | N/A |
|  | Uncorrected venDBS | 7.30 ± 1.65 (N = 79) | 2.54, 0–26.52 |
|  | Corrected venDBS | 6.44 ± 1.29 (N = 79) | N/A |

Note: WB = whole blood; ven = venous; cap = capillary; DBS = dried blood spot; SD = standard deviation; CV = coefficient of variation; N/A = not applicable

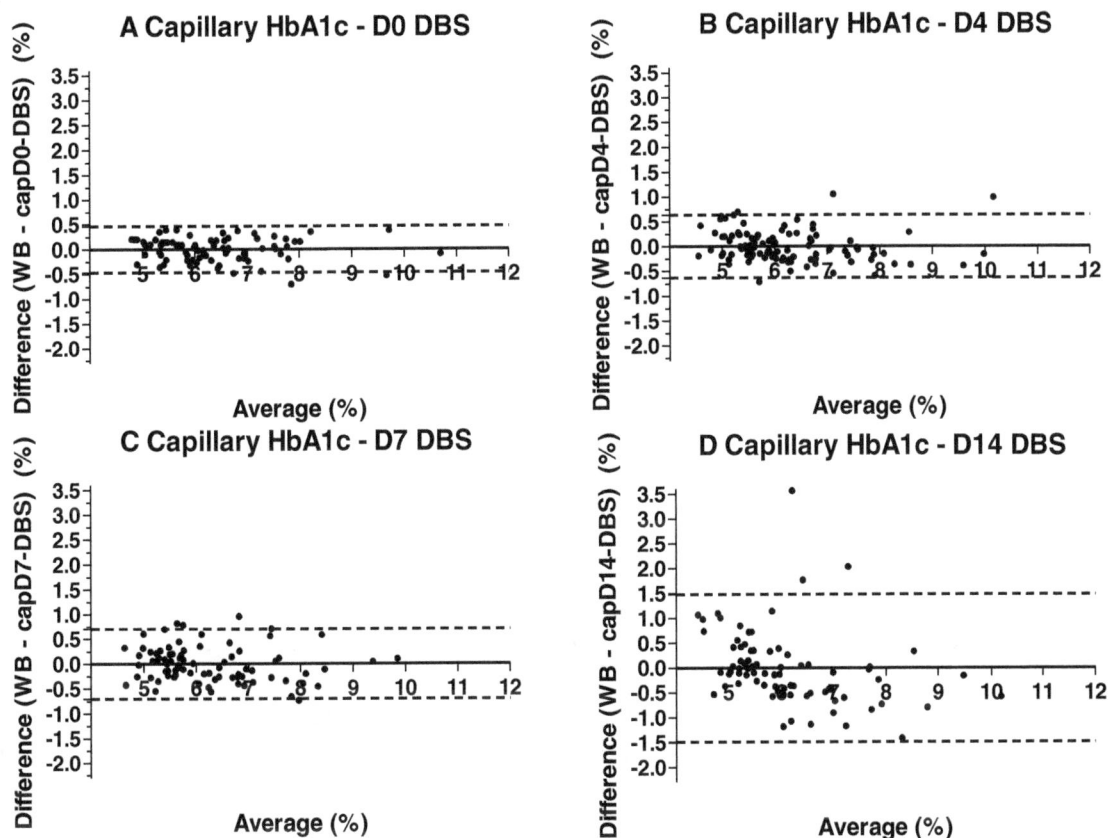

**Fig. 1** Bland-Altman plots of capillary dried blood spot samples from days 0, 4, 7 and 14. Note: Corrected DBS results are represented on D0, D4, D7 and D14; dashed lines represent 95 % limits of agreement; full lines represent biases. WB = whole blood on D0; cap = capillary; DBS = dried blood spot

## Discussion

There is growing demand for human pathology test services in Australia and around the world, driven by the ageing global population and increasing incidence of chronic diseases [13]. Dried blood spot sampling is an alternative to traditional blood sampling, and has been used in clinical and epidemiological studies for several decades [6, 8, 14]. This method provides results that are comparable to those obtained through traditional venipucture [2, 12], without its logistical obstacles regarding sample collection, processing, transportation and storage. For the measurement of HbA1c, DBS has also been shown to produce results that are comparable to those obtained through venous sampling [15–25]. In our study, we showed that HbA1c levels from DBS samples collected via finger pricking from volunteers with and without diabetes were comparable to those measured from venous samples, when measured up to seven days after collection.

In our study, DBS samples collected from finger pricking (capDBS) were analysed on the same day (D0), four (D4), seven (D7) and fourteen (D14) days after collection. High correlation and agreement between capDBS results on D0 and venous blood HbA1c values showed that the analysis of samples collected on matrix paper and analysed immediately provides results that are similar to those obtained and processed by traditional methods.

In a real-life scenario, DBS samples are mailed or shipped to the pathology laboratory that performs the assays. Therefore, DBS samples are not analysed immediately. To assess whether this gap between collection and analysis may interfere with the results, we performed analyses also four, seven and fourteen days after collection. We observed that, over time, the correlation between DBS and venous blood results becomes weaker, and the 95 % limits of agreement become wider, especially for D14 results, which may be clinically unacceptable. It is noteworthy that WB samples also degrade over time when not analysed immediately, particularly if not kept refrigerated. Haemoglobin degradation products may show up in

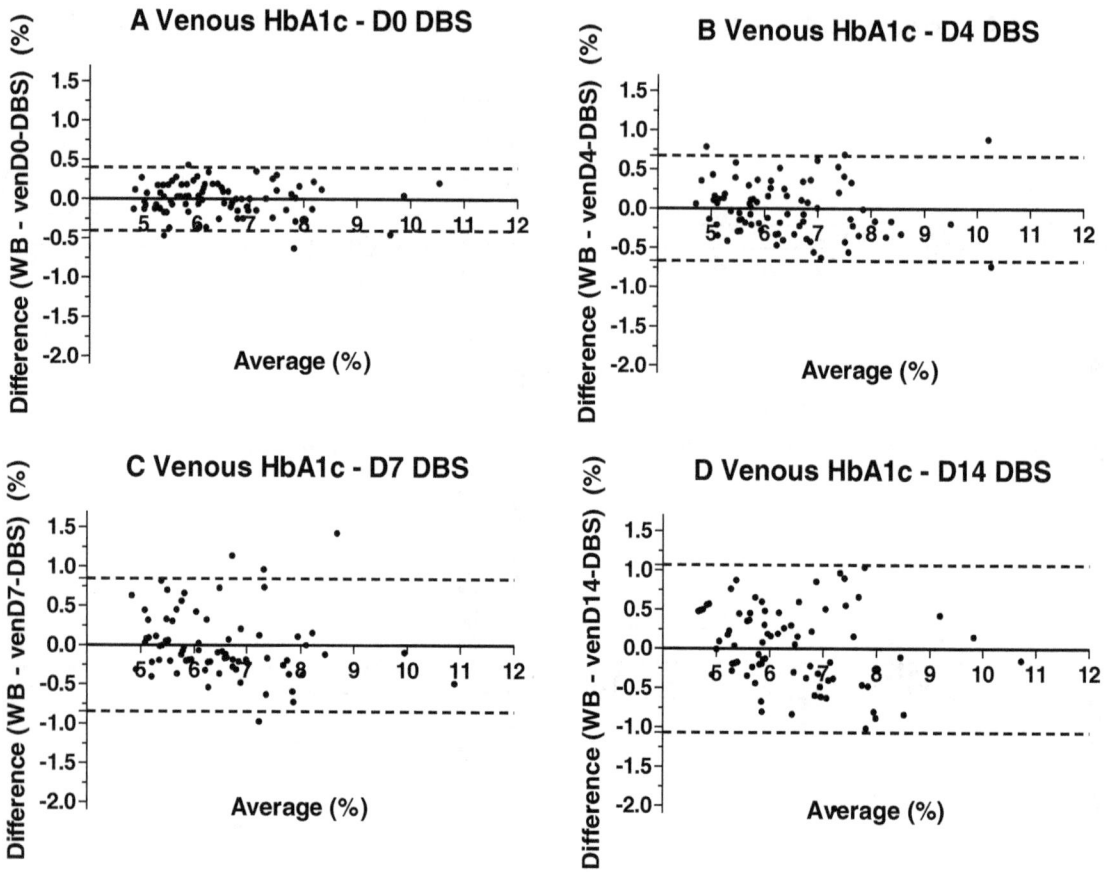

**Fig. 2** Bland-Altman plots of venous dried blood spot samples from days 0, 4, 7 and 14. Note: Corrected DBS results are represented on D0, D4, D7 and D14; dashed lines represent 95 % limits of agreement; full lines represent biases. WB = whole blood on D0; cap = capillary; DBS = dried blood spot

**Table 3** 95% limits of agreement for capillary and venous DBS results, uncorrected and corrected

|     |           | Upper limit | | Lower limit | |
| --- | --- | --- | --- | --- | --- |
|     |           | Uncorrected | Corrected | Uncorrected | Corrected |
| D0  | Capillary | 0.2308 | 0.462 | −0.6828 | −0.463 |
|     | Venous    | 0.1174 | 0.404 | −0.7051 | −0.402 |
| D4  | Capillary | 0.1117 | 0.638 | −1.428  | −0.636 |
|     | Venous    | 0.1203 | 0.671 | −1.567  | −0.666 |
| D7  | Capillary | 0.2383 | 0.668 | −1.436  | −0.668 |
|     | Venous    | 0.2345 | 0.845 | −1.943  | −0.845 |
| D14 | Capillary | 1.111  | 1.484 | −2.151  | −1.485 |
|     | Venous    | 0.6642 | 1.065 | −2.373  | −1.069 |

samples that have coagulated and aged. These products may co-elute with, or be incompletely separated from, HbA1c. In these cases, the HbA1c value obtained may be reported as higher than it actually is [26]. This effect is particularly evident for venDBS samples, which were collected without anticoagulant.

We used a linear regression model for cross-validation, to ensure unbiased measures of goodness-of-fit and prediction intervals for WB. In that model, capD0-DBS results were closer to the predicted WB values for all evaluated HbA1c steps (4 %, 7 %, 7.5 %, and 10 %), and the prediction intervals were narrower. On the remaining days, capDBS results were further away from the predicted WB values, and the prediction intervals broadened over time. In the clinics, capD0-DBS samples would provide the most accurate HbA1c results, closer to the predicted WB results and with a narrower prediction interval. However, the difference between predicted WB and both capD4- and capD7-DBS results

**Table 4** Prediction intervals for WB from capillary DBS values of 4 %, 7 %, 7.5 % and 10 %, obtained through linear regression models

| | capDBS 4 % | | | capDBS 7 % | | | capDBS 7.5 % | | | capDBS 10 % | | | MSE | Adjusted $R^2$ |
|---|---|---|---|---|---|---|---|---|---|---|---|---|---|---|
| | pWB | Lower 95 % CI | Upper 95 % CI | pWB | Lower 95 % CI | Upper 95 % CI | pWB | Lower 95 % CI | Upper 95 % CI | pWB | Lower 95 % CI | Upper 95 % CI | | |
| D0 | 3.84 | 3.36 | 4.32 | 6.76 | 6.30 | 7.23 | 7.25 | 6.78 | 7.72 | 9.69 | 9.20 | 10.18 | 0.0554 | 0.9463 |
| D4 | 3.86 | 3.22 | 4.51 | 6.33 | 5.70 | 6.95 | 6.74 | 6.11 | 7.36 | 8.79 | 8.14 | 9.43 | 0.0992 | 0.9064 |
| D7 | 3.97 | 3.26 | 4.67 | 6.37 | 5.68 | 7.06 | 6.77 | 6.08 | 7.46 | 8.77 | 8.06 | 9.49 | 0.1247 | 0.8267 |
| D14 | 4.48 | 3.20 | 5.76 | 6.33 | 5.08 | 7.59 | 6.64 | 5.38 | 7.90 | 8.19 | 6.89 | 9.48 | 0.3905 | 0.5268 |

Note: pWB = predicted whole blood; capDBS = capillary dried blood spot; MSE: mean standard error; CI: confidence interval

may be clinically acceptable, as well as their prediction intervals. In the case of capD14-DBS results, their prediction intervals may be too wide to be clinically acceptable. We applied four different capDBS values to the model, but any result can be applied to it (R program available upon request), providing similar behaviour.

In some cases, patients may have difficulty in collecting sufficient amount of blood samples from finger pricking on the matrix paper. That difficulty was evidenced by the fact that the sample size for each day was not equal to the total number of recruited participants. Therefore, we assessed whether venous blood collected through standard methods and spotted on the matrix paper would produce similar results. In those analyses, venous DBS samples were correlated to traditionally-processed venous blood samples in a similar way as capillary DBS. Also, there was high correlation and agreement between capDBS and venDBS results.

In our study, we recruited 67 diabetic patients. Most of them had type 2 diabetes, and had HbA1c levels that are considered adequate (particularly among participants with type 2 diabetes). Only three participants had HbA1c levels higher than 9 %. Therefore, results might have been different should more participants with decompensated diabetes had been recruited. Samples were measured at least in duplicates, and the median intra-assay coefficients of variation were clinically acceptable, lower than 3 % at all times. However, some participants had heterogeneous results. It is unclear why results using the same sample and assay method may vary in some participants.

One of the key issues to be considered for the employment of DBS sampling is the standardization of the analysis of the DBS measurements. It is essential to predict, with the highest possible level of accuracy, the concentration of HbA1c in WB from the values measured in the DBS tests. In a recent study, a meta-analysis of seventeen heterogeneous studies (employing different methods for measuring HbA1c) was performed by Affan *et al.*, and a correction formula to approximate the DBS results to the WB values was

published (12). We employed their correction formula in our current studies (results not presented), but the outcomes of the corrected DBS values resulted in a poorer approximation to the WB values. It appears that the time elapsed between sample collection and processing is a key component of the variability observed in the DBS sampling. Indeed, we found that there are significant differences among the Bland-Altman plots constructed from data on each particular day (*e.g.* D0, D4, D7 and D14) between DBS vs. WB. Thus, in our current analytical method, we analysed the data of each processed day independently by proposing mean values and prediction intervals for each particular processing day. Additionally, we corrected capillary DBS results by applying a correction formula that derived from regression analyses for each particular day, to approximate the regression line to the equality line. Thus, we obtained a different formula for each day, and observed that corrected capillary DBS results were closer to the predicted WB ones on all days except D14, when MSE was higher (*i.e.*, WB results were less precisely predicted).

We acknowledge that our study is limited by the fact that participants were evaluated in a controlled research setting, and results may be different when capillary HbA1c is evaluated in a real-life scenario. Future studies need to evaluate samples from participants who collect their capillary DBS samples on their own, and mail them to the testing laboratory via standard postal services (subjected to confounding factors such as delays and temperature variations). Furthermore, future studies should evaluate the prediction intervals for other elapsed times such as D1, D2, and D3, and also determine how these prediction intervals can be applied in the management of diabetes. To answer those questions, future studies should evaluate healthy individuals and those with diabetes who are treatment-naïve, and compare their DBS values and their prediction intervals with their WB HbA1c outcomes. By considering their WB values as the gold-standard, a more accurate clinical interpretation of the prediction intervals, as proposed here, could be established.

## Conclusion

In conclusion, HbA1c measured from DBS samples collected via finger pricking provided results that were comparable to those obtained from venous samples and measured by standard procedures. When results from DBS samples (processed up to 7 days after their collection) were applied to correction equations, HbA1c results with the most accuracy and the least clinically-acceptable variability were obtained, with high correlation and agreement to HbA1c results from whole venous blood, and with narrow 95 % limits of agreement. Those findings were further confirmed by a cross-validation model, which provided prediction intervals that were narrow enough to be clinically acceptable. In order for the measurement of HbA1c through DBS sampling to be considered in situations where traditional venipuncture is not available, further studies need to evaluate the effects of external factors, in a broader population.

### Competing interests

This study was funded by MyHealthTest Pty. MyHealthTest Pty funded the article-processing charge; MyHealthTest Pty staff instructed participants how to collect their capillary blood samples. MyHealthTest Pty had no role in study design, data analysis and interpretation of data, writing of the manuscript, and decision to submit the manuscript for publication. All authors had and have full access to the study data.

### Authors' contributions

BW performed samples collection, developed the DBS elution protocol, performed samples assays, performed data analysis, wrote the manuscript; CAM designed the study, performed data analysis, wrote the manuscript. RT performed samples collection, developed the DBS elution protocol, performed samples assays. TN designed the study, performed data analysis, wrote the manuscript. GP-F designed the study, performed samples collection, performed data analysis, wrote the manuscript. All authors read and approved the final manuscript.

### Authors' information

Claudio A. Mastronardi and Belinda Whittle considered co-first authors.

### Acknowledgements

We thank MyHealthTest Pty staff, Dr. Marianne Gould (for logistical assistance), and Ms. Jennifer Orr (for her assistance with capillary blood samples collection). We also thank DiabetesACT for their assistance with the recruitment of volunteers. This study was funded by MyHealthTest Pty, including the article-processing charge.

### Author details

[1]Department of Genome Sciences, The John Curtin School of Medical Research, The Australian National University, 131 Garran Rd, Canberra, Acton ACT 2601, Australia. [2]Australian Phenomics Facility, The Australian National University, 117 Garran Rd, Canberra, Acton ACT 2601, Australia. [3]Statistical Consulting Unit, The Australian National University, 27 Union Lane, Canberra, Acton ACT 2601, Australia.

### References

1. American Diabetes A. Standards of medical care in diabetes–2014. Diabetes Care. 2014;37 Suppl 1:S14–80.
2. McDade TW. Development and validation of assay protocols for use with dried blood spot samples. Am J Hum Biol. 2014;26(1):1–9.
3. Bang I. Ein verfahren zur mikrobestimmung von blutbestandteilen. Biochem Ztschr. 1913;49:19–39.
4. Guthrie R, Susi A. A Simple Phenylalanine Method for Detecting Phenylketonuria in Large Populations of Newborn Infants. Pediatrics. 1963;32:338–43.
5. Mei JV, Alexander JR, Adam BW, Hannon WH. Use of filter paper for the collection and analysis of human whole blood specimens. J Nutr. 2001;131(5):1631S–6.
6. Parker SP, Cubitt WD. The use of the dried blood spot sample in epidemiological studies. J Clin Pathol. 1999;52(9):633–9.
7. Bhatti P, Kampa D, Alexander BH, McClure C, Ringer D, Doody MM, et al. Blood spots as an alternative to whole blood collection and the effect of a small monetary incentive to increase participation in genetic association studies. BMC Med Res Methodol. 2009;9:76.
8. Wilcken B, Wiley V. Newborn screening. Pathology. 2008;40(2):104–15.
9. Corran PH, Cook J, Lynch C, Leendertse H, Manjurano A, Griffin J, et al. Dried blood spots as a source of anti-malarial antibodies for epidemiological studies. Malar J. 2008;7:195.
10. Sherman GG, Stevens G, Jones SA, Horsfield P, Stevens WS. Dried blood spots improve access to HIV diagnosis and care for infants in low-resource settings. J Acquir Immune Defic Syndr. 2005;38(5):615–7.
11. Xu YY, Pettersson K, Blomberg K, Hemmila I, Mikola H, Lovgren T. Simultaneous quadruple-label fluorometric immunoassay of thyroid-stimulating hormone, 17 alpha-hydroxyprogesterone, immunoreactive trypsin, and creatine kinase MM isoenzyme in dried blood spots. Clin Chem. 1992;38(10):2038–43.
12. Affan ET, Praveen D, Chow CK, Neal BC. Comparability of HbA1c and lipids measured with dried blood spot versus venous samples: a systematic review and meta-analysis. BMC Clin Pathol. 2014;14:21.
13. Britt H. An analysis of pathology test use in Australia. Australian Association of Pathology Practices Inc. 2008. Available from http://pathologyaustralia.com.au/wp-content/uploads/2013/03/DOD-paper-+-append.pdf. Accessed 7 May 2015.
14. Williams SR, McDade TW. The use of dried blood spot sampling in the national social life, health, and aging project. J Gerontol B Psychol Sci Soc Sci. 2009;64 Suppl 1:i131–6.
15. Anjali, Geethanjali FS, Kumar RS, Seshadri MS. Accuracy of filter paper method for measuring glycated hemoglobin. J Assoc Physicians India. 2007;55:115–9.
16. Egier DA, Keys JL, Hall SK, McQueen MJ. Measurement of hemoglobin A1c from filter papers for population-based studies. Clin Chem. 2011;57(4):577–85.
17. Fokkema MR, Bakker AJ, de Boer F, Kooistra J, de Vries S, Wolthuis A. HbA1c measurements from dried blood spots: validation and patient satisfaction. Clin Chem Lab Med. 2009;47(10):1259–64.
18. Gay EC, Cruickshanks KJ, Chase HP, Klingensmith G, Hamman RF. Accuracy of a filter paper method for measuring glycosylated hemoglobin. Diabetes Care. 1992;15(1):108–10.
19. Jeppsson JO, Jerntorp P, Almer LO, Persson R, Ekberg G, Sundkvist G. Capillary blood on filter paper for determination of HbA1c by ion exchange chromatography. Diabetes Care. 1996;19(2):142–5.
20. Jones TG, Warber KD, Roberts BD. Analysis of hemoglobin A1c from dried blood spot samples with the Tina-quantR II immunoturbidimetric method. J Diabetes Sci Technol. 2010;4(2):244–9.
21. Lacher DA, Berman LE, Chen TC, Porter KS. Comparison of dried blood spot to venous methods for hemoglobin A1c, glucose, total cholesterol, high-density lipoprotein cholesterol, and C-reactive protein. Clin Chim Acta. 2013;422:54–8.
22. Lakshmy R, Gupta R. Measurement of glycated hemoglobin A1c from dried blood by turbidimetric immunoassay. J Diabetes Sci Technol. 2009;3(5):1203–6.
23. Little RR, McKenzie EM, Wiedmeyer HM, England JD, Goldstein DE. Collection of blood on filter paper for measurement of glycated hemoglobin by affinity chromatography. Clin Chem. 1986;32(5):869–71.
24. Lomeo A, Bolner A, Scattolo N, Guzzo P, Amadori F, Sartori S, et al. HPLC analysis of HbA1c in dried blood spot samples (DBS): a reliable future for diabetes monitoring. Clin Lab. 2008;54(5–6):161–7.
25. Wikblad K, Smide B, Bergstrom A, Wahren L, Mugusi F, Jeppsson JO. Immediate assessment of HbA1c under field conditions in Tanzania. Diabetes Res Clin Pract. 1998;40(2):123–8.
26. Selvin E, Coresh J, Jordahl J, Boland L, Steffes MW. Stability of haemoglobin A1c (HbA1c) measurements from frozen whole blood samples stored for over a decade. Diabet Med. 2005;22(12):1726–30.

# 8

# Ruptured hepatic metastases of cutaneous melanoma during treatment with vemurafenib

Takuto Nosaka[1], Katsushi Hiramatsu[1], Tomoyuki Nemoto[1], Yasushi Saito[1], Yoshihiko Ozaki[1], Kazuto Takahashi[1], Tatsushi Naito[1], Kazuya Ofuji[1], Hidetaka Matsuda[1], Masahiro Ohtani[1], Hiroyuki Suto[1], Yoshiaki Imamura[2] and Yasunari Nakamoto[1*]

## Abstract

**Background:** The spontaneous rupture of hepatic metastases is rare compared to that of primary hepatic tumors. In addition, vemurafenib, a selective inhibitor of the mutant BRAF protein or gene product, has been reported to be extremely effective in patients with metastatic melanoma who harbor a *BRAF V600E* mutation.

**Case presentation:** A 44-year-old female had previously undergone surgery for resection of a malignant melanoma in the lower right leg. Four years later, hepatic metastases became apparent, and transcatheter arterial embolization (TAE) was performed. Then she underwent treatment with vemurafenib. The size of the hepatic metastases markedly decreased. Two months later, they enlarged rapidly and ruptured, requiring emergency TAE. However, the patient developed hemorrhagic shock and died of renewed intra-abdominal bleeding on the 26th postoperative day.

**Conclusions:** This is a rare case of ruptured hepatic metastases of malignant melanoma during treatment with vemurafenib. Postmortem examination and immunohistochemical analysis indicated reactivation of the mitogen-activated protein kinase pathway in the metastatic tumor, suggesting secondary resistance to vemurafenib as the possible underlying mechanism.

## Background

Hepatic metastases are observed in 68 % of all patients with malignant melanoma at autopsy [1]. However, few cases of ruptured hepatic metastases of melanoma have been reported [2–9]. Recently, it has been reported that treatment with vemurafenib results in complete or partial tumor regression in >80 % of melanoma patients with the *BRAF V600E* mutation [10]. The following case report describes a rare complication of ruptured hepatic melanoma that occurred during treatment with vemurafenib. The postmortem examination of the present case may provide insight into the mechanism underlying this tumor's secondary resistance to vemurafenib and the subsequently fatal rupture.

## Case presentation

In August 2008, a 44-year-old female had undergone surgery for resection of a malignant melanoma in the right lower leg and a right inguinal metastatic lymph node (Fig. 1), followed by chemotherapy with doxorubicin, adriamycin, vincristine, and interferon beta (DAV-feron). In March 2012, computed tomography (CT) revealed brain and lung metastases, so the patient began radiation therapy to treat these lesions.

In September 2012, the patient was admitted to our hospital for back pain. Abdominal CT and magnetic resonance imaging detected new multiple hepatic metastases of melanoma. A transcatheter arterial infusion of cisplatin was administered, and transcatheter arterial embolization (TAE) was performed. In October 2012, she began treatment with vemurafenib, based on the finding of a positive *BRAF V600E* mutation in the resected primary site of the skin, which was analyzed by direct sequencing analysis using DNA from the paraffin-embedded primary cutaneous melanoma. She tolerated the treatment

* Correspondence: nakamoto-med2@med.u-fukui.ac.jp
[1]Second Department of Internal Medicine, Faculty of Medical Sciences, University of Fukui, Fukui, Japan
Full list of author information is available at the end of the article

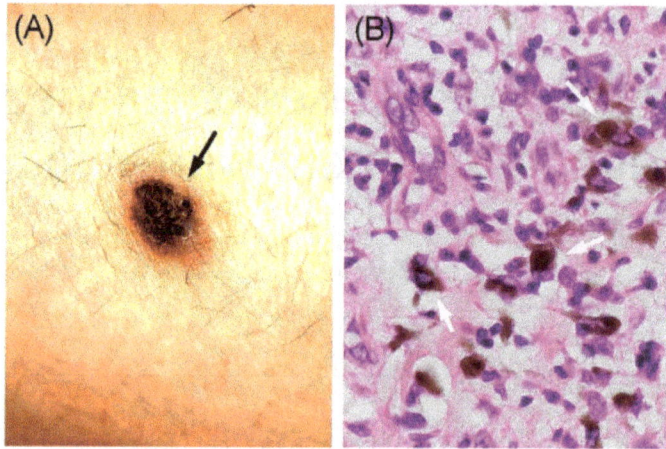

**Fig. 1** Gross examination and histologic finding of the cutaneous melanoma. The pigmented skin is located on the lower right leg (*black arrow*) (**a**). The resected specimen contained granular, brown, cytoplasmic pigmented cells (*white arrow*) (hematoxylin-eosin stain, ×400) (**b**)

remarkably well, and the size of the multiple hepatic and lung metastases decreased, while the size of the brain metastases did not. In addition, the serum concentration of 5-S-cysteinyldopa (5-S-CD), a biological marker of melanoma progression, was also decreased from 40.1 ng/mL to 5.2 ng/mL.

In December 2012, she suddenly developed severe abdominal pain. Abdominal CT revealed ruptured hepatic metastases accompanied by massive intra-peritoneal hemorrhage. A retrospective and sequential analysis of the CT images suggested that a part of the liver metastases had enlarged rapidly and then ruptured with intratumoral hemorrhage during vemurafenib treatment (Fig. 2). An emergency TAE was performed by selective occlusion of the right hepatic artery using gelatin sponge particles. The postoperative course was uneventful for several days.

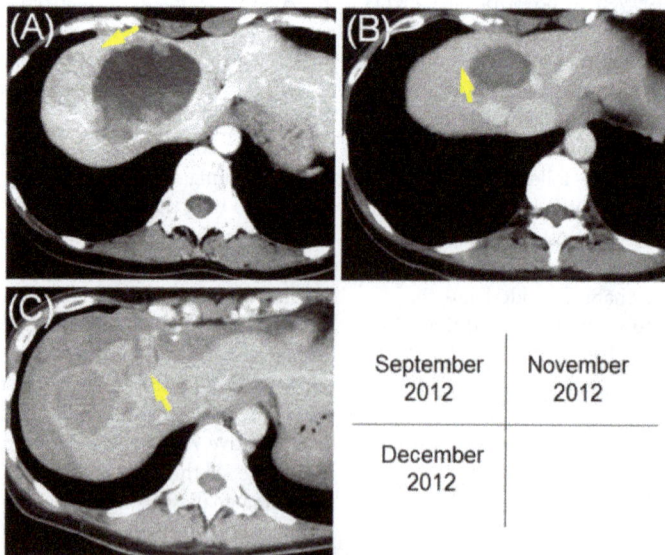

**Fig. 2** Sequential images of abdominal computed tomography (CT). These images are from September 2012 (**a**), November 2012 (**b**), and December 2012 (**c**). There is a metastatic tumor in the right lobe of the liver (**a**). Initially, the hepatic metastases considerably respond to vemurafenib treatment, and they become almost invisible (**b**). Later, they grow rapidly and rupture, resulting in a large amount of free fluid within the peritoneal cavity surrounding the liver (**c**). The *yellow arrow* demonstrates the same tumor in each image

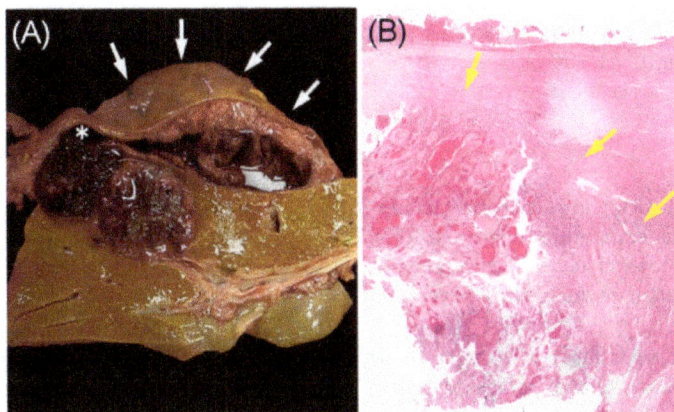

**Fig. 3** Cross-sectional and histologic findings of the liver at autopsy. The ruptured region (*white asterisk*) and subcapsular hematoma surrounding the liver (*white arrow*) (**a**). The metastatic tumor is well demarcated by a fibrous capsule (*yellow arrow*) (hematoxylin-eosin stain, ×40) (**b**)

However, on the 26th postoperative day, she developed hemorrhagic shock and died of renewed intra-abdominal bleeding.

An autopsy examination revealed hemoperitoneum due to rupture of the liver metastases. Metastases were also discovered in the brain and lungs as well as in the kidneys, adrenal gland, and lymph nodes, although these had not been detected on imaging while she was alive. There was also massive bloody ascites (1700 mL). The background liver was completely normal, whereas exposed necrotic tissue and intratumoral hemorrhage were observed at the site of tumor rupture (Fig. 3). We concluded that the cause of death was hemorrhagic shock from ruptured hepatic metastases of malignant melanoma. Finally, for improved understanding of the mechanism of refractory metastasis, we conducted an immunohistochemical analysis of the signal transduction molecules, phosphorylated extracellular signal-regulated kinase (p-ERK), and phosphorylated Akt (p-Akt), as well as the melanocyte marker Melan-A and Ki-67 in tumor cells of the primary malignant melanoma obtained from the right lower leg and in hepatic and lymph node

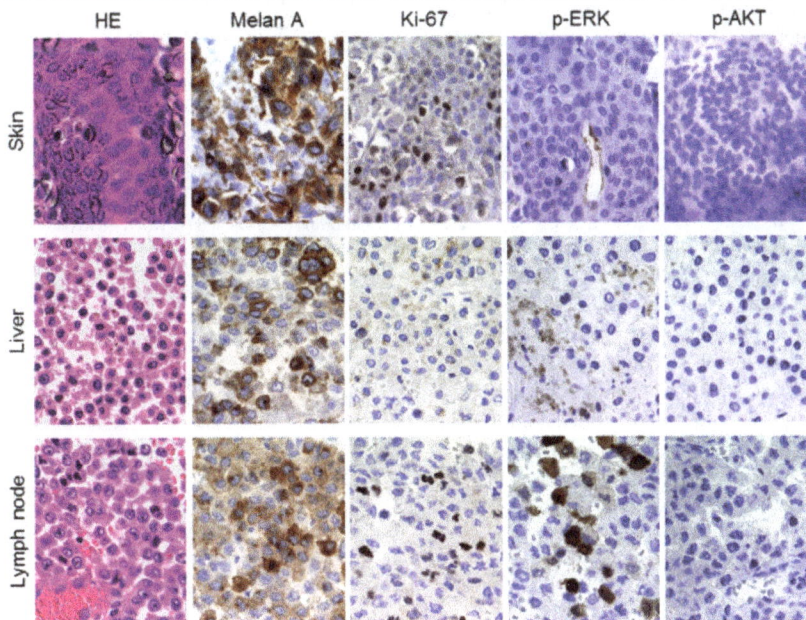

**Fig. 4** Microscopic findings of the skin, liver, and lymph node specimen. The skin lesion and the liver and lymph node metastases are stained to detect Melan-A, Ki-67, phosphorylated extracellular signal regulated kinase, and phosphorylated Akt (×400)

metastases obtained on autopsy (Fig. 4). Our findings showed that hepatic and lymph node metastases were positive for p-ERK and negative for p-AKT, even though the primary tumor was negative for both.

## Conclusions

Compared to primary hepatic tumors, hepatic metastases that result in spontaneous rupture are rare [6]. Furthermore, only eight reports describing rupture of hepatic metastases of malignant melanoma have been published [2–9].

The rupture of hepatic metastases is thought to be derived from tumor necrosis and increased intra-abdominal pressure due to straining upon defecation and forceful palpation [11–13]. In our autopsy case, gross examination and a microscopic study of the liver suggested that the increased intratumoral pressure by rapid growth, acute intratumoral bleeding, and the subsequent tumor necrosis resulted in rupture (Fig. 3).

The recently developed vemurafenib, a selective inhibitor of the mutant BRAF protein or gene product, has been reported to be extremely effective in patients with metastatic melanoma who harbor a *BRAF V600E* mutation [14–16]. Davies et al. reported that this mutation is present in approximately 50 % of cutaneous melanoma cases [16]. In our case, since the *BRAF* mutation was positive, we used vemurafenib for treatment, and the patient was responsive to it. In addition, Anker et al. described synergistic toxicity from the combination of radiation and vemurafenib [17], but fortunately, our patient did not experience complications, such as liver and skin toxicity, during the course of radiation and vemurafenib treatment. However, 2 months later, a part of the hepatic metastasis had enlarged and ruptured with an increased 5-S-CD.

The clinical course indicated that secondary resistance occurred during treatment with vemurafenib. As for the mechanism of secondary resistance to vemurafenib, tumor re-proliferation requires reactivation of the mitogen-activated protein kinase (MAPK) pathway (intrinsic pathway) or activation of the phosphatidylinositiol 3-kinase/AKT/mammalian target of rapamycin (PI3K/AKT/mTOR) pathway (extrinsic pathway), both of which have been reported [18, 19]. Therefore, we conducted an immunohistochemical analysis of the signal transduction molecules, p-ERK, and p-Akt, as well as the melanocyte marker Melan-A and Ki-67 (Fig. 4). Our findings showed that hepatic and lymph node metastases obtained on autopsy were positive for p-ERK and negative for p-AKT, even though the primary tumor was negative for both. These findings suggested the strong possibility that reactivation of the MAPK pathway had occurred without activation of the PI3K/AKT/mTOR pathway in the hepatic and lymph node metastases. This type of secondary resistance is thought to be derived from various causes such as *NRAS* or *MEK* mutations.

This case suggested that secondary resistance of vemurafenib, confirmed by an immunohistochemical study, may cause rapid tumor growth and subsequent rupture. In addition, immunohistochemical studies may clarify the mechanism underlying secondary resistance, and they may provide important information regarding the future treatment of vemurafenib-resistant metastatic melanoma.

## Consent

Written informed consent was obtained from the patient for publication of this Case report and any accompanying images. A copy of the written consent is available for review by the Editor of this journal.

**Abbreviations**

TAE: Transcatheter arterial embolization; MAPK: Mitogen-activated protein kinase; DAV-feron: Doxorubicin, adriamycin, vincristine, and interferon beta; CT: Computed tomography; 5-S-CD: 5-S-cysteinyldopa; PI3K/AKT/mTOR: Phosphatidylinositiol 3-kinase/AKT/mammalian target of rapamycin; p-ERK: Phosphorylated extracellular signal regulated kinase; p-Akt: Phosphorylated Akt.

**Competing interests**

The authors declare that they have no competing interests.

**Authors' contributions**

TN and TN managed the patient. TN and KH wrote the manuscript. YN reviewed the manuscript and provided critical revisions. All authors approved the final manuscript.

**Author details**

¹Second Department of Internal Medicine, Faculty of Medical Sciences, University of Fukui, Fukui, Japan. ²Department of Pathology, University of Fukui Hospital, Fukui, Japan.

**References**

1. Dasgupta T, Brasfield R. Metastatic melanoma. A clinicopathological study. Cancer. 1964;17:1323–38.
2. Cooperman AM, Weiland LH, Welch JS. Massive bleeding from a ruptured metastatic hepatic melanoma treated by hepatic lobectomy. Case report and review of the literature. Mayo Clin Proc. 1976;51:167–70.
3. Mokka R, Seppälä A, Huttunen R, Kairaluoma M, Sutinen S, Larmi TK. Spontaneous rupture of liver tumours. Br J Surg. 1976;63:715–7.
4. Foster JH. Survival after liver resection for secondary tumors. Am J Surg. 1978;135:389–94.
5. Wagner WH, Lundell CJ, Donovan AJ. Percutaneous angiographic embolization for hepatic arterial hemorrhage. Arch Surg. 1985;120:1241–9.
6. Dousei T, Miyata M, Yamaguchi T, Nagaoka M, Takahashi E, Kawashima Y. Rupture of liver metastasis of malignant melanoma–a case of hepatic resection. Jpn J Surg. 1991;21:480–4.
7. Welch M. Spontaneous hepatic rupture due to metastatic malignant melanoma. Postgrad Med J. 1991;67:1028–9.
8. Chun HJ, Osuga K, Fahrni M, Nakamura H. Massive bleeding of ruptured metastatic hepatic melanoma treated by transarterial embolization. Jpn J Radiol. 2010;28:395–7.
9. Wolfson RM, Romsa J. Ruptured liver metastasis with active hemorrhage has the classic appearance of a giant cavernous hemangioma on 99mTc-labeled RBC scintigraphy. Clin Nucl Med. 2012;37:984–5.
10. Murakami R, Taniai N, Kumazaki T, Kobayashi Y, Ogura J, Ichikawa T. Rupture of a hepatic metastasis from renal cell carcinoma. Clin Imaging. 2000;24:72–4.

11.  Sakai M, Oguri T, Sato S, Hattori N, Bessho Y, Achiwa H, et al. Spontaneous hepatic rupture due to metastatic tumor of lung adenocarcinoma. Intern Med. 2005;44:50–4.

12.  Okazaki M, Higashihara H, Koganemaru F, Nakamura T, Kitsuki H, Hoashi T, et al. Intraperitoneal hemorrhage from hepatocellular carcinoma: emergency chemoembolization or embolization. Radiology. 1991;180:647–51.

13.  Ong GB, Taw JL. Spontaneous rupture of hepatocellular carcinoma. Br Med J. 1972;4:146–9.

14.  Flaherty KT, Puzanov I, Kim KB, Ribas A, McArthur GA, Sosman JA, et al. Inhibition of mutated, activated BRAF in metastatic melanoma. N Engl J Med. 2010;363:809–19.

15.  Chapman PB, Hauschild A, Robert C, Haanen JB, Ascierto P, Larkin J, et al. Improved survival with vemurafenib in melanoma with BRAF V600E mutation. N Engl J Med. 2011;364:2507–16.

16.  Davies H, Bignell GR, Cox C, Stephens P, Edkins S, Clegg S, et al. Mutations of the BRAF gene in human cancer. Nature. 2002;417:949–54.

17.  Anker CJ, Ribas A, Grossmann AH, Chen X, Narra KK, Akerley W, et al. Severe liver and skin toxicity after radiation and vemurafenib in metastatic melanoma. J Clin Oncol. 2013;31:e283–7.

18.  Shi H, Hugo W, Kong X, Hong A, Koya RC, Moriceau G, et al. Acquired resistance and clonal evolution in melanoma during BRAF inhibitor therapy. Cancer Discov. 2014;4:80–93.

19.  Van Allen EM, Wagle N, Sucker A, Treacy DJ, Johannessen CM, Goetz EM, et al. The genetic landscape of clinical resistance to RAF inhibition in metastatic melanoma. Cancer Discov. 2014;4:94–109.

# 9

# Comparing gene expression data from formalin-fixed, paraffin embedded tissues and qPCR with that from snap-frozen tissue and microarrays for modeling outcomes of patients with ovarian carcinoma

William H. Bradley[1]*, Kevin Eng[2,4], Min Le[3], A. Craig Mackinnon[3], Christina Kendziorski[2] and Janet S. Rader[1]

## Abstract

**Background:** Previously, we have used clinical and gene expression data from The Cancer Genome Atlas (TCGA) to model a pathway-based index predicting outcomes in ovarian carcinoma. This data were obtained from snap-frozen tissue measured with the Affymetrix U133 platform. In the current study, we correlate the data used to model with data derived from TaqMan qPCR both snap frozen and paraffin embedded (FFPE) samples.

**Methods:** To compare the effect of preservation methods on gene expression measured by qPCR, we assessed 18 patient and tumor sample matched snap-frozen and FFPE ovarian carcinoma samples. To compare gene measurement technologies, we correlated qPCR data from 10 patients with tumor sample matched snap-frozen ovarian carcinoma samples with the microarray data from TCGA. We normalized results to the average expression of three housekeeping genes. We scaled and centered the data for comparison to the Affymetrix output.

**Results:** For the 18 specimens, gene expression data obtained from snap-frozen tissue correlated highly with that from FFPE samples in our TaqMan assay (r > 0.82). For the 10 duplicate TCGA specimens, the reported microarray data correlated well (r = 0.6) with our qPCR data, and ranges of expression along pathways were similar.

**Conclusions:** Gene expression data obtained by qPCR from FFPE serous ovarian carcinoma samples can be used to assess in the pathway-based predictive model. The normalization procedures described control variations in expression, and the range calculated along a specific pathway can be interpreted for a patient's risk profile.

## Background

Using gene expression and clinical data from The Cancer Genome Atlas (TCGA), we previously developed a model that predicts variations in response of high-grade serous ovarian cancer to cytotoxic chemotherapies. In that publication [1], we described a method for reducing the list of genes needed to predict clinical outcomes to fewer than 100. We selected those genes from more than 10,000 possibilities by identifying genes within a core group of 12 cancer pathways [2, 3] whose variation in expression had the greatest effect on disease progression. Predictions of response to specific chemotherapeutic agents were suggested by the cumulative levels of gene expression among the 91 genes selected from the 12 pathways. Three of the pathways did not have genes identified, leaving 9 core pathways informative. We defined the predictions made by gene expression within these pathways as the Patient-Specific Risk Profile (PSRP).

Gene expression levels reported by Affymetrix microarrays and qPCR may differ significantly, creating potential difficulties for models developed on one platform and utilized in the other [4]. For example, measurements of reference RNAs from commercial sets of ~1000 genes

* Correspondence: wbradley@mcw.edu
[1]Department of Obstetrics and Gynecology, Medical College of Wisconsin, 8701 Watertown Plank Road, Milwaukee, WI 53226, USA
Full list of author information is available at the end of the article

from human brain, liver, and lung showed correlations (r) ranging from 0.45 to 0.75 when TaqMan measurements were compared with Applied Biosystems and Agilent microarray technologies [5]. The MicroArray Quality Control (MAQC) project showed correlations of $r = \geq 0.9$ between Affymetrix and TaqMan data [6], but those measurements and correlations were made with reference RNA from a large gene set, undirected by model building or clinical practice. Moreover, the technology used to measure expression may have a greater or lesser influence on output, depending on how the genes of interest are selected. A predictive model that features only highly differentially expressed genes may more easily translate from microarray to qPCR than a model not based on large changes in expression [7]. A requirement of highly differentiated genes may not represent the biology of the disease, and the modeling we have done includes lower expressed genes in the set.

TCGA derives gene expression by placing RNA from snap-frozen tissue on an Affymetrix U133 Array platform [8]. To migrate to a more clinically functional platform, we evaluated the reliability of gene expression inputs derived by using qPCR to analyze formalin-fixed, paraffin-embedded tumor samples. Because FFPE blocks are readily available from primary debulking surgery, whereas snap-frozen tissue is not, this modified approach increases the number of patients who can potentially benefit from this profiling technique.

Two factors could significantly affect the clinical utility of our profiles when FFPE tissue samples are used: (i) differences in tissue preservation techniques altering the RNA quality and expression detection between snap-frozen and FFPE and (ii) gene expression levels differing due to alterations in technology between Affymetrix Microarray and TaqMan qPCR. Although either or both changes could have a major effect on predictive capability, the effect might be modified depending on the number of genes measured or the ways the data are analyzed for prediction. For example, the impact of variance in expression measurements could be ameliorated by aggregating multiple data points when using multiple genes for prediction [9].

In this study, we compared gene expression measurements for individual genes selected by our PSRP 91 gene assay (gene by gene) and for those same genes aggregated into the pathways of our model (pathway by pathway). We derived correlations between snap-frozen and FFPE tissue preparations and between Affymetrix U133 Microarrays and TaqMan qPCR. In addition, we used techniques for normalizing qPCR gene expression that allows us to directly compare qPCR assays with the TCGA microarray data. The result is that our PSRP 91 model developed from snap-frozen tissue on an Affymetrix platform can be tested using a qPCR outputs and FFPE specimens.

## Methods

### Study subjects

To compare tissue preservation methods, we measured gene expression from 18 patients who had both snap-frozen ovarian carcinoma samples in the Medical College of Wisconsin (MCW) gynecologic tissue bank and a case-matched FFPE sample archived by the Department of Pathology. All samples were taken during debulking surgery of patients diagnosed with Stage IIIC or IV, grade 3 serous ovarian carcinoma. Tissue samples were taken to pathology immediately after extirpation. Once assessed by a pathologist, the portion acquired for tissue banking was excised, and snap frozen in the pathology lab. The remainder was fixed in formalin and processed per standard pathology protocol. Prior to analysis, the tissues had been stored as FFPE blocks or snap frozen sections for up to 3 years. The pathology for each MCW patient was reviewed with hematoxylin and eosin (H&E) to confirm both the diagnosis and a tumor content of at least 75 % [8]. Approval from the Institutional Review Board (IRB) of the Human Research Protection Office and Medical College of Wisconsin was obtained, and all patients signed an informed consent for tissue banking.

To compare two methods of assaying gene expression, we used TCGA identification numbers to identify 10 snap-frozen tumor samples submitted to the TCGA from the tissue bank at Washington University in St. Louis. Approval from the institutional Human Research Protection Office was obtained. For each patient's sample, TCGA had reported gene expression and annotated pathology. All of these samples were from patients with Stage IIIC, grade 3 serous ovarian carcinoma, and microarray analysis had been performed by TCGA. A qPCR expression level of the 91 genes was measured in the 10 snap frozen samples.

### Gene list

The genes whose expression we assayed were selected from a gene set constituting the 9 core pathways described previously [1]. 91 genes were chosen from our previously published PSRP results. Analysis was performed according to the 9 core pathways as well as a revised six-gene set representing the neurotrophin pathway, making a total of 10 pathways available for analysis (Additional file 1: Table S1). The subsets of genes used to define a pathway's expression are listed in the Supplement as well (Additional file 1: Table S2). We used the housekeeping genes glyceraldehyde 3-phosphate dehydrogenase (GAPDH), hypoxanthine phosphoribosyltransferase 1 (HPRT1), and beta-D-glucuronidase (GUSB) to normalize gene expression.

### RNA isolation, cDNA, and qPCR

RNA from the snap-frozen tissue samples was extracted using an RNAqueous Kit from Life Technologies

(Carlsbad, CA, USA). RNA from FFPE blocks was extracted using a RecoverAll™ Total Nucleic Acid Isolation Kit, also from Life Technologies. All RNAs were treated with Ambion TURBO DNase. RNA concentrations were determined with a Qubit™ RNA Assay Kit (Carlsbad, CA, USA), and integrity was checked on an Experion Automated Electrophoresis Station (Hercules, CA, USA).

All reagents used in cDNA synthesis and qPCR were obtained from Applied Biosystems (Carlsbad, CA, USA). RNA concentration was adjusted to 40 ng/μl for the reverse transcription reaction. cDNA synthesis was carried out with a High-Capacity cDNA Reverse Transcription Kit. About 200 ng of RNA was used in a final 10-μl RT reaction. The TaqMan® Array Plates 96 Plus were custom-made to include TaqMan Gene Expression Assays of 91 target genes and the three endogenous control genes. Best Coverage probes from Applied Biosystems were used to target the genes of interest. The assays of 91 target genes and 3 housekeeping genes were pooled at 0.2X concentration for the PreAmp reaction. cDNAs (2 μl) were preamplified in a 20-μl reaction for 10 cycles, using TaqMan PreAmp Master Mix and pooled assays. The reaction products were diluted 5-fold with 1X TE and mixed with 500 μl of TaqMan Fast Advanced Master Mix. Water was added to give a final mixture volume of 1 ml. A 10 μl aliquot of the assay mixture was added to each well of the TaqMan Gene Expression Assay Plate, and amplification was carried out on a 7500 Fast Real Time PCR System. Genes that were not detected within 34 cycles (Ct > 34) were considered unexpressed for the purpose of our evaluation.

### Normalization of affymetrix and TaqMan data

TCGA derives gene expression by extracting RNA from snap-frozen tissue and aggregating data from three different array platforms (Affymetrix U133a 2.0, Digital Gene Expression from Illumina, and a custom high-density Agilent array). We evaluated the Affymetrix results only as these were the most complete reported and had fully accessible probe information.

To compare gene expression across the two technologies (Affymetrix Microarray and TaqMan qPCR) we used the following normalization techniques for data output. For the Affymetrix data, we took the Robust Multi-array Average (RMA; Affymetrix) for each gene, and then normalized to the average of the endogenous housekeeping genes GAPDH, HPRT1 and GUSB.

For TaqMan qPCR, we used two techniques to normalize gene measurements. First, we used the average of the cycles from the same three housekeeping genes as the control within the array. We then subtracted the number of cycles of a target gene from the average of the housekeeping genes. Reported Ct values of

34 or greater were considered to be unidentified or unexpressed genes. This method is demonstrated in Fig. 1 was used to correlate gene expression levels for each of the 91 genes measured by the two different technologies – Affymetrix and TaqMan.

TaqMan qPCR-based expression levels passed through a quality control step and were normalized using housekeeping genes. Reported Ct values of 34 or greater were considered to be unexpressed and therefore were not considered in the analysis of a given pathway on a subject-by-subject basis. The average of the housekeeping genes GAPDH, HPRT1 and GUSB served as an endogenous control for the assay. Noting that large Ct values imply less gene sample expression, we subtracted each probe's ΔCt value from the control to obtain a Ct score that rises with expression consistent with the array-based expression measurement.

### Calibration and PSRP 91 gene computation

Each TaqMan qPCR assay is normalized so it requires no control outside of its own assay. However there are technology-specific differences between the Affymetrix and TaqMan probes. We accounted for this in a calibration step: In deriving the array-based measurements we relied on mean zero, standard deviation one (scaled and centered) values for constructing the risk indexes that comprise the Patient-Specific Risk Profile (PSRP)[1]. We also normalized the TaqMan qPCR expression values by scaling and centering using the observed probe average and standard deviation (Additional file 1: Table S3). Thus a new sample can be normalized and calibrated and the PSRP 91 gene indexes can be computed.

### Statistical methods

For each sample, we used Pearson and Spearman's rank correlation to compare measurements. The curves for each patient's 91 gene expression measurements are provided in Fig. 1. We used a locally weighted scatterplot smoothing (LOWESS) to obtain a summary of the relationship between gene expression derived by one technology and that derived by the other.

### Results

#### RNA quality metrics and dropped genes

The quality of the RNA derived from the snap-frozen tissues was uniformly high with a RNA quality indicator (RQI) of >7 for 20 of the 28 specimens. The remaining 8 specimens were all 6.2 or greater, except a single outlier with a RQI of 2.9. The FFPE samples had predictably low RQI levels ranging from 1.9 to 3.1. The range of storage time of the tissue samples did not correla te with RQI for the FFPE samples. TaqMan probes for WNT16, WNT3, and DNTT had ΔCt of >34 and were considered unexpressed in most assays (84 %

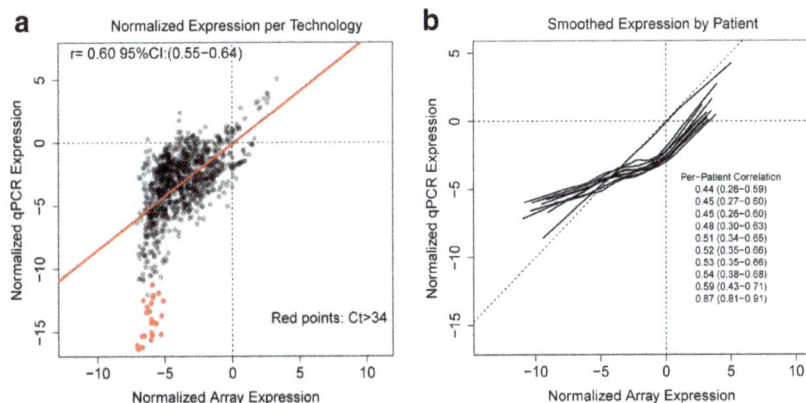

**Fig. 1** Correlation of gene expression of 91 genes from 10 snap-frozen TCGA samples measured with Affymetrix U133 microarray (X-axis) and, in the current study, with TaqMan qPCR (Y-axis). The 91 probes from the 10 samples were each normalized to the average of three housekeeping genes (GUSB, GAPDH, and HPRT1). **a** The scatterplot shows that gene-to-gene expression has similar ranges across both technologies when normalized to the same three-gene average (r = 0.60). **b** Lowess smoothing curves. Red dots signify Ct values >34 which are not included in final index measurements

unexpressed, 94 % unexpressed, and 100 % unexpressed respectively); *PLA2G2D* and *CACNG1* were not expressed in 37 % and 46 % of assays respectively, and 15 other probes were not expressed at least once in 68 total TaqMan assays (Additional file 1: Table S4). These findings are consistent with the data showing that these were among the lowest expressing genes in TCGA samples. Samples with low RQI levels still exhibited reportable gene expression levels. Probes considered unexpressed (Ct >34) were removed from samples on a per-assay basis and were not included in the denominator for the index calculation.

### Gene-to-gene comparison of expression levels measured by Affymetrix microarrays and TaqMan qPCR

From TCGA, we obtained gene expression levels in snap-frozen ovarian cancer samples from patients treated at Washington University (St. Louis, MO). To evaluate the concordance of expression measured by array-based probes and qPCR-based probes we acquired ovarian carcinoma samples extracted from the same patient and case, using TCGA numbers for identification. When the microarray and qPCR outputs were plotted against each other and matched gene for gene across the patients, the overall correlation was r = 0.60 (Fig. 1). The plotted slope confirms that the two techniques gave equivalent expression levels and that higher expression of a target gene resulted in a higher number (arbitrary value) on the y-axis. Taking the 10 specimens individually and performing a per-patient smooth estimate of the output (Fig. 1) showed a consistent correlation across the various genes measured. Using housekeeping genes to normalize expression of both technologies also demonstrated that the expression levels of the 91 genes of interest were similar across the two measurement platforms.

### Validating TaqMan assay profiles between matched paraffin-embedded and snap frozen samples

To gauge whether our PSRP 91 gene TaqMan qPCR assay provides equivalent expression measurements from both snap-frozen and paraffin-embedded samples, we measured gene expression in the tumor-matched samples of the 18 patients at the Medical College of Wisconsin who had tumor tissue preserved by both snap- freezing and the standard FFPE. The expression outputs were correlated for each gene between the two preservation techniques for each patient. Intra-patient gene expression was higher than any inter-patient gene expression (Fig. 2). Eight of the patients are highlighted in Fig. 2, and the degree of correlation across genes is noted. The correlation between preservation techniques was excellent: > = 0.82 per pair of matched samples. The range of correlation among the 18 sample sets was from 0.82 to 0.96 when comparing snap frozen to FFPE samples. A qPCR was repeated on a second cut from the snap frozen specimens, and the correlation ranged from 0.84 to 0.97 for the 18 samples demonstrating a high level of reproducibility.

### Distribution of pathway expression from 18 FFPE samples measured with qPCR and mapped to the TCGA cohort

Plotting the distribution of Affymetrix pathway expression for patients from the TCGA gave a normal curve. Samples measured by qPCR (noted with red ticks in Fig. 3) centered under these normal curves. Figure 3 shows the TCGA-generated expression distribution for each pathway. The distribution of each of the 18 samples we measured by qPCR falls within the normal curves, and does not appear biased when we observe their position under the Affymetrix-generated

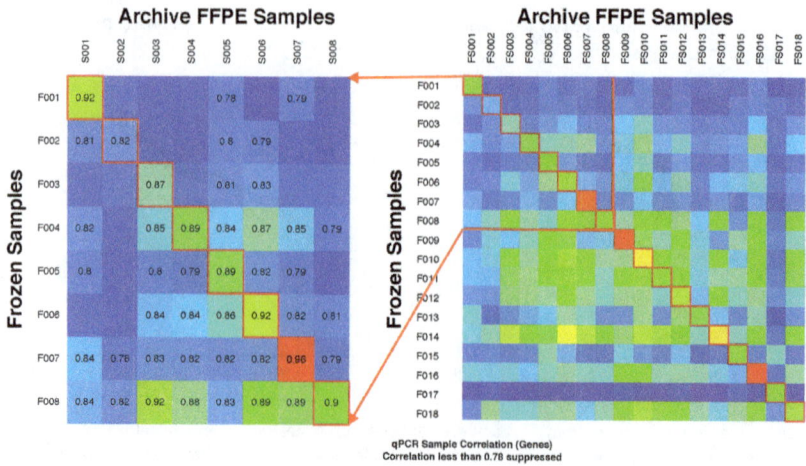

**Fig. 2** Correlation of gene expression from 18 matched serous ovarian cancer samples. F-labeled samples represent snap-frozen tissue; S represents each patient's matched FFPE tissue block. All samples were obtained from an initial surgical procedure, and gene outputs were measured with qPCR. Blue represents lower correlation, red higher. An expansion of samples 001 through 008 with absolute level of correlation is provided. Levels of correlation <0.79 are not displayed

curves for each of the 10 pathways. The PSRP 91 gene assay utilizes gene expression aggregated within a pathway to stratify outcomes. Distribution of these aggregations is not biased by changes in technology or preservation.

## Discussion

This manuscript demonstrates the feasibility of comparing measurements of gene expression used to model clinical outcomes in ovarian cancers from alternative technology and tissue preservation. We demonstrated

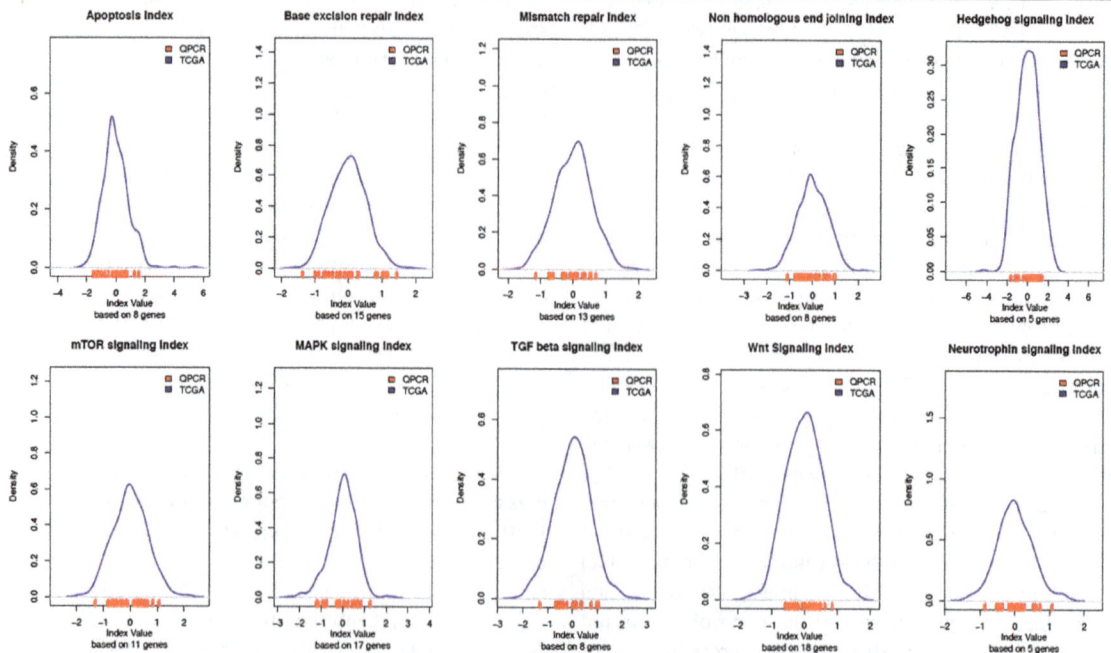

**Fig. 3** Range of gene expression measured from the selected pathways. The bell curve represents the distribution of expression across the entire TCGA cohort, using Affymetrix array. The red ticks on the x-axis represent gene expression levels aggregated within a pathway from the 18 patients whose FFPE samples were measured using qPCR. The range of expression can be normalized across the Affymetrix and TaqMan qPCR platforms. Patient samples measured with qPCR have a range of expression that does not appear biased within the normal curve

that qPCR outputs of high-grade serous ovarian carcinoma specimens were nearly identical whether tissue was preserved by snap freezing or fixed with formalin and embedded in a paraffin block. This work was driven by the discovery of a gene panel that is predictive of ovarian cancer patient survival and response to therapy. The correlations described here will enable us to better test our modeling in archived FFPE tissue samples.

A similar correlation between fresh-freezing and FFPE has been observed with breast cancer samples, but a cDNA-mediated annealing, selection, extension, and ligation (DASL) platform was used for gene measurement [10]. That correlation was observed across an unselected whole genome assay when the data was median centered, a technique similar to ours. Interestingly, these authors noted a high level of concordance between tissue types when they applied a selected predictive model that used 291 genes. When ovarian tissue gene expression in 240 FFPE samples was measured using DASL, the correlation was 0.618 to gene signatures described by Tothill and a TCGA working group [9], a high enough level to allow for preservation of the predictive value of the gene sets. Our predictive technique relies less on direct gene-to-gene comparison, as a group of genes is evaluated within a pathway. However, we observed a similar gene-to-gene correlation for our selected set (r = 0.60). A second qPCR run of the snap frozen samples against the FFPE demonstrated that the measurements were stable.

Large variations in expression have been noted to provide confidence in cross-technological measurements. Fedorowicz found correlation between fresh- frozen and FFPE ovarian cancer samples, but that study was confined to the top 100 differentially expressed genes [7]. In contrast, our PSRP 91 gene TaqMan assay did not require genes to have high levels of differential. Although we observed lower expression genes drop out occasionally (e.g., 16 % of the WNT16 assays), this did not seem to offer significant changes at the level of pathway expression. The degree this drop out effects the overall prediction capacity of the model needs further clarification.

We used a combination of two techniques to normalize gene expression across the two technological platforms. First, we averaged housekeeping genes and simply subtracted the result from the target gene in both technologies. Second, we used the scale and center technique that is commonly used in Affymetrix analyses. To ensure the expression levels of the TaqMan data were on the same scale as those from the TCGA Affymetrix data, TaqMan qPCR outputs were centered and scaled. After that normalization they showed comparable ranges of expression.

Variations in expression levels reported from this study are within previously described tolerances [11–14], and the range of differences over an entire pathways appears to have a potentially small or negligible effect on predictive power. Thus, our method for applying the Patient-Specific Risk Profile that was derived with snap-frozen tissue and large-scale Affymetrix microarrays can be effectively applied to a limited gene set measured by qPCR, using RNA extracted from FFPE tissues. Our PSRP 91 gene assay uses measurements aggregated within a cellular pathway, with unbiased selection techniques. This allows poorly expressed genes to be weighted as much as highly expressed genes in the predictive model.

Our work was limited by the small sample size of the snap-frozen tissues we obtained to compare to outputs provided by TCGA. Moreover, we did not measure gene expression in samples preserved for more than 3 years when we compared the FFPE blocks to the snap-frozen samples. The inability to detect expression changes as FFPE blocks age has been a concern in prior reports, but improved techniques and choices in housekeeping genes appear to have reduced its potential impact [15]. Variations in pathologic processing and the ischemia in the tissue sample may be a source of noise in the FFPE gene measurements. Thus far, our assessment of RQI showed lower quality for these specimens, which is expected. This did not seem to effect the quality of measurement for a plurality of the genes assayed. Fixation for snap frozen and FFPE samples occurred simultaneously after surgical removal. Another concern is intra-tumor heterogeneity in duplicate patient samples. Variation in a single patient's tumor profiling has been identified by groups measuring expression arrays from multiple tumor sites. Our comparisons were from the same tumor excised at the same time, but variation in location may affect the correlation of the two tumor sites [16]. The loss of detection of some lower expressing genes in the qPCR (e.g., WNT16) is a concern for future modeling. Alternative technologies may need to be considered depending on the weighted importance of specific genes.

In summary, this study validated the use of FFPE tissue and qPCR—instead of snap-frozen tissue and microarrays—to obtain gene expression data for core cellular pathways. This supports the use these tissue samples when predictive modeling of ovarian cancer was done in larger data sets such as the TCGA. The variation in expression noted between our different samples does not appear to significantly distort expected outputs, leading us to believe that a model derived from expression reported using one approach could be used with a more convenient and "real world" approach when evaluating clinical samples. Our assay will be tested in a recurrent disease setting to more definitively evaluate predictive capacity prospectively.

## Conclusion

This study offers evidence that a predictor model based on a large data set generated from Affymetrix microarray and snap frozen ovarian carcinoma samples can be applied to paraffin embedded clinical samples from a local pathology lab. Our predictive model used a "pathway" approach, and we observed that these local samples had pathway measurements across 10 separate pathways that fell within expected ranges. Normalization with scaling and centering was used for this in the qPCR data generated.

## Additional file

Additional file 1: Table S1. Gene list. Table S2. Pathway list and genes in the pathway. Table S3. Scale and center data used for qPCR. Table S4. Genes unexpressed in at least one TaqMan assay. (DOCX 54 kb)

## Abbreviations

TCGA: The Cancer Genome Atlas; qPCR: Quantitative real-time reverse transcription polymerase chain reaction; FFPE: Formalin fixed, paraffin embedded; PSRP: Patient specific risk profile; MAQC: Microarray quality control; GAPDH: Glyceraldehyde 3-phosphate dehydrogenase; HPRT1: Hypoxanthine phosphoribosyltransferase 1; GUSB: beta-D-glucuronidase; LOWESS: Locally weighted scatterplot smoothing; DASL: cDNA-mediated Annealing, Selection, extension, and Ligation.

## Competing interests

The authors declare that we have no competing interests

## Authors' contributions

WB conceived the study, collected the tissue samples, and drafted the manuscript. KE ran statistical correlations. ML ran tissue microarrays and quality control. AM evaluated tumor density and quality of tissue samples, supervised tissue control, and microarrays. CK reviewed the statistical correlations. JR helped conceive the study and draft the manuscript. All authors read and approved the final manuscript.

## Authors' information

Not applicable.

## Acknowledgements

David G. Mutch, MD generously provided tissue samples from Washington University. The results published here are in part based upon data generated by the TCGA research network: http://cancergenome.nih.gov/.

## Funding

Support and funding was received by the Froedtert Foundation, the Women's Health Research Program, Falk Medical Trust, The Heitz Foundation, and National Center for Research Resources and the National Center for Advancing Translational Sciences, National Institutes of Health, through Grant Numbers 8UL1TR000055 and GM102756. Its contents are solely the responsibility of the authors and do not necessarily represent the official views of the NIH.

## References

1. Eng KH, Wang S, Bradley WH, Rader JS, Kendziorski C. Pathway index models for construction of patient-specific risk profiles. Stat Med. 2013; 32(9):1524-1535
2. Jones D. Pathways to cancer therapy. Nat Rev Drug Discov. 2008;7:875–6.
3. Jones S, Zhang X, Parsons DW, Lin JC, Leary RJ, Angenendt P, et al. Core signaling pathways in human pancreatic cancers revealed by global genomic analyses. Science. 2008;321:1801–6.
4. Irizarry RA, Warren D, Spencer F, Kim IF, Biswal S, Frank BC, et al. Multiple-laboratory comparison of microarray platforms. Nat Methods. 2005;2:345–50.
5. Wang Y, Barbacioru C, Hyland F, Xiao W, Hunkapiller KL, Blake J, et al. Large scale real-time PCR validation on gene expression measurements from two commercial long-oligonucleotide microarrays. BMC Genomics. 2006;7:59.
6. Consortium M, Shi L, Reid LH, Jones WD, Shippy R, Warrington JA, et al. The MicroArray Quality Control (MAQC) project shows inter- and intraplatform reproducibility of gene expression measurements. Nat Biotechnol. 2006;24:1151–61.
7. Fedorowicz G, Guerrero S, Wu TD, Modrusan Z. Microarray analysis of RNA extracted from formalin-fixed, paraffin-embedded and matched fresh-frozen ovarian adenocarcinomas. BMC Med Genomics. 2009;2:23.
8. Cancer Genome Atlas Research Network. Integrated genomic analyses of ovarian carcinoma. Nature. 2011;474: 609–15.
9. Sfakianos GP, Iversen ES, Whitaker R, Akushevich L, Schildkraut JM, Murphy SK, et al. Validation of ovarian cancer gene expression signatures for survival and subtype in formalin fixed paraffin embedded tissues. Gynecol Oncol. 2013;129:159–64.
10. Mittempergher L, de Ronde JJ, Nieuwland M, Kerkhoven RM, Simon I, Rutgers EJ, et al. Gene expression profiles from formalin fixed paraffin embedded breast cancer tissue are largely comparable to fresh frozen matched tissue. PLoS One. 2011;6:e17163.
11. Farragher SM, Tanney A, Kennedy RD, Paul HD. RNA expression analysis from formalin fixed paraffin embedded tissues. Histochem Cell Biol. 2008;130:435–45.
12. Arikawa E, Sun Y, Wang J, Zhou Q, Ning B, Dial SL, et al. Cross-platform comparison of SYBR Green real-time PCR with TaqMan PCR, microarrays and other gene expression measurement technologies evaluated in the MicroArray Quality Control (MAQC) study. BMC Genomics. 2008;9:328.
13. Shi L, Jones WD, Jensen RV, Harris SC, Perkins RG, Goodsaid FM, et al. The balance of reproducibility, sensitivity, and specificity of lists of differentially expressed genes in microarray studies. BMC Bioinformatics. 2008;9 Suppl 9:S10.
14. Canales RD, Luo Y, Willey JC, Austermiller B, Barbacioru CC, Boysen C, et al. Evaluation of DNA microarray results with quantitative gene expression platforms. Nat Biotechnol. 2006;24:1115–22.
15. Walter RF, Mairinger FD, Wohlschlaeger J, Worm K, Ting S, Vollbrecht C, et al. FFPE tissue as a feasible source for gene expression analysis–a comparison of three reference genes and one tumor marker. Pathol Res Pract. 2013;209:784–9.
16. Gerlinger M, Rowan AJ, Horswell S, Larkin J, Endesfelder D, Gronroos E, et al. Intratumor heterogeneity and branched evolution revealed by multiregion sequencing. N Engl J Med. 2012;366:883–92.

## Author details

[1]Department of Obstetrics and Gynecology, Medical College of Wisconsin, 8701 Watertown Plank Road, Milwaukee, WI 53226, USA. [2]Department of Biostatistics and Medical Informatics, University of Wisconsin-Madison, Madison, WI 53792, USA. [3]Department of Pathology, Medical College of Wisconsin, Milwaukee, WI 53226, USA. [4]Current Address: Department of Biostatistics and Bioinformatics, Roswell Park Cancer Institute, Buffalo, NY, USA.

# 10

# Membranous CD24 expression as detected by the monoclonal antibody SWA11 is a prognostic marker in non-small cell lung cancer patients

Michael Majores[1], Anne Schindler[1], Angela Fuchs[1], Johannes Stein[1], Lukas Heukamp[2], Peter Altevogt[3,4] and Glen Kristiansen[1*]

## Abstract

**Background:** Lung cancer is one of the most common malignant neoplasms worldwide and has a high mortality rate. To enable individualized therapy regimens, a better understanding of the molecular tumor biology has still to be elucidated. The expression of the cell surface protein CD24 has already been claimed to be associated with shorter patient survival in non-small cell lung cancer (NSCLC), however, the prognostic value and applicability of CD24 immunostaining in paraffin embedded tissue specimens has been questioned due to the recent acknowledgement of restricted epitope specificity of the commonly used antibody SN3b.

**Methods:** A cohort of 137 primary NSCLC cases was immunostained with a novel CD24 antibody (clone SWA11), which specifically recognizes the CD24 protein core and the resulting expression data were compared with expression profiles based on the monoclonal antibody SN3b. Furthermore, expression data were correlated to clinico-pathological parameters. Univariate and multivariate survival analyses were conducted with Kaplan Meier estimates and Cox regression, respectively.

**Results:** CD24 positivity was found in 34 % resp. 21 % (SN3b) of NSCLC with a membranous and/or cytoplasmic staining pattern. Kaplan-Meier analyses revealed that membranous, but not cytoplasmic CD24 expression (clone SWA11) was associated with lympho-nodular spread and shorter overall survival times (both $p < 0.05$). CD24 expression established by SN3b antibodies did not reveal significant clinicopathological correlations with overall survival, neither for cytoplasmic nor membranous CD24 staining.

**Conclusions:** Membranous CD24 immunoreactivity, as detected with antibody clone SWA11 may serve as a prognostic factor for lymphonodular spread and poorer overall survival. Furthermore, these results corroborate the importance of a careful distinction between membranous and cytoplasmic localisation, if CD24 is to be considered as a potential prognostic biomarker.

**Keywords:** Non-small cell lung cancer, NSCLC, CD24, Immunohistochemistry, Prognostic marker

* Correspondence: glen.kristiansen@ukb.uni-bonn.de
Michael Majores and Anne Schindler shared first authorship.
[1]Institute of Pathology, University of Bonn, Sigmund-Freud-Str. 25, D-53127 Bonn, Germany
Full list of author information is available at the end of the article

## Background

Lung cancer is a major cause of carcinoma related death, being responsible for 17.8 % of all cancer deaths and accounting for more than a million deaths worldwide per year [1]. Despite intense studies to improve therapy options, its prognosis has remained poor with a 5-year overall survival rate of less than 15 % [2].

In the past decade, the largest subgroup of lung cancer, i.e. non-small cell lung cancer (NSCLC), has been subjected to exerted research for a better understanding of the underlying molecular biology of lung cancer. More than ten years ago, CD24 has already been suggested as a novel and promising biomarker for carcinoma progression in NSCLC [3] and several groups have confirmed this finding on protein and transcript level [2, 4]. CD24 is a highly glycosylated protein, that binds to the cell surface through a GPI (glycosyl-phosphatidylinositol)-anchor and functions as a cell adhesion molecule and is involved in cell-cell-interaction via its P-selectin binding site [5]. CD24 has been found to be expressed by pre-B-lymphocytes [5]. It is assumed that CD24-positive cells can attach more easily to platelets and activated endothelial cells [6, 7]. Notably, CD24 has also been observed in many human carcinomas, such as ovarian cancer, renal cell cancer, breast cancer and NSCLC [3, 8–12]. In epithelial ovarian cancer high scores of cytoplasmic CD24 were highly predictive of shorter patient survival times (mean 97.8 vs. 36.5 months), whereas membranous CD24 expression seemed to have no influence on survival times. Interestingly, CD24 positivity (membranous or cytoplasmic) of prostate cancer samples was significantly associated to younger patient age and higher pT stages and a higher 3-year prostate-specific antigen (PSA) relapse rate compared with CD24-negative tumours.

In patients with gallbladder carcinoma, tumors with up-regulation of CD24 revealed lymph node metastasis and lymphovascular invasion more frequently. Moreover, up-regulation of CD24 tended to show deeper invasion depth and higher TNM stage [13]. Together, these findings support CD24 as a prognostic marker for carcinoma progression and poorer survival.

Despite these intriguing findings, major concerns regarding a lack of epitope specificity of the commonly used monoclonal antibody SN3b have been raised [14]. Recent findings indicate that the mAb (monoclonal antibody) SN3b does not bind to the protein core itself, but binds to a glycan structure that decorates the CD24 molecule. On the one hand, this motif is not present on all forms of CD24 and—on the other hand—it can be present in other epitopes irrespective of CD24 [14]. These limitations underline the need for more specific CD24 antibodies, such as the mAb SWA11 antibody that has been suggested to be more specific as it binds to the protein core [14].

As CD24 is a promising biomarker for the risk assessment of disease progression, the goal of the present study was to investigate CD24 expression in NSCLC using the novel, more specific monoclonal antibody (mAb) SWA11. Special emphasis was put on the comparison of SN3b- and SWA11-mediated CD24 detection regarding a) the subcellular distribution of CD24 expression (i.e. membranous versus cytoplasmic expression) and b) its correlation with various clinicopathological features including patient survival times.

## Methods
### Patient characteristics/ tumor samples

A cohort of 137 primary NSCLC patients, who had undergone surgery between 1995 and 2009 and who were all diagnosed in the Institute of Pathology, University of Bonn, was compiled. Tumor samples were available as formalin-fixed, paraffin-embedded tissue. According to the current WHO classification the NSCLC were classified as adenocarcinoma (AC) ($n = 102$) or squamous cell carcinoma (SCC) ($n = 35$). The male:female ratio (5:2) and mean age at diagnosis (64y; SD +/– 9y; range 24–86y) in our cohort was in accordance with the published epidemiologic distribution [1] (Table 1). No neoadjuvant radiotherapy or chemotherapy were applied before surgery. All cases were subjected to a central review based on the current WHO guidelines [1].

**Table 1** Clinicopathological characteristics of the NSCLC cohort

| | | AC | SCC |
|---|---|---|---|
| | | N (%) | N (%) |
| Tumour stage (pT) | | | |
| | 1 | 29 (21.2 %) | 5 (3.6) |
| | 2 | 51 (37.2 %) | 23 (16.8 %) |
| | 3 | 6 (4.4 %) | 6 (4.4 %) |
| | 4 | 1 (0.7 %) | 0 (0 %) |
| Nodal Status (pN) | 0 | 37 (27.0 %) | 15 (10.9 %) |
| | 1 | 15 (10.9 %) | 9 (6.6 %) |
| | 2 | 14 (10.2 %) | 3 (2.2 %) |
| | 3 | 1 (0.7 %) | 0 (0.0 %) |
| Grading (G) | 1 | 5 (3.6 %) | 0 (0.0 %) |
| | 2 | 41 (29.9 %) | 16 (11.6 %) |
| | 3 | 44 (32.1 %) | 17 (12.4 %) |
| Mean age at surgery | | 64,2 | 64,56 |
| (median age) | | (65) | (67) |
| Sex (m:w) | | 68:34 | 30:5 |
| Median OS (months) | | 52 | 24 |
| (SD; 95 % CI [months]) | | (±23.7; 5.5– 98.5) | (± 12.8;0.0– 49.0) |

*SD* standard deviation; *CI* confidence interval; *n* number of cases; *OS* overall survival

## Ethics statement

This study was accomplished under the consent of the independent ethics committee of the University of Bonn (approval number 188/14).

## Tissue microarray (TMA) assembly

For construction of the tissue microarrays, suitable areas for extraction of tissue were selected and marked on haematoxylin-eosin (HE) specimen slides. A senior pathologist conducted the microscopic selection of suitable areas. The selected areas were then punched out of the corresponding paraffin donor block and inserted into the recipient block. The tissue arrayer (LD 120 Sm5-x) was purchased from Alphalys, Paris, France. All punch diameters were 0.8 mm (corresponding to an spot area of 0.79 mm$^2$). Each case was represented by 3 tumor samples and 1 peritumoral non-neoplastic tissue sample.

## Immunohistochemistry

Formalin-fixed TMA sections were freshly cut (2–3 μm) and mounted on superfrost specimen slides (Thermo Fisher). Next, dewaxing was carried out with xylene and the tissue sections were gradually rehydrated. Antigen retrieval was achieved by pressure cooking in the autoclave at pH6 and under hyperfrequency wave of 360 W at 125 °C for 8 min. MAb SWA11 was diluted 1:100 and SN3b was diluted 1:50, each using a modul buffer from Medac (TA-250-PM). The immunohistochemical reaction was visualized using the detection system C-DPVB 500 HRP by Medac (all procedures were conducted according to the instructions of the manufacturer).

Positive controls, consisting of tissue samples with known positivity for the antibody, and negative controls (i.e. reactions lacking the primary antibody), were performed in parallel for each TMA slide. Expression intensity was examined in a semiquantitative manner (score 0: no staining, score 1: weak, score 2: moderate and score 3: strong staining). For statistical analyses, cases with moderate to strong expression were bundled in a 'high expression' and cases with negative or weak expression in a 'low expression' group.

## Follow-up analyses

Follow-up data were available in 93 cases. Patients suffered from primary malignant tumors of the lung and were subjected to surgical resection or diagnostic sampling between 1995 and 2009 Cases with sufficient availability of formalin-fixed, paraffin-embedded tissue entered the cohort. Survival data were obtained by the analysis of surgical and oncological medical reports as well as written request for data of the local registration offices. The survival time was defined as the time period between the date of surgery and the date of death resp. the date of the documentation as "still alive" at the last available time point.

The median survival of AC cases was 52 months (SD 23.7; 95 % CI: 5.5–98.5; $n = 67$), compared to SCC with 24 months (SD 12; 95 % CI: 0–49.0; $n = 26$). 62 patients died within the follow-up period. The remaining 31 patients were documentes as "still alive" at the last available time point. Only in 13 patients without documentation of death the follow-up period was less than 60 months.

## Statistical analysis

For statistical analysis the SPSS software v. 21.0 was used. For evaluation of the correlation between expression of CD24 and clinicopathological parameters Fisher's exact test was used. Univariate survival analysis included Kaplan-Meier-analyses with log-rank testing for the estimation of differences in survival times. For multivariate survival analysis, the Cox regression model was used. All cutoff values of significance were set $p < 0.05$ with two-sided testing.

## Results

### Immunohistochemical detection of CD24 expression using clone SWA11 and SN3b

Using the mAb SWA11, 47 of 137 (34.3 %) NSCLC revealed CD24 expression (either cytoplasmic or membranous) (Table 2). CD24 expression was observed more frequently in adenocarcinomas (AC) than in squamous cell carcinomas (SCC). In AC cytoplasmic expression was observed more frequently than membranous expression. In SCC, both cyptoplasmic and membranous expression was rare. Normal lung parenchyma (i.e. alveolar surface cells) showed no expression of CD24. Bronchial epithelium showed a strong membranous and cytoplasmic staining of the brush border (Fig. 1).

*Using* the mAb *SN3b*, 29 of 137 (21.2 %) NSCLC revealed CD24 expression (either cytoplasmic or membranous) (Table 2). As above, CD24 expression was observed more frequently in adenocarcinomas (AC) than in squamous cell carcinomas (SCC). However, in contrast to mAb SWA11 cytoplasmic expression was observed less frequently than membranous expression in AC. In SCC, both cytoplasmic and membranous expression was rare. Normal lung parenchyma (i.e. alveolar surface cells) showed a distinct membranous immunoreactivity. Bronchial epithelium revealed both membranous and cytoplasmic staining of CD24.

*Correlation between SWA11 and SN3b:* As SWA11 and SN3b detect different epitopes, we evaluated the correlation of the immunohistochemical staining patterns. Of 132 NSCLC specimens with matched expression data, only 9 specimens (6.8 %) revealed a concordant CD24 expression. Of these cases, 4 cases revealed a concordant cytoplasmic staining and another 5 cases revealed a concordant membranous CD24 expression. Statistically, no significant correlation between the two mAb could be observed (cc = −0.63, $p = 0.470$; Fisher's exact test $p = 0.665$). The correlation of cytoplasmic and membranous expression (for each

**Table 2** Cytoplasmic and membranous expression of CD24

| SWA11 (mAb clone) | | | SN3b (mAB clone) | | |
|---|---|---|---|---|---|
| | AC | SCC | | AC | SCC |
| Cytoplasmic | N (%) | N (%) | Cytoplasmic | N (%) | N (%) |
| 0 | 45 (32.6 %) | 19 (13.8 %) | 0 | 76 (55.1 %) | 31 (22.5 %) |
| 1 | 22 (15.9 %) | 8 (5.8 %) | 1 | 12 (8.7 %) | 1 (0.7 %) |
| 2 | 17 (12.3 %) | 4 (2.9 %) | 2 | 7 (5.1 %) | 2 (1.4 %) |
| 3 | 18 (13.0 %) | 4 (2.9 %) | 3 | 1 (0.7 %) | 0 (0 %) |
| | AC | SCC | | AC | SCC |
| Membranous | N (%) | N (%) | Membranous | N (%) | N (%) |
| 0 | 68 (49.3 %) | 21 (15.2 %) | 0 | 64 (46.4 %) | 30 (21.7 %) |
| 1 | 21 (15.2 %) | 5 (3.6 %) | 1 | 10 (7.2 %) | 2 (1.4 %) |
| 2 | 8 (5.8 %) | 4 (2.9 %) | 2 | 12 (8.7 %) | 2 1.4 %) |
| 3 | 5 (3.6 %) | 5 (3.6 %) | 3 | 10 (7.2 %) | 0 (0 %) |

Staining intensities are determined as follows:
0: negative or equivocal, 1: weak, 2: moderate and 3: strong CD24 staining

antibody) was as follows: cc = 0.475 ($p < 0.05$) for SWA11 ($n = 108$) and cc = 0.140 ($p = 0.11$) for SN3b ($n = 103$).

### Survival analyses
Recent studies indicate that CD24 expression is associated with tumor progression and poorer survival rates. Therefore, we performed follow up analyses with a special emphasis on 1) the prognostic value of mAb SWA11 in dependence on subcellular staining characteristics and 2) the prognostic values of different clinicopathological parameters:

#### Prognostic value of CD24 in Kaplan Meier Analyses
Only membranous CD24 (SWA11) staining revealed significantly poorer survival rates (median overall survival 21 vs. 52 months; $p = 0.005$) as illustrated in Fig. 2. In contrast, cytoplasmic CD24 (SWA11) staining did not affect the survival rates (median OS 34 vs. 35 months; $p = 0.884$) (Table 3). When stratifying the cohort into SCC ($n = 35$) and AC ($n = 102$) in Kaplan Meier analyses, membranous CD24 (SWA11) expression did not affect patients' survival, neither in SCC ($p = 0.243$) nor AC ($p = 0.135$) (Table 3), probably due to the small number of observations (Fisher exact test: $p > 0.05$). After stratification for AC subtypes, membranous CD24 expression (SWA11) showed a tendency towards an association with poorer survival in acinar subtype AC, but failed significance ($p = 0.328$).

CD24 immunoreactivity using the mAb SN3b was not associated with patients' survival: neither the membranous

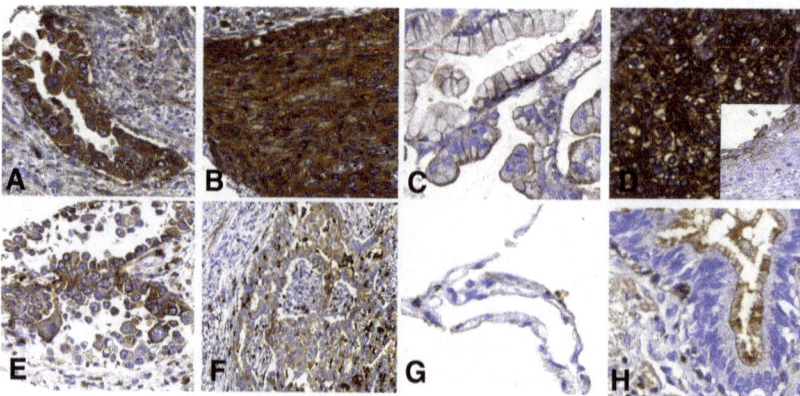

**Fig 1** The immunohistochemical characterization reveals membranous and/or cytoplasmic CD24 (mAb SWA11) expression. Strong cytoplasmic CD24 expression is found in a proportion of both AC (**a**) and SCC (**b**, **d**) specimens. Membranous CD24 expression can be pronounced with only scant or even absent cytoplasmic staining as shown in the AC (**c**). Also, both membranous and cytoplasmic CD24 detection can be found in some instances (**d**), the insert is showing the corresponding squamous carcinoma in-situ with membranous staining. Simultaneous membranous and cytoplasmic CD24 expression is also found in AC specimens (**e**, **f**). In normal tissue, alveolar epithelial cells do not express CD24 (**g**), whereas CD24 staining is found at the apical cell membrane of bronchial respiratory epithelia (**h**)

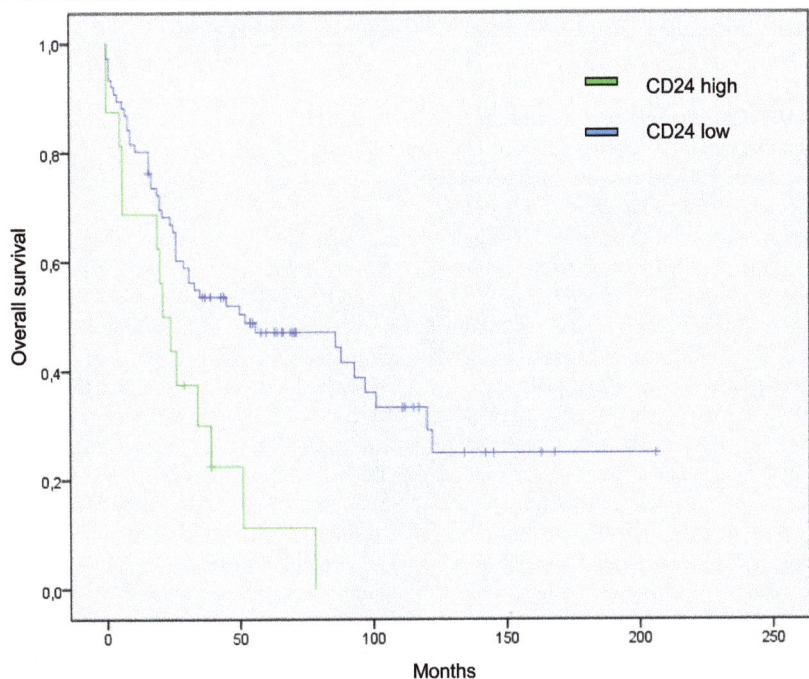

**Fig 2** Survival analysis. Kaplan-Meier curves according to SWA11 expression. Cases with moderate to strong expression were bundled in a 'high expression' and cases with negative or weak expression in a 'low expression' group. Membranous expression of CD24 detected by SWA11 proved to be an independent marker for shorter survival times in NSCLC ($p = 0.005$)

**Table 3** Univariate survival analysis

| SWA11 | No. of cases | Mean survival time (months +/− s.e.) | Median survival time (months +/− s.e.) | p-value |
|---|---|---|---|---|
| Mem CD24 | | | | |
| Negative | 76 | 84.833 +/− 10.395 | 52.000 +/− 27.030 | 0.005 |
| Positive | 16 | 27.925 +/− 6.379 | 21.000 +/− 4.000 | |
| Cyto CD24 | | | | |
| Negative | 66 | 75.209 +/− 10.577 | 35.000 +/− 12.422 | 0.884 |
| Positive | 26 | 60.540 +/− 11.551 | 34.000 +/− 12.196 | |
| Total CD24 | | | | |
| Negative | 64 | 76.972 +/− 10.841 | 35.000 +/− 13.726 | 0.633 |
| Positive | 28 | 57.535 +/− 10.895 | 34.000 +/− 9.303 | |
| SCC | | | | |
| Mem CD24 negative | 16 | 52.063 +/− 14.668 | 16.000 +/− 16.000 | 0.243 |
| Mem CD24 positive | 7 | 21.571 +/− 7.201 | 24.000 +/− 23.568 | |
| AC | | | | |
| Mem CD24 negative | 59 | 88.953 +/− 11.631 | 56.000 +/− 22.885 | 0.135 |
| Mem CD24 positive | 8 | 39.167 +/− 11.674 | 21.000 +/− 8.485 | |
| pN0 | 31 | 103.641 +/− 14.940 | 93.000 +/− 28.224 | 0.012 |
| pN1+ | 30 | 54.911 +/− 10.646 | 26.000 +/− 0.983 | |

staining pattern ($p = 0.9$), nor the cytoplasmic staining pattern ($p = 0.924$) revealed any significant effect on the overall survival.

### Prognostic values of the clinicopathological parameters

To further verify the prognostic values of different clinicopathological parameters, Cox regression analyses were conducted. As expected, positive nodal status (pN > 0) ($p = 0.003$) and disease stage (pT) ($p = 0.006$) were associated with poorer survival rates in univariate analyses (Table 4). Also, membranous CD24 (SWA11) positivity ($p = 0.007$) and histological tumour type ($p < 0.001$) showed a correlation with poorer survival rates. Subjecting the first three criteria to multivariate analyses, only membranous CD24 (SWA11) positivity ($p = 0.014$) and positive nodal status ($p = 0.027$), but not disease stage ($p = 0.185$) maintained independent factors for poorer overall survival (Table 5). In an extended multivariate Cox regression model with inclusion of tumour histology, membranous CD24 expression failed significance, but still showed a trend towards an association with shortened survival times ($p = 0.094$). CD24 expression using the mAb SN3b revealed no association with survival characteristics, neither for total (membranous or cytoplasmic) expression, nor for membranous or cytoplasmic expression alone (all $p > 0.05$, data not shown).

## Discussion

In the present study, we have analyzed immunohistochemical staining characteristics and the prognostic value of CD24 expression in NSCLC with a special emphasis on the comparison of the CD24 antibodies SWA11 and SN3b. The most important result of our study is that the prognostic relevance of CD24 is critically dependent on the careful consideration of subcellular compartments and the epitope specificity of the antibody used.

Overall, about one third of the NSCLC cohort revealed a significant CD24 expression (either cytoplasmic or membranous). These results are in line with the findings of other studies. In another NSCLC cohort, CD24 (SN3b) expression was found in 33 % of the samples (87 of 267 cases) [2]. Consistent with those results, we have found similar rates of high CD24 expression levels (35 % of the cases) for SWA11. Originally, we would have

**Table 4** Univariate survival analysis according to the Cox regression model (mAb SWA11)

|  | Beta | HR (hazard ratio) | 95 % CI of HR | P-value |
|---|---|---|---|---|
| SWA11 mem all | 0.856 | 2.353 | 1.268–4.364 | 0.007 |
| pN | 0.963 | 2.620 | 1.389–4.943 | 0.003 |
| pT | 0.844 | 2.325 | 1.279–4.224 | 0.006 |
| Tumour type | 0.975 | 2.651 | 1.999–3.517 | 0.000 |

**Table 5** Multivariate survival analysis according to the Cox regression model (mAb SWA11)

|  | Beta | HR (hazard ratio) | 95 % CI of HR | P-value |
|---|---|---|---|---|
| SWA11 mem all | 0.944 | 2.571 | 1.211–5.458 | 0.014 |
| pN | 0.737 | 2.091 | 1.087–4.021 | 0.027 |
| pT | 0.587 | 1.799 | 0.755–4.283 | 0.185 |

expected lower rates than those found by Lee et al, as they used the antibody SN3b, that also recognizes yet unidentified other glycoproteins next to CD24. Furthermore, they used whole mount sections instead of tissue microarrays. A possible explanation for rather equal detection rates would be the fact that it has been demonstrated that the epitope recognized by SN3b is indeed present in CD24, but is not found in all glycoforms of CD24 [14]. In contrast to the commonly used mAb SN3b, mAb SWA11 binds to the protein core of CD24 and does not depict other glycan moieties next to CD24. The protein core of CD24 is linear, consisting of the amino acid sequence leucine-proline-alanine (LAP) next to a glycosyl-phosphatidylinositol anchor [15].

CD24 expression has been associated with disease progression and cancer-related death in the majority of malignant tumors [2, 3, 16, 17], although a caveat to these data is that most of these studies are based on the supposedly less specific CD24 clone SN3b. Lee et al demonstrated a significant association between CD24-high expression (SN3b) and shorter patient survival times. Furthermore, Lee and colleagues and ourselves in former studies referred the results to cytoplasmic CD24 expression [2, 3].

In invasive ovarian carcinoma, patients carrying tumors with cytoplasmic CD24 expression showed a significantly shorter mean survival time of 37 months versus patients with tumors without cytoplasmic expression of CD24 (98 months) [16]. Also in NSCLC, expression of CD24 has been claimed to be an independent prognostic marker of shorter patient survival times, especially in AC [3].

Recently, CD24 expression has been addressed as a putative stem cell marker in NSCLC [10]. In that context particular attention has to be paid to the co-expression of CD44. Sterlacci et al. demonstrated that the phenotype CD24−/CD44+ did not show a significant difference in overall survival for the entire NSCLC cohort when compared with the CD24+/CD44 –population. However, when stratified according to histology, AC displaying the putative cancer stem cell (CSC) signature CD24−/CD44+ had a significantly shorter overall survival than CD24+/CD44− AC. However, these findings could not be ascertained as an independent factor, when calculated by multivariable analysis [10]. Since the overwhelming evidence of the pro-tumorigenic properties of CD24 is independent of the CD24low/CD44-high stem cell definition, we focused on

CD24 expression alone and did not include CD44 expression data in the present study.

Our results are only partly consistent with the published data. We were able to demonstrate that membranous staining pattern (using the mAb SWA11) was associated with a poorer overall survival and we revealed an increased risk of lymphonodular spread in the subgroup of CD24-high tumors, being in accordance with the published data. Nonetheless, our results are also partially conflicting with previous immunohistochemical data, as we could not confirm a significant correlation with patient survival for cytoplasmic expression of CD24, neither for SWA11 nor for SN3b.

The underlying biological mechanisms of CD24 promoted tumor progression are still incompletely characterized, although a growing number of studies have contributed to our comprehension [5–7, 17–20]. Expression of CD24 may provide an enhanced capability of tumor cells to adhere to activated endothelial cells mediated by its P-selectin binding site [5] or alter cellular signaling [21]. Aigner and colleagues showed that CD24 functions as a ligand for P-Selectin under physiological flow conditions, using a plate flow chamber assay. In their study, CD24 proved to be necessary for mediation of rolling on P-Selectin, as low expression levels or cleavage of CD24 resulted in inhibition of attachment and rolling, in a breast carcinoma cell line [6]. The precise mechanisms of ligand binding have still to be elucidated. In particular, CD24 does not contain the sulfated tyrosine residue of the P-Selectin glycoprotein ligand 1 (PSGL-1), i.e. another P-Selectin ligand [22]. Another mechanism of CD24 binding focuses on the observed association of CD24 with the sulfate-containing epitope HNK-1 which is also recognized by P-Selectin. This observation may lead to the assumption that HNK-1 mediates CD24 binding [7]. Enhanced disease progression as a result of metastatic spread with poorer survival rates may therefore be reasonable [6, 7]. As known, cells of hematogenously metastasizing tumours attach to platelets in the bloodstream [23–25]. Activated platelets express P-Selectin. Therefore, CD24-positive cells probably attach to activated platelets, containing P-Selectin on their surface, at the point, when the primary tumour invades into the vascular system [6]. Moreover, CD24-mediated tumor propagation has also been associated with an increase of local invasiveness: CD24 mediated invasion of cancer cells has been hypothesized as a result of increased contractile forces as indicated by the findings of A125 human lung cancer cells with different CD24 expression levels using CD24-high and CD24-low transfectants in three-dimensional extracellular matrix (ECM) invasion assays [19]. The percentage of invasive cells and their invasion depth was increased in CD24-high cells compared with CD24-low cells. Conversely,

knockdown of CD24 and of the ß1-integrin subunit in CD24-high cells decreased their invasiveness, indicating that the increased invasiveness is CD24- and ß1-integrin subunit-dependent [19]. Interestingly, besides acting as a ligand for P-Selectin, recently it has been proven that CD24 expression also indirectly stimulates cell adhesion to fibronectin, collagens 1 and 4, and laminin through activation of $\alpha3\beta1$ and $\alpha4\beta1$ integrin activity. Sleeman and colleagues have reported that $\beta1$ integrins colocalize focally with CD24. This suggests a direct interaction between CD24 and $\beta1$-containing integrins. In their study they show that CD24 interacts with c-scr, leading to stabilization of the kinase-active form of c-scr, which is necessary for sufficient activation of integrin adhesion to extracellular matrix components such as fibronectin. Thus, CD24 mediates cell adhesion in a P-Selectin dependent and a P-Selectin independent manner [26]. Next to its influence on cell adhesion, metastasis and on invasion, CD24 also serves as a mediator of proliferation. Apparently, a depletion of CD24 by siRNA leads to a significant decrease of cell numbers in several cell lines as well as to a reduction of their clonogenicity [17]. These experimental results provide a functionally well compatible explanation for the observed clinicopathological correlation of CD24 expression and poorer overall survival resp. increased occurrence of lymphonodular spread in our study.

Notably, CD24 may also provide a promising target for individualized therapy strategies beyond the scope of prediction. For example, CD24 specific antibodies have been applied in the treatment of the transplantation associated B-cell proliferative syndrome [18]. Moreover, mAb SWA11 has recently been shown to have a beneficial effect on anti-cancer treatment when used as addition to gemcitabine treatment in an A549 lung cancer model [20]. Pretreatment with mAb SWA11 led to a significant retardation of carcinoma growth compared to monotherapy with gemcitabine, which was attributed to faster internalisation of tumour antigen-bound therapeutic antibodies and alterations in the intratumoural cytokine milieu. Increased levels of intratumoural chemoattractants such as CXCL9/MIG and CCL2/MCP-1 were observed, in accordance to a heightened infiltration of xenografts by macrophages, possibly gained through the involvement of the antibody-dependent cell-mediated cytotoxicity. [20]

Some parts of our results, however, are conflicting with previous data, as we could not reproduce a significant correlation with patient survival for cytoplasmic expression of CD24 for SWA11. Vice versa, we revealed that only the membranous staining pattern was indicative for poorer overall survival ($p = 0.007$). As a minimal discordance to findings of former NSCLC studies [2, 3], our SWA11 based study could not confirm an especially relevant prognostic value of CD24 for pulmonary adeno-carcinomas. Still, this study demonstrates a small trend towards a subtype-dependent prognostic relevance of membranous CD24 expression. Larger cohorts will be necessary for a more substantial statistical power concerning its prognostic relevance for AC.

## Conclusions

In summary, our data provides further evidence for CD24 as a functionally relevant biomarker with prognostic significance in NSCLC. Methodically, our results underline the necessity to choose a specific antibody and to carefully consider subcellular staining differences of CD24 for robust prognostic conclusions. The use of mAb SWA11 should be favoured for a more specific detection of the cell surface protein CD24 as it allows a good visual distinction between membranous and cytoplasmic staining. A distinction between strongly and less strongly stained cells may be challenging in the light of laboratory-specific variations as well as inevitable inter-observer variability. Further studies should clarify, if an adjuvant therapeutic use of CD24 antibodies may have an additive value in cancer treatment.

**Abbreviations**
NSCLC: Non-small cell lung cancer; GPI: Glycosyl-phosphatidylinositol; PSA: Prostate-specific antigen; mAb: Monoclonal antibody; TMA: Tissue microarray; HE: Haematoxylin-eosin; AC: Adenocarcinomas; SC: Squamous cell carcinomas; LAP: Leucine-proline-alanine; PSGL-1: P-Selectin glycoprotein ligand 1; ECM: Extracellular matrix.

**Competing interests**
The authors declare that they have no competing interests.

**Authors' contributions**
MM, GK - conceived the study, analyzed the data, wrote and revised the manuscript, established follow up data.
AS - conducted the study, evaluated immunohistochemistry, analyzed the data, wrote and revised the manuscript, generation of tissue microarrays, established follow up data.
AF, JS, LH - provided tumor samples, read and revised the paper, established follow up data, generation of tissue microarrays.
PA - provided SWA11-antibody, analyzed the data, read and revised the manuscript.

**Acknowledgements**
We are greatly indebted to Susanne Steiner for excellent technical assistance.

**Author details**
[1]Institute of Pathology, University of Bonn, Sigmund-Freud-Str. 25, D-53127 Bonn, Germany. [2]New Pathology, Cologne, Germany. [3]Skin Cancer Unit, German Cancer Research Center (DKFZ), Heidelberg, Germany. [4]Department of Dermatology, Venereology and Allergology University Medical Center Mannheim, Ruprecht-Karl University of Heidelberg, Mannheim, Germany.

**References**
1. Siegel R, Naishadham D, Jemal A. Cancer statistics, 2013. CA Cancer J Clin. 2013;63(1):11–30.
2. Lee HJ, Choe G, Jheon S, Sung SW, Lee CT, Chung JH. CD24, a novel cancer biomarker, predicting disease-free survival of non-small cell lung carcinomas: a retrospective study of prognostic factor analysis from the viewpoint of forthcoming (seventh) new TNM classification. J Thorac Oncol. 2010;5(5):649–57.
3. Kristiansen G, Schluns K, Yongwei Y, Denkert C, Dietel M, Petersen I. CD24 is an independent prognostic marker of survival in nonsmall cell lung cancer patients. Br J Cancer. 2003;88(2):231–6.
4. Győrffy G, Surowiak S, Budczies B, Lanczky L. Online Survival Analysis Software to Asses the Prognostic Value of Biomarkers Using Transcriptomic Data in Non-Small-Cell Lung Cancer. PLOS One. 2013;18(8(12)):e82241.
5. Sammar M, Aigner S, Hubbe M, Schirrmacher V, Schachner M, Vestweber D, et al. Heat-stable antigen (CD24) as ligand for mouse P-selectin. Int Immunol. 1994;6(7):1027–36.
6. Aigner S, Ramos CL, Hafezi-Moghadam A, Lawrence MB, Friederichs J, Altevogt P, et al. CD24 mediates rolling of breast carcinoma cells on P-selectin. Faseb J. 1998;12(12):1241–51.
7. Aigner S, Sthoeger ZM, Fogel M, Weber E, Zarn J, Ruppert M, et al. CD24, a mucin-type glycoprotein, is a ligand for P-selectin on human tumor cells. Blood. 1997;89(9):3385–95.
8. Burgos-Ojeda D, Wu R, McLean K, Chen Y, Talpaz M, Yoon E, et al. CD24+ Ovarian Cancer Cells Are Enriched for Cancer-Initiating Cells and Dependent on JAK2 Signaling for Growth and Metastasis. Mol Cancer Ther. 2015;14(7):1717–27.
9. Rostoker R, Abelson S, Genkin I, Ben-Shmuel S, Sachidanandam R, Scheinman EJ, et al. CD24+ cells fuel rapid tumor growth and display high metastatic capacity. Breast Cancer Research. 2015;17:78.
10. Sterlacci MD, Savic S, Fiegl M, Obermann E, Tzankov A. Putative Stem Cell Markers in Non-Small-Cell-Lung Cancer A Clinicopathologic Characterization. J Thorac Oncol. 2014;9:41–9.
11. Stuelten CH, Mertins SD, Busch JI, Gowens M, Scudiero DA, Burkett MW, et al. Complex Display of Putative Tumor Stem Cell Markers in the NCI60 Tumor Cell Line Panel. Stem Cells. 2010;28:649–60.
12. Wang G, Zhang Z, Ren Y. TROP-1/Ep-CAM and CD24 are potential candidates for ovarian cancer therapy. Int J Clin Exp Pathol. 2015;8(5):4705–14.
13. Song SP, Zhang SB, Liu R, Yao L, Hao YQ, Liao MM, et al. NDRG2 down-regulation and CD24 up-regulation promote tumor aggravation and poor survival in patients with gallbladder carcinoma. Med Oncol. 2012;29(3):1879–85.
14. Kristiansen G, Machado E, Bretz N, Rupp C, Winzer KJ, Konig AK, et al. Molecular and clinical dissection of CD24 antibody specificity by a comprehensive comparative analysis. Lab Invest. 2010;90(7):1102–16.
15. Weber E, Lehmann HP, Beck-Sickinger AG, Wawrzynczak EJ, Waibel R, Folkers G, et al. Antibodies to the protein core of the small cell lung cancer workshop antigen cluster-w4 and to the leucocyte workshop antigen CD24 recognize the same short protein sequence leucine-alanine-proline. Clin Exp Immunol. 1993;93(2):279–85.
16. Kristiansen G, Denkert C, Schluns K, Dahl E, Pilarsky C, Hauptmann S. CD24 is expressed in ovarian cancer and is a new independent prognostic marker of patient survival. Am J Pathol. 2002;161(4):1215–21.
17. Smith SC, Oxford G, Wu Z. The Metastasis Associated Gene CD24 Is Regulated by Ral GTPase and Is Mediator of Cell Proliferation and Survival in Human Cancer. Cancer Research. 2006;66(4):1917–22.
18. Benkerrou M, Jais JP, Leblond V, Durandy A, Sutton L, Bordigoni P, et al. Anti-B-cell monoclonal antibody treatment of severe posttransplant B-lymphoproliferative disorder: prognostic factors and long-term outcome. Blood. 1998;92(9):3137–47.
19. Mierke CT, Bretz N, Altevogt P. Contractile forces contribute to increased glycosylphosphatidylinositol-anchored receptor CD24-facilitated cancer cell invasion. J Biol Chem. 2011;286(40):34858–71.
20. Salnikov AV, Bretz NP, Perne C, Hazin J, Keller S, Fogel M, et al. Antibody targeting of CD24 efficiently retards growth and influences cytokine milieu in experimental carcinomas. Br J Cancer. 2013;108(7):1449–59.
21. Bretz N, Salnikov A, Perne C, Keller S, Wang X, Mierke C, et al. CD24 controls Src/STAT3 activity in human tumors. Cell Mol Life Sci. 2012;69(22):3863–79.
22. Needham LK, Schnaar RL. The HNK-1 reactive sulfoglucuronyl glycolipids are ligand for L-selectin and P-selectin. Proc Natl Acad Sci USA. 1993;90:1359.
23. Gasic GJ. Role of plasma, platelets, and endothelial cells in tumour metastasis. Cancer Metastasis Rev. 1984;3:99–144.
24. Grigani G, Pacchiarini L, Pagliarino M. The possible role of blood platelets in tumour growth and dissemination. Haematologica. 1986;71:245–55.
25. Honn KV, Tang DG, Crissman JD. Platelets and cancer metastasis-a causal relationship. Cancer Metastasis Rev. 1992;11:325–251.
26. Sleeman JP, Baumann P, Cremers N, Kroese F, Gertraud O, Chiquet-Ehrismann R, et al. CD24 Expression Causes the Aquisition of Multiple Cellular Properties Associated with Tumor Growth and Metastasis. Cancer Research 2005. 2005;65(23):10783–93.

# Comparison of targeted next-generation sequencing and Sanger sequencing for the detection of *PIK3CA* mutations in breast cancer

Ruza Arsenic*, Denise Treue, Annika Lehmann, Michael Hummel, Manfred Dietel, Carsten Denkert and Jan Budczies

## Abstract

**Background:** Phosphatidylinositol-4,5-bisphosphate 3-kinase, catalytic subunit alpha, *PIK3CA*, is one of the most frequently mutated genes in breast cancer, and the mutation status of *PIK3CA* has clinical relevance related to response to therapy.
The aim of our study was to investigate the mutation status of PIK3CA gene and to evaluate the concordance between NGS and SGS for the most important hotspot regions in exon 9 and 20, to investigate additional hotspots outside of these exons using NGS, and to correlate the *PIK3CA* mutation status with the clinicopathological characteristics of the cohort.

**Methods:** In the current study, next-generation sequencing (NGS) and Sanger Sequencing (SGS) was used for the mutational analysis of *PIK3CA* in 186 breast carcinomas.

**Results:** Altogether, 64 tumors had *PIK3CA* mutations, 55 of these mutations occurred in exons 9 and 20. Out of these 55 mutations, 52 could also be detected by Sanger sequencing resulting in a concordance of 98.4 % between the two sequencing methods. The three mutations missed by SGS had low variant frequencies below 10 %. Additionally, 4.8 % of the tumors had mutations in exons 1, 4, 7, and 13 of *PIK3CA* that were not detected by SGS. *PIK3CA* mutation status was significantly associated with hormone receptor-positivity, HER2-negativity, tumor grade, and lymph node involvement. However, there was no statistically significant association between the *PIK3CA* mutation status and overall survival.

**Conclusions:** Based on our study, NGS is recommended as follows: 1) for correctly assessing the mutation status of *PIK3CA* in breast cancer, especially for cases with low tumor content, 2) for the detection of subclonal mutations, and 3) for simultaneous mutation detection in multiple exons.

**Keywords:** Next-generation sequencing, Breast cancer, Sanger sequencing, *PIK3CA*

## Background

Historically, Sanger sequencing (SGS) has been the gold standard for detecting DNA mutations. However, SGS has limitations due to its restricted sensitivity and its inability to perform parallel investigation of multiple targets. Furthermore, somatic cancer mutations can be difficult to detect using SGS without performing micro-dissections because tumors are heterogeneous and often mixed with normal tissue. Recent progress in massive parallel sequencing, termed next-generation sequencing (NGS), has increased the speed and efficiency of mutation testing in molecular pathology [1–9]. NGS allows for the detection of a broad spectrum of mutations, including single nucleotide substitutions, small insertions and deletions, large genomic duplications and deletions, and rare variations [9].

Targeted NGS, which involves the targeted enrichment of a set of DNA regions, is used for the parallel sequencing of amplicons derived from multiplex polymerase chain reaction (PCR) or other amplicon-based

* Correspondence: ruza.arsenic@charite.de
Institute of Pathology, Charité University Hospital Berlin, Berlin, Germany

enrichment approaches, such as hybridization capture. When the amplicon size is kept small (e.g., <175 bp) in the design of the sequencing panel, NGS is also applicable to formalin-fixed tissue samples. Moreover, targeted NGS is more cost efficient than SGS [10]. This high-throughput technology is currently used with several platforms, including the Genome Analyzer/HiSeq/MiSeq (Illumina Solexa), the SOLiD System (Thermo Fisher Scientific), the Ion PGM/Ion Proton (Thermo Fisher Scientific), and the HeliScope Sequencer (Helicos BioSciences) [11, 12].

NGS can be used to detect both somatic and germline mutations in the cancer genome. The somatic genetic changes can be classified as either driver or passenger mutations. The former contribute to tumor development [13, 14], while the latter do not directly contribute to tumor development and may be the product of genomic instability within the tumor. Although SGS and PCR are routinely used to identify clinically relevant mutations and select the best treatment for patients, these techniques are insensitive to changes occurring at an allele frequency lower than 20 %, apart from real-time PCR, which could reach higher sensitivity [15, 16].

However, the more sensitive and cost-effective multiplex NGS testing platforms provide comprehensive genomic information, and thus allow for the implementation of targeted therapies and improved treatment decisions [17]. TP53 and PIK3CA are the most frequently mutated genes in breast cancer (BC), both being mutated in about one-third of all primary breast carcinomas [18, 19]. In recent years, several studies identified the clinical relevance of PIK3CA mutations in terms of decreasing the benefits of anti-HER2 therapies and poly-chemotherapies in patients with PIK3CA mutations [20–22] . In the present study, we investigated the PIK3CA status of 186 primary BC patients from the Berlin area using targeted NGS and SGS. Recent studies have analyzed mutations in hot spots (i.e., exon 9 and 20) and only a few studies have analyzed mutations in other exons [23] Consequently, our aims were to evaluate the concordance between NGS and SGS for the most important hotspot regions in exon 9 and 20, to investigate additional hotspots outside of these exons using NGS, and to correlate the PIK3CA mutation status with the clinicopathological characteristics of the cohort.

# Methods

### Patient cohort and histopathological evaluation

Tissue samples were collected from 186 patients with a diagnosis of primary BC at the Department of Pathology, University Hospital Charité and the Breast Cancer Center at the DRK Klinikum Koepenick in Berlin, Germany. The median follow-up time was 38 months. Data on tumor histology and tumor grade were evaluated at the time of primary diagnosis and extracted from pathology reports. Tumors were graded according to the Bloom-Richardson

grading system modified by Elston and Ellis [24]. HER2 status was determined by immunohistochemistry (IHC) using the Dako HercepTest kit (Dako, Carpinteria, CA, USA). Chromatic in situ hybridization (CISH) was also performed on samples with a HER2 score of 2+. The estrogen receptor (ER) monoclonal antibody clone SP1 (NeoMarkers, Fremont, CA, USA) was used to identify the ER status, and the progesterone receptor (PR) status was determined with the PR monoclonal antibody PgR 636 (Dako, Wiesentheid, Germany). Only nuclear labeling was scored as positive. Negative ER and PR status was defined as positivity in <1 % of tumor cells according to ASCO/CAP guidelines [25]. HER2 negativity (HER2-) was defined as the absence of membranous staining or weak, discontinuous membranous staining. Cases with moderate membranous staining in >10 % of the tumor cells were examined by CISH according to ASCO/CAP guidelines [26]. A proliferation index was not available for all samples. Representative tumor samples containing at least 30 % tumor cells were selected for molecular studies.

### Sample cohort and clinical parameters

Median patient age at the time of diagnosis was 65 years, with a range of 34–95 years.

A total of 149 patients (80.1 %) had ductal carcinoma and 20 (10.7 %) had lobular carcinoma. Seventeen patients (9.1 %) had carcinoma of another histological type, such as mucinous ductal carcinoma with squamous differentiation, mixed-ductal and lobular carcinoma, medullary carcinoma, or invasive papillary adenocarcinoma. None of the patients received any medical treatment related to BC before surgery. After diagnosis, most (93 %) of the hormone receptor-positive (HR+) cases were administered hormonal therapy alone or in combination with other therapies according to relevant guidelines.

### Ethics approval

Patients provided written informed consent for use of their biomaterial samples in biomarker studies. Consent was obtained using the standardized informed consent forms of the participating institutions. The project and consent process was approved by the ethics board of the Charité Hospital, Berlin (reference number EA1/139/05, last amendment 2013).

### DNA extraction, PCR, and PIK3CA semiconductor next-generation sequencing

Briefly, 10 consecutive 10-µm thick sections were prepared. The first section was stained with hematoxylin/eosin and the tumor area was marked by a pathologist. The corresponding area was manually microdissected from each of the consecutive unstained sections and transferred to 180 µl of lysis buffer (QIAamp® DNA Mini

Comparison of targeted next-generation sequencing and Sanger sequencing for the detection...

83

Kit, Qiagen, Venlo, Niederlande) for 10 min at 95 °C. Enzymatic lysis was carried out with 20 μl of Proteinase K for 1 h at 56 °C. Subsequent DNA preparation was performed according to the manufacturer's instructions, and the DNA was eluted in 80 μl of elution buffer. Total nucleic acid concentrations were measured with a Qubit fluorometer HS DNA Assay (Life Technologies, Carlsbad, CA, USA) and a TaqMan RNase P Detection Reagents Kit (Life Technologies). Ten nanograms of genomic DNA were utilized for the library preparation. The final library was quantified using an Ion AmpliSeq Library Kit 2.0 (Life Technologies). The samples were 8-fold multiplexed and amplified on Ion Spheres Particles using the Ion One-Touch™ 200 Template Kit v2 DL (Life Technologies). After library enrichment and quality control on a Qubit instrument (Ion Sphere Quality Control Kit, Life Technologies), the samples were sequenced using the Ion 318 chip v2 according to the standard protocol of the chip manufacturer.

A customized sequencing panel consisting of 154 amplicons from 48 genes was designed using the Ion AmpliSeq Designer to cover the most frequent somatic mutations found in BC. The panel included six amplicons located in *PIK3CA* exons 1, 4, 7, 9, 13, and 20. The genomic positions and primer sequences can be found in the well plate data sheet generated by the Ion AmpliSeq Designer (Additional file 1: Table S1). Only samples with at least 30 % tumor cells within the dissected area were included in the study.

Base calling and alignment to the human genome (hg19) were executed with the Torrent Suite Software 4.0.3. The mean coverages (minimum – maximum) of the amplicons were 4128 bp (1315–22668 bp) for exon 1, 5237 bp (1962–25371 bp) for exon 4, 2044 bp (347–12066 bp) for exon 7, 3588 bp (278–20808 bp) for exon 9, 3742 bp (1386–20063 bp) for exon 13, and 1552 bp (438–9901 bp) for exon 20. Variant calling was executed using the Torrent Variant Caller 4.2 and the low stringency somatic variant calling protocol. Only non-synonymous nucleotide exchanges were considered for the analysis of single nucleotide polymorphisms.

### Sanger sequencing primers and sequencing parameters

Primers were designed using the Primer Design Tool from NCBI. The primers were as follows:

exon 9 forward 5′-
GGGAAAAATATGACAAAGAAAGC-3′,
exon 9 reverse 5′-GAGATCAGCCAAATTCAGTT-3′,
exon 20 part 1 forward 5′-
CATTTGCTCCAAACTGACCA-3′,
exon 20 part 1 reverse 5′-
TgTgCATCATTCATTTgTTTCA-3′,

exon 20 part 2 forward 5′-
TTGATGACATTGCATACATTCG-3′,
and exon 20 part 2 reverse 5′-
GGTCTTTGCCTGCTGAGAGT-3′.

The sequencing reactions were loaded on the 3730xl DNA Analyzer from Hitachi (Applied Biosystems). Sequence traces from tumor DNA samples were aligned to the genomic reference sequence and analyzed using Seq-Pilot software (Applied Biosystems).

### Statistical evaluation

Statistical analyses were conducted using the SPSS 19 statistical software (SPSS Inc., Chicago, IL, USA) and the statistical language R (Foundation for Statistical Computing, Vienna, Austria). Significance of associations between *PIK3CA* status and age, ER/PR status, tumor stage, and histological grade were assessed using a Fisher's exact test, a chi-squared test, and a chi-squared test for trends. Overall survival was analyzed using the Kaplan-Meier method and the log-rank test. All tests were two-tailed, and results were considered significant when $p < 0.05$. Barplots and beeswarm plots were produced using the R package graphics and beeswarm [27, 28].

### Results

#### Prevalence of different types of *PIK3CA* mutations using NGS

Using NGS to sequence the *PIK3CA* gene in each of the 186 tissue samples identified a total of 64 tumors with exon mutations (34.4 %), which agreed with the 36 % *PIK3CA* mutation rate in BC reported by the Cancer Genome Atlas (TCGA) [18, 19]. As shown in Fig. 1, the mutations were distributed as follows: exon 20 (34 cases; 18.3 %), exon 9 (19 cases; 10.2 %), and other exons (1, 4, 7, or 13) (9 cases; 4.8 %). In very few samples (2 cases; 1.1 %), we found mutations in two exons. The majority of mutations were base pair substitutions (60 cases, 93.8 %). Additionally, we detected deletions (4 cases, 6.3 %). Sixty of the tumors (93.7 %) had a single mutation in the *PIK3CA* gene, while three tumors had two mutations in the *PIK3CA* gene. The most frequent mutations were p.H1047R (31 cases, 48.4 %), p.E545K (11 cases, 17.2 %), and p.E542K (6 cases, 9.4 %) (Table 1).

Three mutations, p.N347T, p.G451_D454del, and p.L456V, were not described in any of the studies reported in COSMIC (http://cancer.sanger.ac.uk/cancergenome/projects/cosmic), TCGA [18, 19], or any other large genomic database [29, 30]. Thus, they are being described for the first time in our study. Additionally, a single nucleotide polymorphism (rs3729674) (NC_000003.11:g.178917005A > G) was found in 33 cases. Out of a total of 55 mutations in exons 9 and 20 that were detected using NGS, 49 were also detected by SGS. By resequencing

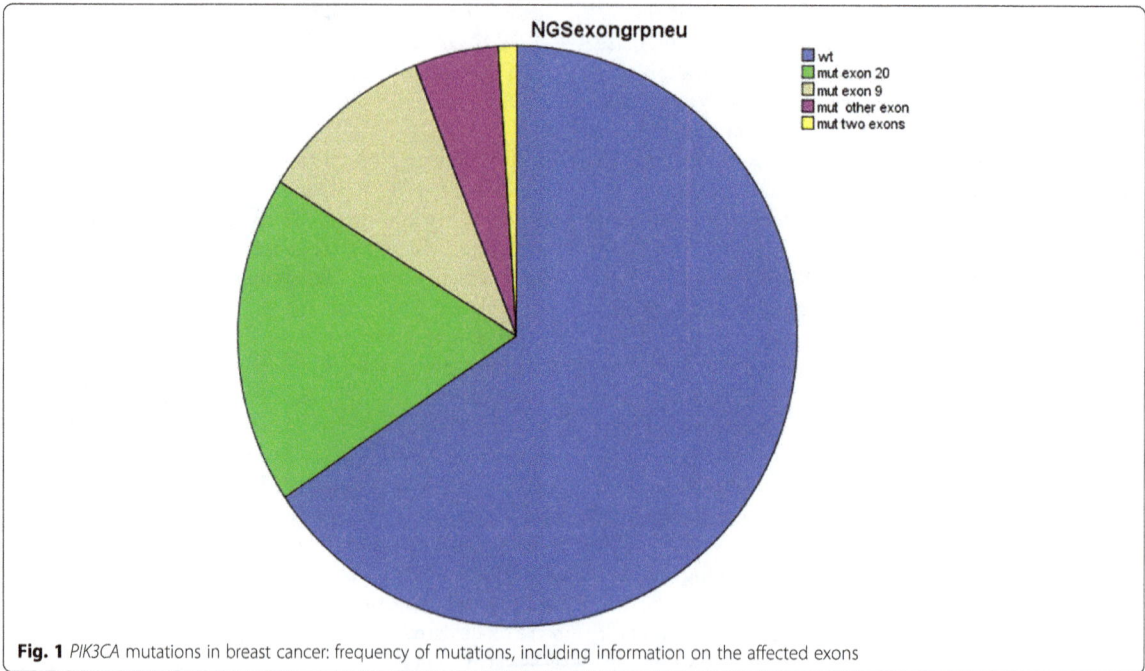

**Fig. 1** *PIK3CA* mutations in breast cancer: frequency of mutations, including information on the affected exons

discrepant cases using SGS, we found an additional three cases with mutations with small peak heights that could be detected by analyzing the electropherograms manually. A comparison of the NGS and SGS results is shown in Fig. 2. The three mutations in exon 9 and exon 20 that were missed by SGS had low variant frequencies of 4 % (twice) and 7 %.

### PIK3CA mutations and clinical characteristics

*PIK3CA* mutations were analyzed for correlation with several clinicopathological parameters at the time of the diagnosis: age, tumor size, tumor grade, nodal status, HR status, HER2 expression, and histological subtype (Table 2). *PIK3CA* mutations were most frequently found in HR+, HER2- ($p = 0.002$), and well-differentiated (G1; $p < 0.001$) cases (Fig. 3a and b). Furthermore, there was a statistically significant difference between cases with

different nodal statuses; there were more cases with *PIK3CA* mutations in the N1 group ($p = 0.042$). We found no statistically significant correlation between mutation status and age, tumor size, or histological tumor type.

When we compared mutations in the other exons (1, 4, 7, and 13) with the clinicopathological parameters, we found a trend toward enrichment of the mutations in lower grade tumors, but this trend did not reach statistical significance ($p = 0.104$). There was no statistically significant difference between *PIK3CA* mutation status in these other exons and cases that were HR+, HR-, HER2+, or HER2-. Also, we could not detect differences in nodal status, tumor size, or age.

An overall survival analysis was performed on 184 patients with available follow-up data. In this group, no statistically significant association was found between long-term survival and the *PIK3CA* mutation status

**Table 1** Hotspots of *PIK3CA* mutations in breast cancer

| Exon | Mutation | Number | Frequency (%) | Total number |
|------|----------|--------|---------------|--------------|
| 1 | R108del, R109del | 1, 2 | 1.6, 3.1 | 3 |
| 4 | N345K, N347T (new), D350N | 3,1,1 | 4.7, 1.6, 1.6 | 5 |
| 7 | G451_D454del (new), p.L456V (new) | 1,1 | 1.6, 1.6 | 2 |
| 9 | E542K, E545K, Q546K, Q546R | 6, 11, 1, 1 | 9.4, 17.2 | 19 |
| 13 | E726K | 2 | 3,1 | 2 |
| 20 | D1029H, N1044K, H1047L, H1047R, G1049R | 1, 1, 3, 31, 1 | 1.6, 1.6, 48.4, 4.7, 1.6 | 37 |
| | | total: 68 | | |

Using semiconductor NGS, we identified a total of 68 non-silent mutations in 186 breast cancer samples (34.4 %). The most frequent aberrations were p.H1047R, p.E545K, and p.E542K

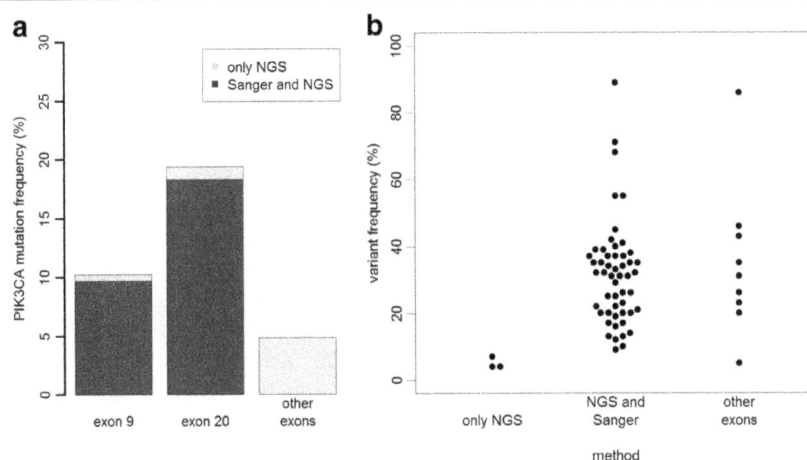

**Fig. 2** Detection sensitivity of semiconductor NGS compared to Sanger sequencing. **a** Barplot showing the number of mutations detected by both Sanger sequencing and NGS and the mutations detected only by NGS. **b** Beeswarm plot showing the variant frequencies of the mutations detected only by NGS and those detected by both methods

(Fig. 4a). There was also no difference in overall survival related to the mutational status of different *PIK3CA* exons (Fig. 4b).

## Discussion

The precise identification of genomic alterations is crucial for personalized cancer therapy. Molecular testing for mutations in cancer susceptibility genes is mainly performed using SGS of individual exons after PCR. The detection threshold of SGS requires an allele frequency of approximately 20 % [31], but BC tissue is heterogeneous, consisting of tumor, stromal, and inflammatory cells, leading to a varying proportion of tumor cells ranging from 20-95 % [32]. Therefore, we speculated that a significant proportion of *PIK3CA* mutations are missed by SGS. There are studies available from other organ systems, including the lung, which report a higher detection rate of mutations using NGS rather than SGS [33, 34]. In general, the detection sensitivity of NGS reported in previous studies ranges from 94–99.9 % [35–39], which is above the sensitivity of Sanger Sequencing. Accordingly, the aim of the present study was to use NGS for the analysis of *PIK3CA* mutations to determine whether additional changes could be identified that might lead to better correlation of the clinicopathological characteristics of breast tumors with *PIK3CA* mutations. We also sought to evaluate the prognostic significance of *PIK3CA* mutation status as previously reported by several authors [40–44]. To this end, we compared the performance of NGS and SGS in the same cohort of patients, and identified *PIK3CA* mutations in 34.4 % of breast tumors using NGS, which is in agreement with the mutation rate reported in TCGA [45].

Overall, we were able to report a good degree of concordance between the two sequencing methods. Only three mutations that were detected by NGS could not be found by SGS due to low variant frequencies below 10 %. Nevertheless, this finding indicates that NGS is more sensitive than SGS, particularly for the detection of low frequency mutations. This has also been reported in previous studies. Rohlin et al. [46] showed that Sanger-based sequencing techniques have problems picking out "minority" gene sequences (mutations below 15 %). Meanwhile, Walsch et al. performed a study on 300 high-risk BC families that screened for mutations in hotspots, and found previously undetected changes in 52 probands [47]. These results clearly support the use of targeted sequencing because it is more sensitive than SGS when it comes to identifying low frequency mutations. Our study, which is the first to compare NGS and SGS for sequencing the *PIK3CA* gene in BC, adds support for this viewpoint. Additionally, the results of our study showed that ~5 % of the mutations were in other exons, and the best and most cost-effective method for detecting these mutations was to use parallel sequencing or targeted NGS. Due to the low mutation rate in these other exons (1, 4, 7, and 13) and a lack of statistical significance when correlated with clinicopathological data, we abstained from validating these mutations by SGS. The clinical relevance of *PIK3CA* mutations outside exon 9 and 20 should be further investigated in future studies.

The *PIK3CA* mutations detected by NGS in our study clustered in two previously reported "hotspot" regions in exons 9 and 20, with most of the mutations clustering in exon 20, which is in agreement with the SGS results reported in our previous study [48]. The consequences of

**Table 2** Correlation of *PIK3CA* mutation status with the clinicopathological characteristics of breast cancer

| Clinicopathological parameters | Mutated (%) | Wild type (%) | P |
|---|---|---|---|
| All Tumor Cases | 64 (34.4) | 122 (65.6) | NS |
| Histological Type | | | NS |
| Ductal/Other Carcinoma | 53 (32.5) | 110 (67.5) | |
| Lobular Carcinoma | 11 (47.8) | 12 (52.2) | |
| Tumor Stage | | | NS |
| T1 | 13 (30.2) | 28 (65.1) | |
| T2 | 37 (34.9) | 69 (65.1) | |
| T3 | 9 (42.9) | 12 (57.1) | |
| T4 | 5 (41.7) | 7 (58.3) | |
| Node Status | | | 0.042 |
| N0 | 25 (27.8) | 65 (72.2) | |
| N+ | 37 (42.5) | 50 (57.5) | |
| Tumor Grade | | | <0.001 |
| G1 | 16 (80.0) | 4 (20.0) | |
| G2 | 35 (36.5) | 61 (63.5) | |
| G3 | 13 (18.8) | 56 (81.2) | |
| Hormone Receptor Status | | | 0.002 |
| HR+ | 58 (40.3) | 86 (59.7) | |
| HR- | 6 (14.3) | 36 (85.7) | |
| HER2 Status | | | 0.032 |
| HER2+ | 3 (13.6) | 19 (86.4) | |
| HER2- | 61 (37.2) | 103 (62.8) | |
| Age | | | NS |
| <50 years | 6 (26.1) | 17 (73.9) | |
| >50 years | 58 (35.6) | 105 (64.4) | |
| Molecular Type | | | 0.003 |
| HR+/HER2- | 57 (42.5) | 77 (57.5) | |
| HR+/HER2+ | 1 (10.0) | 9 (90.0) | |
| HR-/HER2+ | 2 (16.7) | 10 (83.3) | |
| HR-/HER2- | 4 (13.3) | 26 (86.7) | |

The mutation frequency, as determined by NGS, decreased with increasing tumor grade: 85 % for G1, 37 % for G2, and 20 % for G3. *PIK3CA* mutations were more frequently detected (42 %) in HR+ breast cancer than in HR- breast cancer (14 %). *PIK3CA* mutations were more frequently detected in HER2- breast cancer (38 %) than in HER2+ breast cancer (14 %)

each mutation on the function and regulation of *PIK3CA* requires further consideration. The three novel mutation detected in our study are located in the C2 domain of the PIK3CA gene. The C2 is often involved in phospholipid membrane binding, consequently it is possible that these mutations lead to increased membrane binding, as extensively discussed in the study by Ikenoue at al. [49]. In the study by Gymnopoulos at al, the authors showed that the mutants in C2 domain increase basic positive surface charge of that domain and may therefore mediate improved recruitment of p110α to the cell membrane,

making lipid kinase activity independent of signals transmitted through the regulatory subunit, p85 [50]. One of these three mutations, p.L456V is predicted to be probably damaging with a score of 0.988 (sensitivity: 0.27; specificity: 0.99) when analyzed with polyPhen-2 prediction programe.

The goal of our previous study was to analyse only exon 9 and 20 mutations, hence we could not detect these three mutations in this study.

We also noted the presence of multiple mutations in four cases, which has not been reported previously. The significance of these double mutants is unknown, but it is possible that these tumors are multiclonal, and a second hit was required to provide a selective growth advantage if the first mutation was a less potent activator of the kinase.

We found that *PIK3CA* was most frequently mutated in cases that were HR+ and HER2-, which agrees with previously published data [51, 52]. We found significantly more *PIK3CA* mutations in G1 tumors suggesting that theses mutations occur early in BC development, which has also been shown in other studies [53]. Additionally, *PIK3CA* mutations were highly correlated with lymph node status (N+), which is one of the clinical markers associated with patient survival and response to therapy [54, 55]. The finding that *PIK3CA* mutations are more commonly found in HR+ tumors may point to differences in pathogenesis and disease progression between HR+ and HR- tumors. Furthermore, the correlation between *PIK3CA* mutations and lymph node metastasis suggests that activation of the PI3K/Akt pathway may increase the invasion of cancer cells into the lymph nodes. This is supported by the fact that PIP3 regulates cell mobility [56].

There is controversy regarding the prognostic significance of *PIK3CA* mutations. Cizkova et al. [57] described more favorable metastasis-free survival in patients with *PIK3CA* mutations, but Jensen et al. [22] and Baselga et al. [58] reported reduced survival rates and worse outcomes. The largest published study evaluated the *PIK3CA* genotype in 687 tumor samples from patients enrolled in a prospective phase III clinical trial. Those with *PIK3CA* mutations had a better prognosis for the first three years compared to those carrying wild type *PIK3CA* alleles, but this difference disappeared with a longer follow-up [59,60]. In our study, there was no significant association between *PIK3CA* mutational status and overall survival, indicating that an activated *PIK3CA* pathway alone is not a prognostic factor for BC.

An interesting finding by Fu at al. showed that *PIK3CA*-activating mutations are associated with better outcomes in ER+ patients receiving endocrine therapy [61]. This agrees with the observation that *PIK3CA* mutations are more frequent in luminal A tumors compared

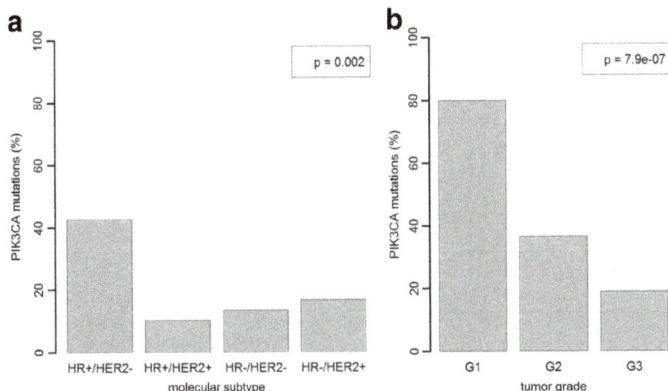

**Fig. 3** Strong association of *PIK3CA* status with molecular subtype and tumor grade in breast cancer. **a** *PIK3CA* mutations were more frequent in HR+/HER2- breast cancer (40 %) compared with the other subtypes (11 %-20 %). **b** The mutation frequency decreased with increasing tumor grade: 80 % in G1, 36 % in G2, and 19 % in G3

with luminal B tumors (e.g., 45 % vs. 29 % in the TCGA cohort) [45]. In contrast, in HER2+ BC, several reports show that *PIK3CA* mutations predict adverse outcomes after treatment with trastuzumab [20, 21]. As such, the impact of *PIK3CA* mutations on the clinical outcome of BC seems to vary with the background of other genomic alterations such as HER2 status.

*PIK3CA* mutations also appear to have a significant interest in the prediction of response to targeted therapies, as many drugs specifically targeting PI3K or other effectors of the PI3K/AKT pathway are intended to be administered only to patients with tumor bearing a mutation of *PIK3CA*, which makes the somatic mutations detection more and more important [62].

In summary, our results show that NGS is more sensitive than SGS for detecting *PIK3CA* mutations in BC samples, and that *PIK3CA* mutations are significantly related to HR and HER2 expression status and tumor grade. Further studies are needed to systematically explore the functional relevance of *PIK3CA* mutations and the contribution of PIK3CA mediated activation of the downstream and upstream signaling pathways in breast tumor development and progression.

## Conclusions

1. This is the first paper in which NGS and SGS were compared sequencing PIK3CA gene in breast cancer.

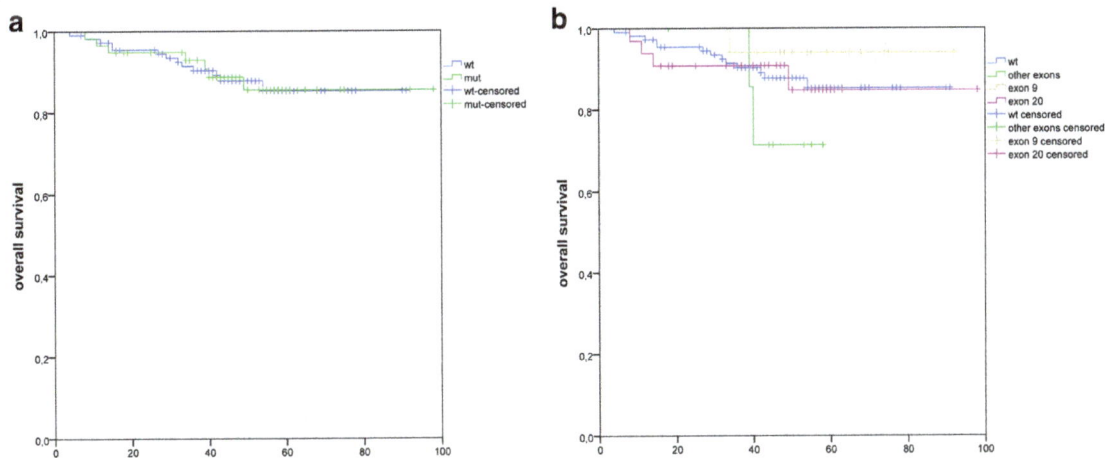

**Fig. 4** Correlation of overall survival with the *PIK3CA* mutation status in breast cancer. **a** Kaplan-Meier analysis comparing patients with mutated *PIK3CA* (green line) and wild type *PIK3CA* (blue line) did not reveal a statistically significant difference in survival. **b** Kaplan-Meier analysis of the *PIK3CA* mutation status stratified for the affected exon did not reveal a statistically significant difference in survival, but there was a trend toward better survival for the cases with a mutation in exon 9. Exon 9 mutation ($p = 0.39$) vs. exon 20 mutation ($p = 0.41$) vs. other exon mutations ($p = 0.16$)

2. We found overall a good concordance between the two methods (98,4 %), but better sensitivity of NGS when it comes to identifying low frequency mutations(<10 %).

3. *PIK3CA* mutation status in breast cancer correlated strongly with HR+ and HER2-, and N1 + .

## Additional file

**Additional file 1: Table S1.** Genomic positions and the primer sequences. (XLS 45 kb)

**Competing interests**
The authors declare that they have no competing interests.

**Authors' contributions**
Each of the authors contributed to the manuscript. AR and JB wrote the manuscript and performed the analysis. JB performed the statistics. AL, DT, MH, CD and MD corrected the manuscript. All authors are responsible for the overall content of the manuscript. All authors read and approved the final manuscript.

**Acknowledgments**
We would like to thank Ines Koch for the excellent technical assistance.

## References

1. Chan M, Ji SM, Yeo ZH, Gan L, Yap E, Yap, YS et al. Development of a next-generation sequencing method for BRCA mutation screening a comparison between a high-throughput and a benchtop platform. J Mol Diagn. 2012; 14(6):602–12.

2. Chou LS, Liu CS-J, Boese B, Zhan X, Mao R. DNA Sequence Capture and Enrichment by Microarray Followed by Next-Generation Sequencing for Targeted Resequencing: Neurofibromatosis Type 1 Gene as a Model. Clin Chem. 2010;56(1):62–72.

3. De Leeneer, KHellemans J, De Schrivjer J, Baetens M, Poppe B., Van Criekinge W, et al. Massive parallel amplicon sequencing of the breast cancer genes BRCA1 and BRCA2: opportunities, challenges, and limitations. Hum Mutat. 2011;32(3):335–44.

4. Goossens D, Moens LN, Nelis E, Lenaerts AS, Glassee W, Kalbe A, et al. Simultaneous mutation and copy number variation (CNV) detection by multiplex PCR-based GS-FLX sequencing. Hum Mutat. 2009;30(3):472–6.

5. Hernan I, Borràs E, de Sousa Dias M, Gamundi MJ, Mañé B, Llort G, et al. Detection of genomic variations in BRCA1 and BRCA2 genes by long-range PCR and next-generation sequencing. J Mol Diagn. 2012;14(3):286–93.

6. Mamanova L, Coffey AJ, Scott CE, Kozarewa I, Turner EH, Kumar A, et al. Target-enrichment strategies for next-generation sequencing. Nat Methods. 2010;7(2):111–8.

7. Ozcelik H, Shi X, Chang MC, Tram E, Vlasschaert M, Di Nicola N, et al. Long-range PCR and next-generation sequencing of BRCA1 and BRCA2 in breast cancer. J Mol Diagn. 2012;14(5):467–75.

8. Pritchard CC, Smith C, Salipante SJ, Lee MK, Thornton AM, Nord AS, et al. ColoSeq provides comprehensive lynch and polyposis syndrome mutational analysis using massively parallel sequencing. J Mol Diagn. 2012;14(4):357–66.

9. Walsh T, Lee MK, Casadei S, Thornton AM, Stray SM, Pennil C, et al. Detection of inherited mutations for breast and ovarian cancer using genomic capture and massively parallel sequencing. Proc Natl Acad Sci U S A. 2010;107(28):12629–33.

10. Walsh T, Casadei S, Lee MK, Pennil CC, Nord AS, Thornton AM, et al. Mutations in 12 genes for inherited ovarian, fallopian tube, and peritoneal carcinoma identified by massively parallel sequencing. Proc Natl Acad Sci U S A. 2011;108(44):18032–7.

11. Rothberg JM, Hinz W, Rearick TM, Schultz J, Mileski W, Davey M, et al. An integrated semiconductor device enabling non-optical genome sequencing. Nature. 2011;475(7356):348–52.

12. Voelkerding KV, Dames SA, Durtschi JD. Next-generation sequencing: from basic research to diagnostics. Clin Chem. 2009;55(4):641–58.

13. Hanahan D, Weinberg RA. The hallmarks of cancer. Cell. 2000;100(1):57–70.

14. Hanahan D, Weinberg RA. Hallmarks of cancer: the next generation. Cell. 2011;144(5):646–74.

15. MacConaill LE. Existing and emerging technologies for tumor genomic profiling. J Clin Oncol. 2013;31(15):1815–24.

16. Bustin SA. Absolute quantification of mRNA using real-time reverse transcription polymerase chain reaction assays. J Mol Endocrinol. 2000;25(2):169–93.

17. Meyerson M, Gabriel S, Getz G. Advances in understanding cancer genomes through second-generation sequencing. Nat Rev Genet. 2010; 11(10):685–96.

18. Forbes SA, Bindal N, Bamford S, Cole C, Kok CY, Beare D, et al. COSMIC: mining complete cancer genomes in the Catalogue of Somatic Mutations in Cancer. Nucleic Acids Res. 2011;39(Database issue):D945–50.

19. Robbins DE, Grüneberg A, Deus HF, Tanik MM, Almeida SJ. A self-updating road map of The Cancer Genome Atlas. Bioinformatics. 2013;29(10):1333–40.

20. Chandarlapaty S, Sakr RA, Giri D, Patil S, Heguy A, Morrow M, et al. Frequent mutational activation of the PI3K-AKT pathway in trastuzumab-resistant breast cancer. Clin Cancer Res. 2012;18(24):6784–91.

21. Cizkova M, Cizkova M, Dujaric ME, Lehmann-Che J, Scott V, Tembo O, et al. Outcome impact of *PIK3CA* mutations in HER2-positive breast cancer patients treated with trastuzumab. Br J Cancer. 2013;108(9):1807–9.

22. Jensen JD, Knoop A, Laenkholm AV, Grauslund M, Jensen MB, Santoni-Rugiu E, et al. *PIK3CA* mutations, PTEN, and pHER2 expression and impact on outcome in HER2-positive early-stage breast cancer patients treated with adjuvant chemotherapy and trastuzumab. Ann Oncol. 2012;23(8):2034–42.

23. Bai X, Zhang E, Ye H, Nandakumar V, Wang Z, Chen L, et al. PIK3CA and TP53 gene mutations in human breast cancer tumors frequently detected by ion torrent DNA sequencing. PLoS One. 2014;9(6):e99306.

24. Frierson Jr HF, Wolber RA, Berean KW, Franquemont DW, Gaffey MJ, Boyd JC, et al. Interobserver reproducibility of the Nottingham modification of the Bloom and Richardson histologic grading scheme for infiltrating ductal carcinoma. Am J Clin Pathol. 1995;103(2):195–8.

25. Hammond ME, Hayes DF, Dowsett M, Allred DC, Hagerty KL, Badve S, et al. American Society of Clinical Oncology/College of American Pathologists guideline recommendations for immunohistochemical testing of estrogen and progesterone receptors in breast cancer. Arch Pathol Lab Med. 2010; 134(6):907–22.

26. Wolff AC, Hammond ME, Hicks DG, Dowsett M, McShane LM, Allison KH, et al. Recommendations for human epidermal growth factor receptor 2 testing in breast cancer: American Society of Clinical Oncology/College of American Pathologists clinical practice guideline update. Arch Pathol Lab Med. 2014;138(2):241–56.

27. A.E. beeswarm: The bee swarm plot, an alternative to stripchart. R package version 0.1.6. 2013. http://CRAN.R-project.org/package=beeswarm.

28. R.C.T. R: A language and environment for statistical computing. R Foundation for Statistical Computing, Vienna, Austria. 2014. URL http://www.R-project.org/.

29. Cerami E, Gao J, Dogrusoz U, Gross BE, Sumer SO, Aksoy BA, et al. The cBio cancer genomics portal: an open platform for exploring multidimensional cancer genomics data. Cancer Discov. 2012;2(5):401–4.

30. Fokkema IF, Taschner PE, Schaafsma GC, Celli J, Laros JF, den Dunnen JT, et al. LOVD v. 2.0: the next generation in gene variant databases. Hum Mutat. 2011;32(5):557–63.

31. Kohlmann A, Klein HU, Weissmann S, Bresolin S, Chaplin T, Cuppens H, et al. The Interlaboratory RObustness of Next-generation sequencing (IRON) study: a deep sequencing investigation of TET2, CBL and KRAS mutations by an international consortium involving 10 laboratories. Leukemia. 2011; 25(12):1840–8.

32. Cleator SJ, Powles TJ, Dexter T, Fulford L, Mackay A, Smith IE, et al. The effect of the stromal component of breast tumours on prediction of clinical outcome using gene expression microarray analysis. Breast Cancer Res. 2006;8(3):R32.

33. Buttitta F, Felicioni L, Del Grammastro M, Filice G, Di Lorito A, Malatesta S, et al. Effective assessment of egfr mutation status in bronchoalveolar lavage and pleural fluids by next-generation sequencing. Clin Cancer Res. 2013; 19(3):691–8.

34. Moskalev EA, Stöhr R, Rieker R, Hebele S, Fuchs F, Sirbu H, et al. Increased detection rates of EGFR and KRAS mutations in NSCLC specimens with low tumour cell content by 454 deep sequencing. Virchows Arch. 2013;462(4):409–19.

35. Chin ELH, C da Silva, M Hegde. Assessment of clinical analytical sensitivity and specificity of next-generation sequencing for detection of simple and complex mutations. BMC Genet. 2013;14:14-6

36. Guan YF, Hu H, Peng Y, Gong Y, Yi Y, Shao L, et al. Detection of inherited mutations for hereditary cancer using target enrichment and next generation sequencing. Fam Cancer. 2015;14(1):9–18.

37. Hadd AG, Houghton J, Choudhary A, Sah S, Chen L, Marko AC, et al. Targeted, high-depth, next-generation sequencing of cancer genes in formalin-fixed, paraffin-embedded and fine-needle aspiration tumor specimens. J Mol Diagn. 2013;15(2):234–47.

38. Lin MT, Mosier SI, Thiess M, Beierel KF, Debeljak M, Tseng LH, et al. Clinical Validation of KRAS, BRAF, and EGFR mutation detection using next-generation sequencing. Am J Clin Pathol. 2014;141(6):856–66.

39. Nijman IJ, van Montfrans JM, Hoogstraat M, Boes ML, van de Corput L, Renner ED, et al. Targeted next-generation sequencing: a novel diagnostic tool for primary immunodeficiencies. J Allergy Clin Immunol. 2014;133(2):529–34.

40. Barbareschi M, Buttitta F, Felicioni L, Cotrupi S, Barassi F, Del Grammastro M, et al. Different prognostic roles of mutations in the helical and kinase domains of the PIK3CA gene in breast carcinomas. Clin Cancer Res. 2007; 13(20):6064–9.

41. Lai YL, Mau BL, Cheng WH, Chen HM, Chiu HH, Tzen CY. et al. PIK3CA exon 20 mutation is independently associated with a poor prognosis in breast cancer patients. Ann Surg Oncol. 2008;15(4):1064–9.

42. Li SY, Rong M, Grieu F, Iacopetta B. PIK3CA mutations in breast cancer are associated with poor outcome. Breast Cancer Res Treat. 2006;96(1):91–5.

43. Mangone FR, Bobrovnitchaia IG, Salaorni S, Manuli E, Nagai MA.PIK3CA exon 20 mutations are associated with poor prognosis in breast cancer patients. Clinics (Sao Paulo). 2012;67(11):1285–90.

44. Saal LH, Holm K, Maurer M, Memeo L, Su T, Wang X, et al. PIK3CA mutations correlate with hormone receptors, node metastasis, and ERBB2, and are mutually exclusive with PTEN loss in human breast carcinoma. Cancer Res. 2005;65(7):2554–9.

45. Koboldt DC, Fulton RS, McLellan, MD, Schmidt H, Kalicki-Veizer J, McMichael, JF, et al. Comprehensive molecular portraits of human breast tumours. Nature. 2012;490(7418):61–70.

46. Rohlin A, Wernersson J, Engwall Y, Wiklund L, Bjoerk J, Nordling M, et al. Parallel sequencing used in detection of mosaic mutations: comparison with four diagnostic DNA screening techniques. Hum Mutat. 2009;30(6): 1012–20.

47. Walsh T, Casadei S, Coats KH, Swisher E, Stray SM, Higgins J, et al. Spectrum of mutations in BRCA1, BRCA2, CHEK2, and TP53 in families at high risk of breast cancer. JAMA. 2006;295(12):1379–88.

48. Arsenic R, Lehmann A, Budczies J, Koch I, Prinzler J, Kleine-Tebbe A, et al. Analysis of PIK3CA mutations in breast cancer subtypes. Appl Immunohistochem Mol Morphol. 2014;22(1):50–6.

49. Ikenoue T, Kanai F, Hikiba Y, Obata T, Tanaka Y, Imamura J, et al. Functional analysis of PIK3CA gene mutations in human colorectal cancer. Cancer Res. 2005;65(11):4562–7.

50. Gymnopoulos M, Elsliger MA, Vogt PK. Rare cancer-specific mutations in PIK3CA show gain of function. Proc Natl Acad Sci U S A. 2007;104(13):5569–74.

51. Boyault S, Drouet Y, Navarro C, Bachelot T, Lasset C, Treilleux I, et al. Mutational characterization of individual breast tumors: TP53 and PI3K pathway genes are frequently and distinctively mutated in different subtypes. Breast Cancer Res Treat. 2012;132(1):29–39.

52. Kalinsky K, Jacks LM, Heguy A, Patil S, Drobnjak M, Bhanot UK, et al. PIK3CA mutation associates with improved outcome in breast cancer. Clin Cancer Res. 2009;15(16):5049–59.

53. Dunlap J, Le C, Shukla A, Patterson J, Presnell A, Heinrich MC, et al. Phosphatidylinositol-3-kinase and AKT1 mutations occur early in breast carcinoma. Breast Cancer Res Treat. 2010;120(2):409–18.

54. Hutter RV. Pathological parameters useful in predicting prognosis for patients with breast cancer. Monogr Pathol. 1984;25:175–85.

55. McGuire WL, Clark, GM, Dressler LG and Owens, MA. Role of steroid hormone receptors as prognostic factors in primary breast cancer. NCI Monogr. 1986;1:19–23.

56. Huang YE, Iijima M, Parent CA, Funamoto S, Firtel RA,Devreotes P, et al. Receptor-mediated regulation of PI3Ks confines PI(3,4,5)P3 to the leading edge of chemotaxing cells. Mol Biol Cell. 2003;14(5):1913–22.

57. Cizkova M, Susini A, Vacher S, Cizeron-Clairac G, Andrieu C, Driouch K, et al. PIK3CA mutation impact on survival in breast cancer patients and in ER alpha, PR and ERBB2-based subgroups. Breast Cancer Res. 2012;14(1):R28.

58. Baselga J, Cortés J, Im SA, Clark E, Ross G, Kiermaier A, et al. Biomarker analyses in CLEOPATRA: a phase III, placebo-controlled study of pertuzumab in human epidermal growth factor receptor 2-positive, first-line metastatic breast cancer. J Clin Oncol. 2014;32(33):3753–61.

59. Joensuu H, Kellokumpu-Lehtinen PL, Bono P, Alanko T, Kataja V, Asola R, et al. Adjuvant docetaxel or vinorelbine with or without trastuzumab for breast cancer. N Engl J Med. 2006;354(8):809–20.

60. Loi S, Michiels S, Lambrechts D, Fumagalli D, Claes B, Kellokumpu-Lehtinen PL, et al. Somatic mutation profiling and associations with prognosis and trastuzumab benefit in early breast cancer. J Natl Cancer Inst. 2013;105(13): 960–7.

61. Fu X, Osborne CK, Schiff R. Biology and therapeutic potential of PI3K signaling in ER+/HER2-negative breast cancer. Breast. 2013;22 Suppl 2:S12–8.

62. Harle A, Lion M, Lozano N, Merlin JL. Clinical, diagnostic significance and theranostic interest of PIK3CA gene mutations in breast cancer. Bull Cancer. 2013;100(10):947–54.

# Quantitative assessment of placental morphology may identify specific causes of stillbirth

Imogen Ptacek[1,2], Anna Smith[3], Ainslie Garrod[1,2], Sian Bullough[1,2], Nicola Bradley[1,2], Gauri Batra[3], Colin P. Sibley[1,2], Rebecca L. Jones[1,2], Paul Brownbill[1,2] and Alexander E. P. Heazell[1,2*]

## Abstract

**Background:** Stillbirth is frequently the result of pathological processes involving the placenta. Understanding the significance of specific lesions is hindered by qualitative subjective evaluation. We hypothesised that quantitative assessment of placental morphology would identify alterations between different causes of stillbirth and that placental phenotype would be independent of post-mortem effects and differ between live births and stillbirths with the same condition.

**Methods:** Placental tissue was obtained from stillbirths with an established cause of death, those of unknown cause and live births. Image analysis was used to quantify different facets of placental structure including: syncytial nuclear aggregates (SNAs), proliferative cells, blood vessels, leukocytes and trophoblast area. These analyses were then applied to placental tissue from live births and stillbirths associated with fetal growth restriction (FGR), and to placental lobules before and after perfusion of the maternal side of the placental circulation to model post-mortem effects.

**Results:** Different causes of stillbirth, particularly FGR, cord accident and hypertension had altered placental morphology compared to healthy live births. FGR stillbirths had increased SNAs and trophoblast area and reduced proliferation and villous vascularity; 2 out of 10 stillbirths of unknown cause had similar placental morphology to FGR. Stillbirths with FGR had reduced vascularity, proliferation and trophoblast area compared to FGR live births. Ex vivo perfusion did not reproduce the morphological findings of stillbirth.

**Conclusion:** These preliminary data suggest that addition of quantitative assessment of placental morphology may distinguish between different causes of stillbirth; these changes do not appear to be due to post-mortem effects. Applying quantitative assessment in addition to qualitative assessment might reduce the proportion of unexplained stillbirths.

**Keywords:** Stillbirth, Unexplained Stillbirth, Placental Morphometry, Fetal Growth Restriction, Villous vascularity, Avascular villi

* Correspondence: alexander.heazell@manchester.ac.uk
[1]Institute of Human Development, Faculty of Medical and Human Sciences, University of Manchester, Oxford Rd, Manchester M13 9PL, UK
[2]Maternal and Fetal Health Research Centre, 5th floor (Research), St Mary's Hospital, Oxford Road, Manchester M13 9WL, UK
Full list of author information is available at the end of the article

# Background

Histological examination of the placenta is one of the most frequently performed investigations to identify the cause of death in cases of stillbirth [1]; its application in this context is recommended by international guidelines [2–4]. A recent systematic review found large variations in the methodological quality of studies of placental examination after stillbirth, with few studies of high quality [5]. Interpretation of the results of such studies is further complicated by the use of different classification systems and a lack of consensus in terminology used to describe placental lesions which results in a large variation in the proportion of stillbirths attributed to a placental "cause" from 11–65 % [5]. Such qualitative placental assessment, combined with varied terminology, has some deficiencies. Firstly, qualitative assessment of placental lesions may introduce bias, particularly if assessors are not blinded to outcome. Furthermore, qualitative assessment may lead to inter-observer variation in diagnoses, which ranged from 25–91 % in one study [6]. The significance of specific abnormalities to stillbirth has also been questioned by Pathak et al. who describe placental abnormalities in a significant proportion of apparently healthy live-born infants [7]. Finally, identification of a specific lesion does not imply a single cause. For example, appearances of fetal thrombotic vasculopathy have been associated with various pathologies including: cytomegalovirus infection [8], umbilical cord accidents [9] or specific patterns of umbilical cord coiling [10]. Similarly, changes of maternal underperfusion may be related to hypertensive disorders [11] and antiphospholipid syndrome [12].

Recently, significant advances have been made in the development of modern classification systems [13–15] that reduce the proportion of unexplained stillbirths [16]. These classification systems have given greater recognition to the role of placental pathology in the aetiology of stillbirth [13–15] and progress has been made in reducing the variation of placental histological findings [6]. However, these clinically-orientated descriptions of placental phenotype have not yet been adopted into widespread practice, in part due to continued debate about terminology which varies between clinical and research studies [17]. Research studies have employed quantitative descriptions of placental morphology by stereology and morphometry to describe differences in placental structure in clinical conditions related to stillbirth such as fetal growth restriction (FGR) [18] and reduced fetal movements [19]. We aimed to use these quantitative methods to objectively evaluate placental appearances of different causes of stillbirth. Firstly, we hypothesised that specific causes of stillbirth would be associated with a morphometric phenotype. Secondly, we hypothesised that morphological abnormalities associated with stillbirth would differ from live births with the same condition. To be of diagnostic value, any observed changes should not represent artefacts of storage or cessation of fetal blood flow after death. Since we have already described the effects of placental storage on placental structure [20], here we address a third hypothesis that there is an acute effect of post-stillbirth fetoplacental haemostasis on placental morphology.

# Methods

## Placental tissue samples

To address the first hypothesis we obtained placental tissue from cases of stillbirth, defined as the birth of an infant with no signs of life after 24 weeks gestation. Parents gave permission for the use of samples for research at the time of consent for post-mortem examination. A favourable ethical opinion was given by the Greater Manchester South Research Ethics Committee (09/H1012/11) and approval given from the Research and Innovation Division of Central Manchester University Hospitals NHS Foundation Trust to conduct the study. Cases of stillbirth were classified using the ReCoDe system [15] by a multidisciplinary meeting following a full panel of investigations including: post-mortem, histopathological examination of the placenta, chromosomal analysis and maternal biochemical, haematological, immunological and serological tests. We obtained samples from the following classifications of stillbirth: cord accident ($n = 8$), diabetes ($n = 5$), FGR ($n = 10$), hypertension ($n = 8$), infection ($n = 8$) and from stillbirths of an unknown cause ($n = 10$). For comparison, matched placental samples were used from appropriately-grown live born infants and preterm births (26-36 weeks) (demographics shown in Table 1). Samples from live births were collected following written informed consent as part of the Maternal and Fetal Research Centre (MFHRC) Biobank (08/H1010/55). To address the second hypothesis, placental samples were taken from a further cohort of stillbirths attributed to FGR ($n = 13$) and from live births with FGR ($n = 13$) with the same ethical approvals as described above. FGR was defined as a customised birthweight <5th centile (demographics shown in Table 2). To address the final hypothesis, placental tissue was obtained from appropriately grown ($n = 7$) and FGR ($n = 5$) live births following written informed consent as part of the MFHRC biobank previously described. For all cases, maternal and infant demographic information was recorded from medical case notes and post-mortem reports (for stillbirths). An estimate of the duration of in utero retention was made according to

**Table 1** Demographic characteristics of samples from live births and stillbirths from known and unknown causes. Birthweight was significantly lower in stillbirths from FGR and hypertension than live births ($P < 0.01$); all other variables did not significantly differ between groups. Data are presented as median with range in parentheses except for estimated time of retention in utero where number of cases are presented

| | | Live births | Preterm birth | Cord | Diabetes | Hypertension | Infection | FGR | Unknown |
|---|---|---|---|---|---|---|---|---|---|
| Number of Samples | | 10 | 7 | 8 | 5 | 8 | 9 | 10 | 10 |
| Maternal Age (years) | | 32 (28–37) | 27 (18–41) | 28 (21–36) | 34 (31–40) | 33 (27–37) | 30 (25–32) | 30 (22–32) | 28 (21–31) |
| Gravidity | | 1 (1–5) | 3 (1–6) | 1 (1–1) | 4 (2–7) | 1 (1–2) | 1 (1–3) | 1 (1–4) | 1 (1–2) |
| Parity | | 0 (0–4) | 0 (0–4) | 0 (0–0) | 1 (1–2) | 0 (0–0) | 0 (0–2) | 0 (0–2) | 0 (0–0) |
| Gestation at delivery (weeks) | | 37 (37–38) | 31 (26–36) | 30 (27–38) | 28 (28–40) | 31 (26–35) | 38 (24–41) | 34 (26–38) | 31 (27–39) |
| Birthweight (g) | | 3090 (2805–3430) | 1821 (786–2760) | 1300 (702–2750) | 3120 (1473–3590) | 1110 (399–1730) | 2680 (494–2985) | 1065 (564–2230) | 2170 (892–3150) |
| Estimated in utero retention time | 0 h - <24 h | N/A | N/A | 0 | 1 | 4 | 4 | 2 | 2 |
| | ≥24 h - < 48 h | | | 1 | 0 | 2 | 2 | 4 | 3 |
| | ≥48 h - < 96 h | | | 2 | 1 | 0 | 2 | 2 | 1 |
| | ≥96 h - <1 week | | | 3 | 1 | 1 | 0 | 0 | 2 |
| | ≥1 week | | | 2 | 2 | 1 | 1 | 2 | 2 |

**Table 2** Demographic details of samples used for experimental comparisons. The left hand columns relate to samples obtained from cases of FGR that were live or stillborn; all these samples had a birthweight <5th centile. The right hand columns relate to samples used for perfusion experiments. Data are presented as median with range in parentheses

|  | FGR live birth | FGR still birth | Appropriate for gestational age - placental perfusion | FGR - placental perfusion |
|---|---|---|---|---|
| Number of Samples | 13 | 13 | 7 | 5 |
| Maternal Age (years) | 32 (20–40) | 23 (19–42) | 33 (27–36 | 31 (23–39)) |
| Gravidity | 2 (1–9) | 2 (1–3) | 2 (2–4) | 1 (1–5) |
| Parity | 1 (0–8) | 0 (0–2) | 2 (1–2) | 1 (0–5) |
| Gestation at delivery (weeks) | 37 (30–41) | 35 (28–38) | 39 (39–39) | 38 (35–39) |
| Birthweight (g) | 1389 (536–3060) | 1010 (385–2000) | 3740 (2910–3940) | 2262 (1900–2440) |
| Mode of delivery (% Caesarean) | 69 | 0 | 71 | 89 |
| Infant gender (% Female) | 54 | 62 | 57 | 78 |

Genests' descriptions of findings at post-mortem and from histopathological examination of the placenta [21–23].

Tissue from live births was obtained within 30 min of delivery. For assessment of placental morphology biopsies of villous tissue were dissected from the centre, middle and edge of the placenta. Tissue was fixed in 4 % neutral buffered formalin for 24 h before being wax embedded. For stillbirth samples three blocks of placental tissue not obtained from specific lesions were obtained for each placenta.

### Placental perfusion

Unless otherwise stated, all reagents were supplied by Sigma-Aldrich Chemical Company (Poole, UK). To examine the acute impact of continued maternal blood flow in the absence of fetal blood flow single-sided (maternal) ex vivo human placental lobule perfusion was adapted from the dual-sided perfusion model [24]. Perfusion was performed on placentas from normal pregnancy ($n = 7$) and placentas from pregnancies complicated by FGR ($n = 5$). An intact peripheral lobule was selected, devoid of post-partum tears, deep decidual damage and marginal membrane separations. Prior to perfusion two villous biopsies were sampled from neighbouring lobules taken 5 cm apart, and fixed immediately in 4 % neutral buffered formalin forming "pre-perfusion samples". The fetal artery and vein on the chorionic surface, serving the villous trees within the lobule designated for perfusion, were each ligated using sutures (Mersilk 3/0, Ethicon, supplied by NuCare, UK) to confine a static fetal blood pool within the fetal vasculature of the associated cotyledons. The maternal surface was cannulated using five 10 cm lengths of polythene tubing (Smiths Medical, UK) arising from a perfusion manifold (Harvard Apparatus, UK). The distal ends of the cannulae were cut into apices and inserted through the decidual surface of the lobule with an even spatial distribution. The perfusate was modified Earle's bicarbonate buffer (EBB 117 mM NaCl, 10.7 mM KCl, 5.6 mM D-glucose, 3.6 mM CaCl, 1.8 mM NaH$_2$PO$_4$, 13.6 mM NaHCO$_3$, 0.04 mM L-arginine, 0.8 mM MgSO$_4$, 3.5 % (w/v) dextran, 0.1 % (w/v) bovine serum albumin, 5000 IU/L Heparin sodium) equilibrated with 95 % O$_2$ / 5 % CO$_2$ to pH 7.4 and warmed to 37 °C, delivered by a roller pump (Watson Marlow, UK) at 14 ml/min. Lobule preparations were only considered acceptable for experimentation when maternal-side perfusion was established within 30 min of delivery. Open-circuit perfusion was for 6 h, and then the physiological buffer was switched to a 4 % neutral buffered formalin at T = 6 h for a 10 min maternal-side perfusion fixation period. Following this, the lobule was excised and two further full thickness (vertical and horizontal) biopsies slices were taken as the "post-perfusion samples". These wide tissue sections where then immersion fixed in 4 % neutral buffered formalin for 24 h before being wax embedded. Placental structure in these biopsies was examined as described above.

### Immunohistochemistry

Placental cell turnover, structure and vascularity were assessed using antibodies specific for Ki67 (Dako, Ely, Cambridgeshire, UK; 0.16 µg/ml), cytokeratin 7 (Dako; 0.9 µg/ml) and CD31 (Dako; 0.16 µg/ml). The number of leukocytes was assessed by an antibody specific for CD45 (Dako; 0.4 µg/ml). Negative controls were performed using non-immune mouse IgG (Dako) at matching concentrations to the primary antibody. Immunohistochemistry was performed as previously described with antigen retrieval performed by microwaving the sections for 10 min in 0.01 M sodium citrate buffer [19, 20].

Quantification of syncytial nuclear aggregates (SNAs, also known as syncytial knots) was conducted on sections stained with haematoxylin and eosin as previously described [19, 20]. Dewaxed and rehydrated sections were stained with Harris's haematoxylin for 10 min before differentiation in acid-alcohol. Slides were stained with eosin for 2 min, rinsed in cold tap water, and dehydrated and mounted as described above.

For all analyses images were captured using an Olympus BX41 light microscope (Southend-on-Sea, UK) and QIcam Fast 1394 (QImaging, BC, Canada) and Image Pro Plus 6.0 and 7.0 (Media Cybernetics Inc., MD, USA). During image acquisition and analysis the presumed cause of stillbirth was concealed

from the observer. Between images the microscope was taken out of focus to prevent selection bias, if the randomly selected image was not mostly of terminal villi another area was identified. Five random images of terminal villi were taken of each section, giving a total of 15 images per placenta for each component evaluated.

### Assessment of placental structure

The number of SNAs were counted and total villous area measured using image analysis software, expressed

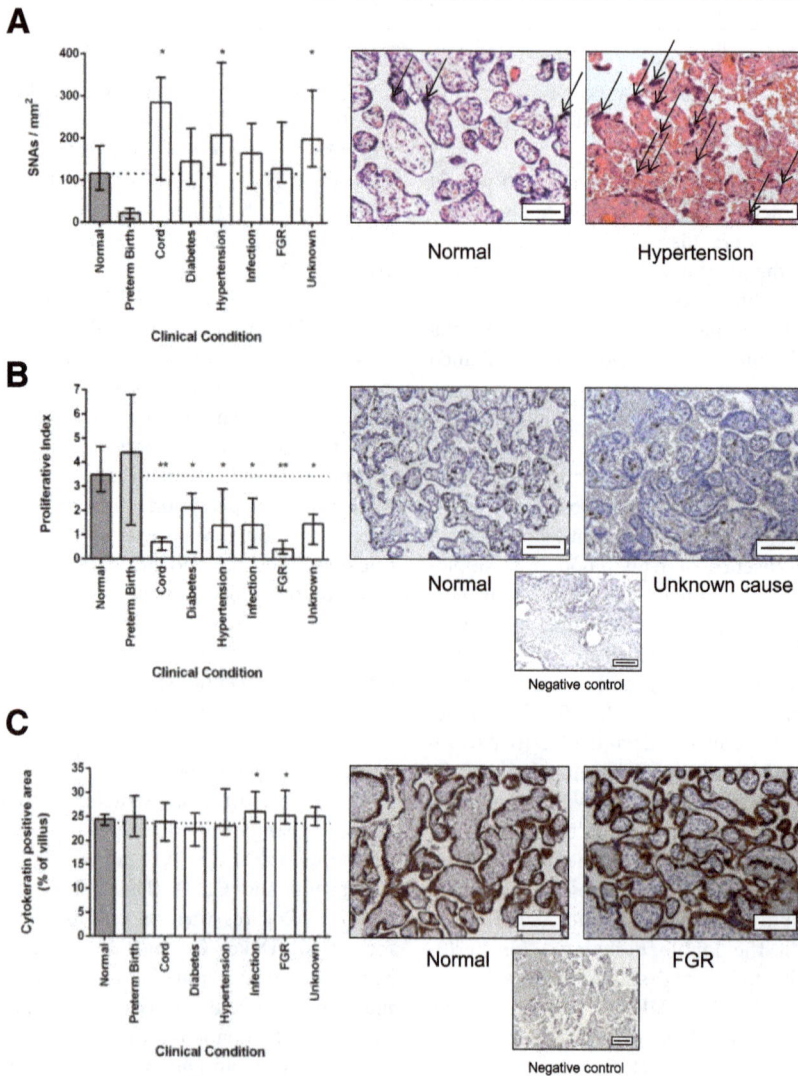

**Fig. 1 a** Assessment of syncytial nuclear aggregates (SNAs) in different causes of stillbirth compared to healthy live births. SNAs are shown by open arrows in representative images from normal pregnancy and stillbirth associated with hypertension. **b** Assessment of proliferation in different causes of stillbirth compared to healthy live births. **c** Assessment of trophoblast area in different causes of stillbirth compared to healthy live births. Negative control images shown in small panel beneath representative images of normal pregnancy and FGR. Scale bar = 50 μm in all images. Graphs show median and range, * $p < 0.05$, ** $p < 0.01$, *** $p < 0.001$. Dotted line indicates median level of healthy control

as the number of SNAs per mm$^2$ of villous tissue as previously described [25]. Proliferative index was the number of Ki67 positive nuclei as a proportion of total nuclei as previously described [19, 20]. Vascularity was expressed as the number of capillaries per terminal villus and the percentage of avascular villi (defined as a villus with no evidence of CD-31 immunostaining or morphological evidence of vessels) [19, 20]. Trophoblast area was expressed as the proportion of villous area positive for CK-7 immunostaining. The number of leukocytes was assessed by the number of CD45 positive cells per 1,000 nuclei.

**Statistical analysis**

For comparison of different causes of stillbirth data from each variable was compared to the median level in healthy controls using Wilcoxon signed rank test. Cases of FGR that were live-born were compared to those who were stillborn using Mann-Whitney $U$ test. Data from pre- and post-perfusion samples were compared using Wilcoxon matched-pairs test. Demographic variables were compared using Kruskal-Wallis test with Dunn's post-hoc test for multiple comparisons and Mann-Whitney $U$ test for single comparisons. For all statistical tests a p-value of 0.05 was considered to be statistically

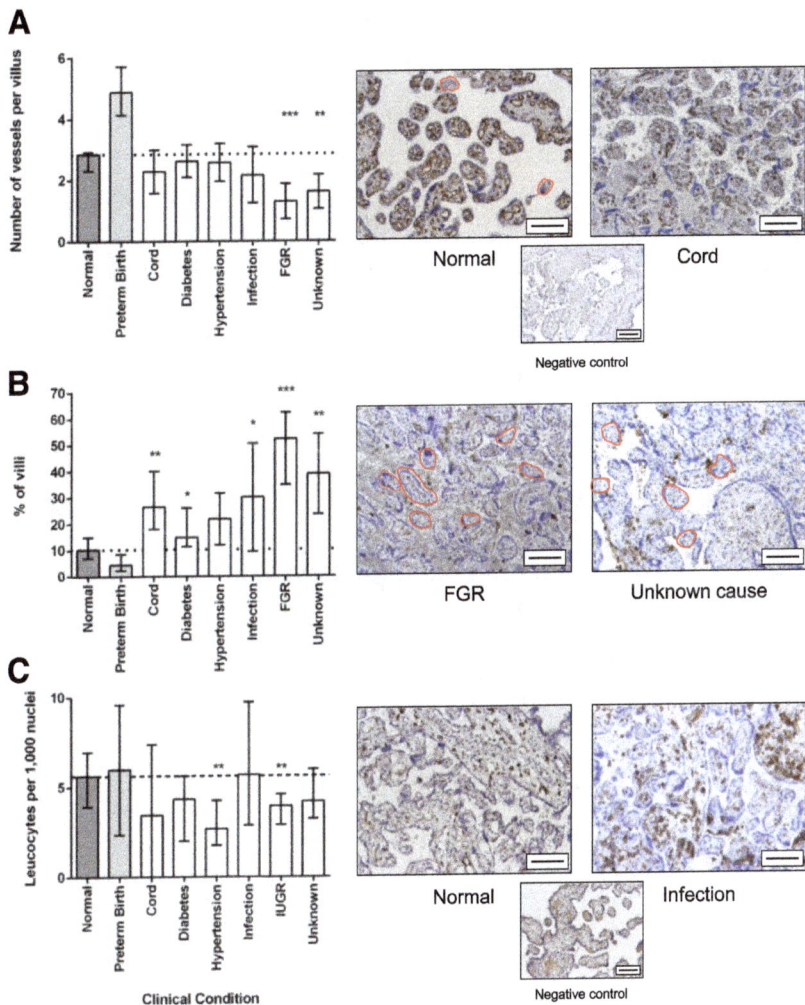

**Fig. 2 a** Assessment of villous vascularity in different causes of stillbirth compared to healthy live births. **b** Proportion of avascular villi in different causes of stillbirth compared to healthy live births. Avascular villi are highlighted in red. **c** Assessment of the number of leukocytes in different causes of stillbirth compared to healthy live births. Negative control images shown in small panel beneath representative images of normal pregnancy and FGR. Scale bar = 50 µm in all images. Graphs show median and range, * $p < 0.05$, ** $p < 0.01$, *** $p < 0.001$. Dotted line indicates median level of healthy control

**Table 3** Pattern of placental morphology in placental samples from stillbirths of unknown cause ($n = 10$) demonstrating two samples with a very similar pattern to samples from FGR (highlighted in grey)

| Sample | SNAs | Proliferation | Vascularity | Avascular villi | Trophoblast | Leukocytes | Profile |
|---|---|---|---|---|---|---|---|
| Unknown 1 | Low | High | Unchanged | High | Low | Low | Not similar |
| Unknown 2 | High | Unchanged | Low | High | Unchanged | Unchanged | Not similar |
| Unknown 3 | High | Low | Low | High | High | Unchanged | Similar to FGR |
| Unknown 4 | High | Unchanged | High | Unchanged | Unchanged | Unchanged | Not similar |
| Unknown 5 | High | Low | Low | High | High | Unchanged | Similar to FGR |
| Unknown 6 | High | Unchanged | Low | High | Unchanged | Unchanged | Not similar |
| Unknown 7 | Unchanged | Unchanged | Low | High | Unchanged | Unchanged | Not similar |
| Unknown 8 | Unchanged | High | Low | High | Increased | Low | Not similar |
| Unknown 9 | High | Unchanged | Low | High | Increased | High | Not similar |
| Unknown 10 | Unchanged | Unchanged | Low | High | Increased | Unchanged | Not similar |

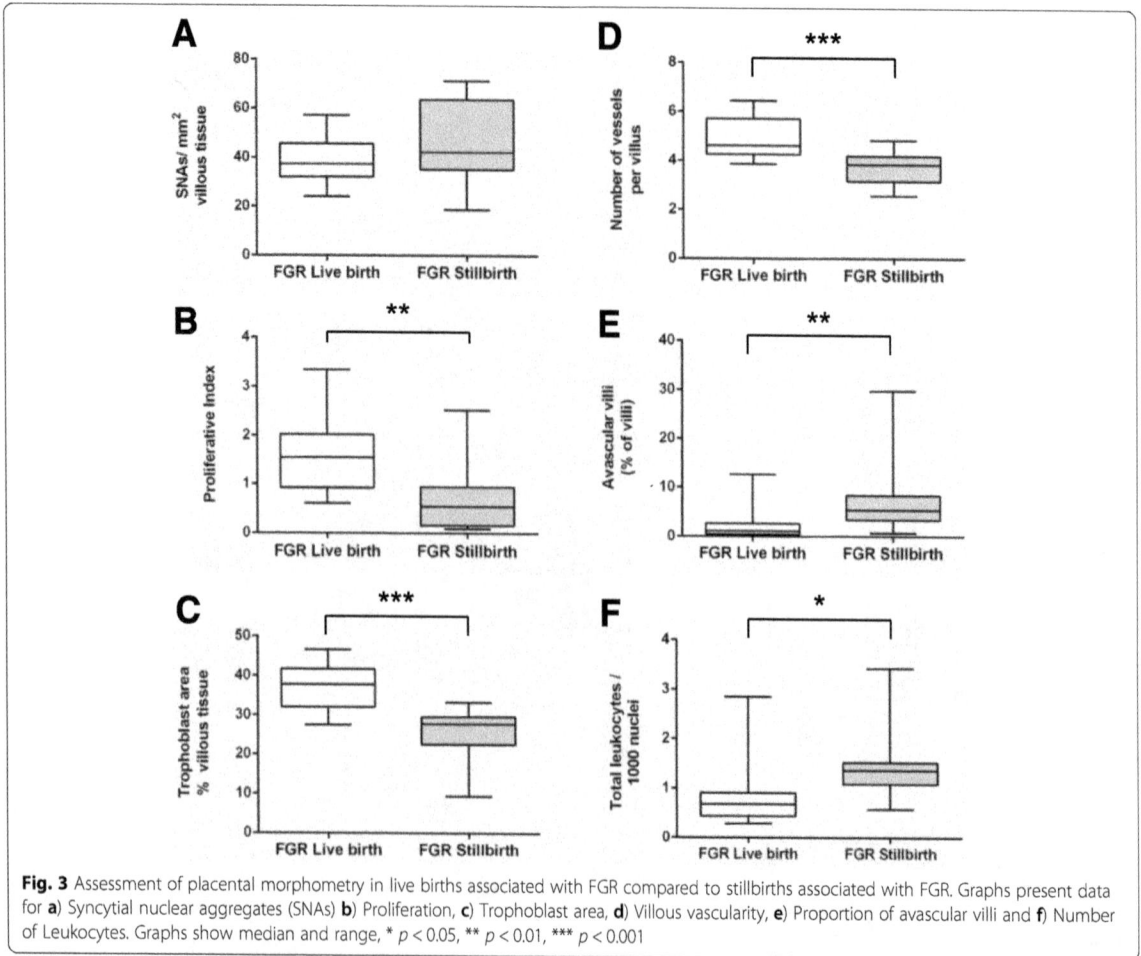

**Fig. 3** Assessment of placental morphometry in live births associated with FGR compared to stillbirths associated with FGR. Graphs present data for **a**) Syncytial nuclear aggregates (SNAs) **b**) Proliferation, **c**) Trophoblast area, **d**) Villous vascularity, **e**) Proportion of avascular villi and **f**) Number of Leukocytes. Graphs show median and range, * $p < 0.05$, ** $p < 0.01$, *** $p < 0.001$

significant. All statistical analyses were carried out using GraphPad PRISM (Version 6, La Jolla, CA).

## Results

### Placental morphology in different causes of stillbirth

In comparison to normal pregnancy, SNAs were increased in stillbirths attributed to cord accident, hypertension, FGR and in stillbirths with an unknown aetiology (Fig. 1a). This was in contrast to fewer SNAs seen in preterm live births. Proliferation was reduced in all cases of stillbirth, but was particularly reduced in those cases attributed to cord accident or FGR (Fig. 1b). The median trophoblast area (measured as cytokeratin-7 positive area) was increased in stillbirths attributed to infection and FGR (Fig. 1c). The median number of blood vessels identified by CD31 immunostaining was significantly reduced in stillbirths attributed to FGR and those with an unknown cause (Fig. 2a). The number of

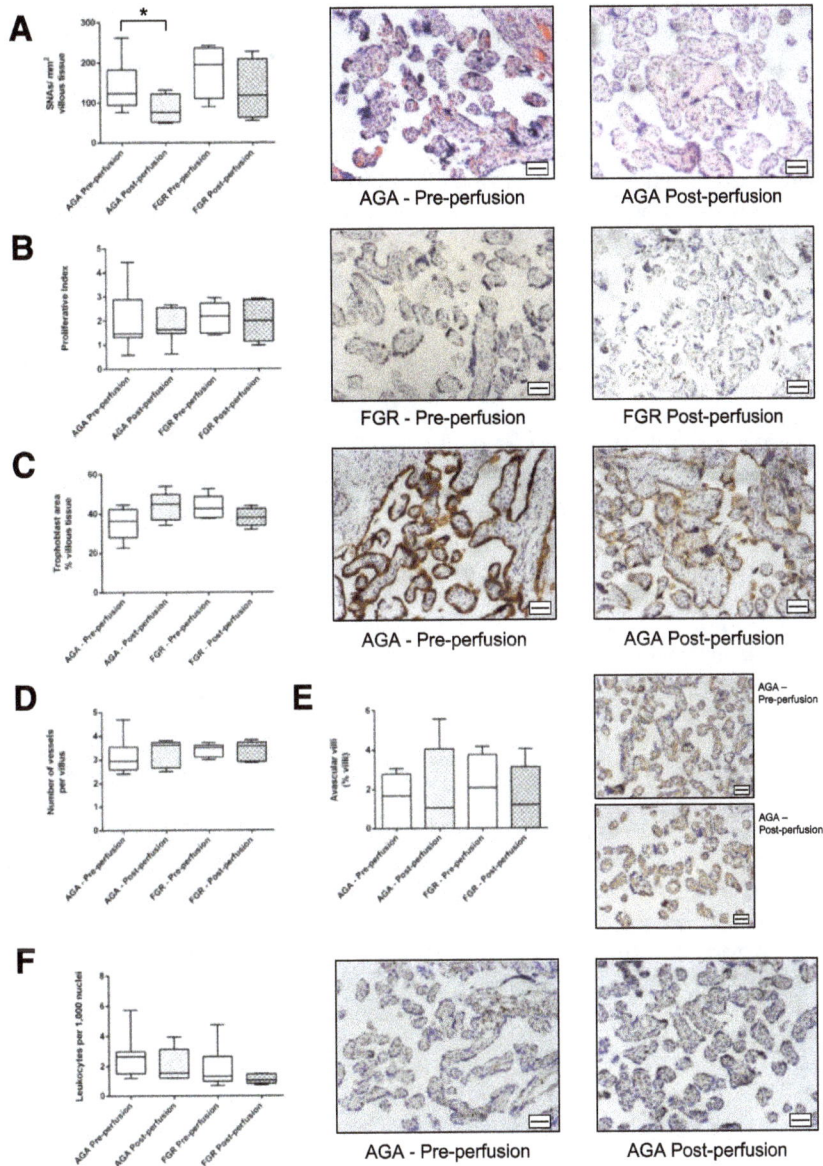

**Fig. 4** Assessment of placental morphometry before and after maternal-side only placental perfusion in normal and FGR placentas. Graphs present data for a reduction in **a**) syncytial nuclear aggregates (SNAs), but no change in **b**) Proliferation, **c**) Trophoblast area, **d**) Villous vascularity, **e**) Proportion of avascular villi and **f**) Number of Leukocytes. Graphs show median and range, * $p < 0.05$. Representative images of each feature are shown. Scale bar = 50 μm in all images

avascular villi was significantly increased in these conditions, although an increase in avascular villi was also seen in stillbirths attributed to cord compression and hypertension (Fig. 2b). These changes were in contrast to an increase in vascularity and reduction in avascular villi observed in preterm live births. The median number of leukocytes was reduced in stillbirths attributed to maternal hypertension and FGR compared to healthy controls (Fig. 2c). It is important to note that in some variables, notably the number of leukocytes in cases of infection, there was a wide range in measurements obtained. The cause of stillbirth with the most placental differences from healthy pregnancies was FGR, which has increased numbers of SNAs, reduced proliferation, increased trophoblast area, fewer blood vessels per villus, more avascular villi and decreased numbers of leukocytes. Interestingly, the condition with next most frequent abnormalities was stillbirths of unknown cause. When the individual profiles of stillbirths from unknown cause are examined, two had a similar profile to those with FGR and others had similar features such as increased density of SNAs and reduced vascularity (Table 3). None of the features examined altered according to the estimated duration of in utero retention (Additional file 1: Figure S1).

When compared to FGR live births, FGR stillbirths did not have increased numbers of SNAs but had reduced proliferation and trophoblast area, fewer blood vessels per villus and a greater proportion of avascular villi. Leukocytes were increased in FGR stillbirths compared to FGR live births (Fig. 3).

### Effect of short-term fetoplacental haemostasis on placental morphology

To assess changes that may happen in utero after cessation of fetal blood flow, placental tissue was examined before and after maternal-side only placental perfusion in placental tissue from healthy and FGR pregnancies. Perfusion in this manner for 6 h was not associated with any changes in proliferation, trophoblast area, villous vascularity or the proportion of avascular villi (Fig. 4). Maternal-side only perfusion was associated with a reduction in the number of SNAs in normal tissue (Fig. 4a). There was a consistent trend towards lower numbers of leukocytes in perfused tissue from both appropriately-grown and FGR pregnancies ($p = 0.08$).

### Discussion

This pilot study demonstrates that objective assessment of placental morphology may provide additional information on placental villous structure in cases of stillbirth and in some cases, such as in FGR, can differentiate between specific causes of stillbirth and healthy live-born infants. In other cases, such as

stillbirths attributed to maternal diabetes, there were no morphological differences from live-born infants, which is consistent with few histopathological abnormalities in stillbirths related to diabetes [26]. When the morphometric profile was applied to ten stillbirths of unknown cause, two had a very similar placental profile to FGR, which suggests that some stillbirths that currently have no identified cause (despite intensive investigation) may actually result from FGR in a fetus that was not small, i.e. infants who have a birthweight >10th centile but whose growth rate was slowing down. These preliminary findings suggest that addition of objective assessment of placental morphology to histological examination with the use of a modern classification system may further decrease the proportion of unexplained stillbirths. However, further research is needed to understand the role that abnormalities of placental structure and function have in the aetiology of stillbirth both in the presence of a small fetus and when the birthweight is within an accepted normal range [27].

The findings in FGR stillbirths are consistent with other stereological and morphometric assessment of FGR placentas including: increased SNAs [25], reduced villous vascularity [28], reduced proliferation [29] and number of cytotrophoblasts [28]. The pattern seen in FGR stillbirths was also consistent with the placental morphology in women with reduced fetal movements [19], who are at increased risk of stillbirth [30]. However, some results differ from other studies, one of which describes a positive relationship between trophoblast area and birthweight [31]. The reduced trophoblast area in stillbirth FGR compared to healthy live births contrasts with an increased area relative to live born FGR infants. This observation may result from thicker syncytiotrophoblast covering hypoplastic villi; application of stereological techniques is required to explore this observation in greater depth.

The findings of this study are consistent with the Stillbirth Collaborative Research Network (SCRN) case-control study which found increased presence of placental lesions in stillbirths, including: diffuse terminal villous immaturity, inflammation, vascular degeneration in the chorionic plate, intra-placental thrombi, avascular villi and parenchymal infarction [32]. The SCRN study found differences in lesions depending on gestation. Avascular villi and fetal vascular thrombi were more frequently seen in term stillbirths than those occurring at earlier gestations. Whereas, chorioamnionitis was seen less frequently in stillbirths than live births at 24 weeks' gestation, but more frequently in term stillbirths compared to matched live births [32]. The SCRN study provides evidence that different causes of stillbirth have a different placental phenotype and addition evidence that gestation may affect the cause of stillbirth. Our study demonstrated that some features (SNAs and villous vascularity) were altered in preterm compared to term live births. Critically, these changes were in the opposite direction to that seen in stillbirth, so the morphology changes seen in cases of stillbirth cannot be attributed to their preterm gestation.

The finding that the placental phenotype of FGR stillbirths had reduced villous vascularity, increased avascular villi and increased leukocyte infiltration compared to live-born FGR may imply that FGR stillbirths result from a more severe placental phenotype. However, these differences must be interpreted cautiously, as differences between live and stillbirth may also result from artefacts from cessation of fetoplacental blood flow after fetal death, differences in mode of delivery or from storage prior to fixation. Our previous experimental data suggest that storage prior to fixation for ≤48 h does not alter any of the indices measured here [20]. Studying the effects of in utero retention is more challenging. We attempted to model this by maternal-side only placental perfusion for 6 h, finding that this did not reproduce any of the differences between FGR stillbirths and live births. However, the duration of perfusion was limited by the experimental technique and it cannot reproduce the in utero environment (e.g. presence of the maternal immune system). Placental changes may be altered by the duration of in utero retention, as evident by changes in histopathological appearances of the placenta in fetal maceration [33]. Thus, further study is needed to determine the effects of potential confounders, particularly in utero retention, on the quantitative measures used in this study. This could be explored by evaluating the morphology of stillbirths with known in utero retention time (e.g. intrapartum events, feticide for structural anomaly). The possibility that morphological changes might arise from differences in mode of delivery should also be considered, as Caesarean section is rarely used in cases of stillbirth, but is frequently employed in live born FGR infants; this can be resolved by detailed study of placental morphology after vaginal delivery and Caesarean section.

The study reported here is strengthened by a detailed assessment of multiple aspects of placental morphology with blinding of assessor to study group or pregnancy outcome. We also have compared cases of stillbirth to appropriately-grown healthy controls and preterm births primarily recruited for research rather than clinical cases with indication(s) for perinatal histology. The use of objective techniques that also have been used to evaluate related conditions allows comparison between different clinical situations. However, this study does have limitations: although 50 samples from well-characterised stillbirths have been analysed, this only amounts to ≤10 samples per group and these were obtained from a single

Paediatric and Perinatal Pathology department. Unfortunately, at the time of collection the collection protocols between the clinical histopathological service and research laboratories were slightly different resulting in different numbers of samples obtained per placenta potentially introducing a bias between samples from stillbirths and live births. However, we believe the chance of selection bias to be low as placental tissue was randomly sampled and blocks of specific lesions were not used in either protocol. Samples were divided into groups based upon the classification of stillbirth determined by multidisciplinary review (involving obstetricians, midwives, sonographers and pathologists) and, although this was made as robust as possible, it is possible that the cause of death was different from that attributed in the perinatal review process.

## Conclusion

Due to the critical role played by the placenta in determining the outcome of pregnancy and the role of placenta failure in the aetiology of stillbirth [34], placental histology is a frequently employed investigation that can provide important information for clinicians and parents regarding the reasons for their child's death [35]. When combined with a modern classification system, histological examination of the placenta reduces the proportion of unexplained stillbirths [36, 37]. Our preliminary findings suggest that addition of objective measurement of placental structure may add to understanding of the cause of stillbirth. These quantitative observations need to be related to established qualitative descriptions; in some cases such as avascular villi and fetal thrombotic vasculopathy this may be straightforward, in others, such as placental maturation disorders, this may be more complex. Prior to clinical application further studies are needed to develop normal ranges for these morphological characteristics at different gestational ages and to determine the effects of in utero retention on these indices. Then blinded studies of randomly sampled cases of stillbirth from multiple populations are needed to ensure the findings presented here are sufficiently sensitive and specific for diagnostic use.

## Additional file

**Additional file 1: Figure S1.** Assessment of placental morphometry in stillbirths (irrespective of cause) grouped by estimated time of in utero retention according to Genest's criteria [21–23]. Graphs present data for A) Syncytial nuclear aggregates (SNAs) B) Proliferation, C) Trophoblast area, D) Villous vascularity, E) Proportion of avascular villi and F) Number of Leukocytes per 1,000 nuclei. Graphs present the median and interquartile range for each group. There is no statistically significant difference of the frequency of the morphological feature and the groups divided by in utero retention. (PPTX 197 kb)

## Abbreviations

EBB: Earles' Bicarbonate Buffer; FGR: Fetal growth restriction; MFHRC: Maternal and Fetal Health Research Centre; ReCoDe: Relevant Condition at Death (Classification System); SCRN: Stillbirth Collaborative Research Network; SNA: Syncytial nuclear aggregate.

## Competing interests

The authors confirm that they have no conflicts of interest to report in relation to this manuscript.

## Authors' contributions

AEPH, GB, CPS, RLJ and PB conceived the study and designed the experiments. IP, SA, AG, SB, NB and AEPH conducted the experiments and completed the analysis. All authors contributed to the development and writing of the manuscript.

## Acknowledgements

This work was funded by Tommy's - The Baby Charity, Holly Martin Stillbirth Research Fund and Tunbridge Wells Sands. The Maternal and Fetal Health Research Centre is supported by funding from Tommy's the Baby Charity, an Action Research Endowment Fund, the Manchester Biomedical Research Centre and the Greater Manchester Comprehensive Local Research Network. The funders did not have any role in the data acquisition, analysis, writing of the manuscript or decision to publish the findings. The authors wish to acknowledge all those who donated placental tissue, particularly bereaved parents who wished to contribute to research efforts to understand stillbirth. The authors wish to thank Mr James Horn for assistance with immunoperoxidase staining.

## Author details

[1]Institute of Human Development, Faculty of Medical and Human Sciences, University of Manchester, Oxford Rd, Manchester M13 9PL, UK. [2]Maternal and Fetal Health Research Centre, 5th floor (Research), St Mary's Hospital, Oxford Road, Manchester M13 9WL, UK. [3]Department of Histopathology, Royal Manchester Children's Hospital, Central Manchester University Hospitals NHS Foundation Trust, Manchester Academic Health Science Centre, Manchester M13 9WL, UK.

## References

1.  Turner K, Sebire NJ, Evans M, on behalf of MBRRACE-UK. Pathological and Histological Investigations. In: Draper ES, Kurinczuk JJ, Kenyon S, on behalf of MBRRACE-UK, editors. MBRRACE-UK Perinatal Confidential Enquiry: Term, singleton, normally formed antepartum stillbirth. Leicester: Department of Health Sciences, University of Leicester; 2015. p. 61–4.
2.  American College of Obstetricians and Gynecologists. ACOG Practice Bulletin No. 102: management of stillbirth. Obstet Gynecol. 2009;113(3): 748–61.
3.  Royal College of Obstetricians and Gynaecologists. Green-Top Guideline 55 - Late Intrauterine Fetal Death and Stillbirth. London: Royal College of Obstetricians and Gynaecologists; 2010.
4.  Flenady V, King J, Charles A, Gardener G, Ellwood D, Day K, McCowan L, Kent A, Tudehope D, Richardson R et al. PSANZ Clinical Practice Guideline for Perinatal Mortality. Version 2.2. 2009. http://www.psanzpnmsig.org
5.  Ptacek I, Sebire NJ, Man JA, Brownbill P, Heazell AE. Systematic review of placental pathology reported in association with stillbirth. Placenta. 2014; 35(8):552–62.
6.  Turowski G, Berge LN, Helgadottir LB, Jacobsen EM, Roald B. A new, clinically oriented, unifying and simple placental classification system. Placenta. 2012;33(12):1026–35.
7.  Pathak S, Lees CC, Hackett G, Jessop F, Sebire NJ. Frequency and clinical significance of placental histological lesions in an unselected population at or near term. Virchows Arch. 2011;459(6):565–72.
8.  Iwasenko JM, Howard J, Arbuckle S, Graf N, Hall B, Craig ME, et al. Human cytomegalovirus infection is detected frequently in stillbirths and is associated with fetal thrombotic vasculopathy. J Infect Dis. 2011;203(11): 1526–33.
9.  Ryan WD, Trivedi N, Benirschke K, Lacoursiere DY, Parast MM. Placental histologic criteria for diagnosis of cord accident: sensitivity and specificity. Pediatr Dev Pathol. 2012;15(4):275–80.
10. Ernst LM, Minturn L, Huang MH, Curry E, Su EJ. Gross patterns of umbilical cord coiling: correlations with placental histology and stillbirth. Placenta. 2013;34(7):583–8.
11. Veerbeek JH, Nikkels PG, Torrance HL, Gravesteijn J, Post Uiterweer ED, Derks JB, et al. Placental pathology in early intrauterine growth restriction associated with maternal hypertension. Placenta. 2014;35(9): 696–701.
12. Viall CA, Chamley LW. Histopathology in the placentae of women with antiphospholipid antibodies: A systematic review of the literature. Autoimmun Rev. 2015;14(5):446–71.
13. Korteweg FJ, Gordijn SJ, Timmer A, Erwich JJ, Bergman KA, Bouman K, et al. The Tulip classification of perinatal mortality: introduction and multidisciplinary inter-rater agreement. BJOG. 2006;113(4):393–401.
14. Flenady V, Froen JF, Pinar H, Torabi R, Saastad E, Guyon G, et al. An evaluation of classification systems for stillbirth. BMC Pregnancy Childbirth. 2009;9:24.
15. Gardosi J, Kady SM, McGeown P, Francis A, Tonks A. Classification of stillbirth by relevant condition at death (ReCoDe): population based cohort study. Br Med J. 2005;331(7525):1113–7.
16. Vergani P, Cozzolino S, Pozzi E, Cuttin MS, Greco M, Ornaghi S, et al. Identifying the causes of stillbirth: a comparison of four classification systems. Am J Obstet Gynecol. 2008;199(3):319 e311–314.
17. Barbaux S, Erwich JJ, Favaron PO, Gil S, Gallot D, Golos TG, et al. IFPA meeting 2014 workshop report: Animal models to study pregnancy pathologies; new approaches to study human placental exposure to xenobiotics; biomarkers of pregnancy pathologies; placental genetics and epigenetics; the placenta and stillbirth and fetal growth restriction. Placenta. 2015;36 Suppl 1:S5–10.
18. Mayhew TM, Manwani R, Ohadike C, Wijesekara J, Baker PN. The placenta in pre-eclampsia and intrauterine growth restriction: studies on exchange surface areas, diffusion distances and villous membrane diffusive conductances. Placenta. 2007;28(2-3):233–8.
19. Warrander LK, Batra G, Bernatavicius G, Greenwood SL, Dutton P, Jones RL, et al. Maternal perception of reduced fetal movements is associated with altered placental structure and function. PLoS One. 2012;7(4):e34851.
20. Garrod A, Batra G, Ptacek I, Heazell AE. Duration and method of tissue storage alters placental morphology - implications for clinical and research practice. Placenta. 2013;34(11):1116–9.
21. Genest DR. Estimating the time of death in stillborn fetuses: II. Histologic evaluation of the placenta; a study of 71 stillborns. Obstet Gynecol. 1992; 80(4):585–92.
22. Genest DR, Singer DB. Estimating the time of death in stillborn fetuses: III. External fetal examination; a study of 86 stillborns. Obstet Gynecol. 1992; 80(4):593–600.
23. Genest DR, Williams MA, Greene MF. Estimating the time of death in stillborn fetuses: I. Histologic evaluation of fetal organs; an autopsy study of 150 stillborns. Obstet Gynecol. 1992;80(4):575–84.
24. Brownbill P, McKeeman GC, Brockelsby JC, Crocker IP, Sibley CP. Vasoactive and permeability effects of vascular endothelial growth factor-165 in the term in vitro dually perfused human placental lobule. Endocrinology. 2007; 148(10):4734–44.
25. Heazell AE, Moll SJ, Jones CJ, Baker PN, Crocker IP. Formation of syncytial knots is increased by hyperoxia, hypoxia and reactive oxygen species. Placenta. 2007;28(Supplement 1):S33–40.
26. Edwards A, Springett A, Padfield J, Dorling J, Bugg G, Mansell P. Differences in post-mortem findings after stillbirth in women with and without diabetes. Diabet Med. 2013;30(10):1219–24.
27. Heazell AE, Whitworth MK, Whitcombe J, Glover SW, Bevan C, Brewin J, et al. Research priorities for stillbirth: process overview and results from UK Stillbirth Priority Setting Partnership. Ultrasound Obstet Gynecol. 2015;46(6): 641–7.
28. Chen C-P, Bajoria R, Aplin JD. Decreased vascularization and cell proliferation in placentas of intrauterine growth-restricted fetuses with abnormal umbilical artery flow velocity waveforms. Am J Obstet Gynecol. 2002;187(3):764–9.
29. Heazell AE, Sharp AN, Baker PN, Crocker IP. Intra-uterine growth restriction is associated with increased apoptosis and altered expression of proteins in the p53 pathway in villous trophoblast. Apoptosis. 2011;16:135–44.

30. Heazell AE, Froen JF. Methods of fetal movement counting and the detection of fetal compromise. J Obstet Gynaecol. 2008;28(2):147–54.
31. Daayana S, Baker P, Crocker I. An image analysis technique for the investigation of variations in placental morphology in pregnancies complicated by preeclampsia with and without intrauterine growth restriction. J Soc Gynecol Investig. 2004;11(8):545–52.
32. Pinar H, Goldenberg RL, Koch MA, Heim-Hall J, Hawkins HK, Shehata B, et al. Placental findings in singleton stillbirths. Obstet Gynecol. 2014;123(2 Pt 1): 325–36.
33. Stanek J, Biesiada J. Relation of placental diagnosis in stillbirth to fetal maceration and gestational age at delivery. J Perinat Med. 2014; 42(4):457–71.
34. Heazell AE, Worton SA, Higgins LE, Ingram E, Johnstone ED, Jones RL, et al. IFPA Gabor Than Award Lecture: Recognition of placental failure is key to saving babies' lives. Placenta. 2015;36 Suppl 1:S20–8.
35. Korteweg FJ, Erwich JJ, Holm JP, Ravise JM, van der Meer J, Veeger NJ, et al. Diverse placental pathologies as the main causes of fetal death. Obstet Gynecol. 2009;114(4):809–17.
36. Heazell AE, Martindale EA. Can post-mortem examination of the placenta help determine the cause of stillbirth? J Obstet Gynaecol. 2009;29(3):225–8.
37. Korteweg FJ, Erwich JJ, Timmer A, van der Meer J, Ravise JM, Veeger NJ, et al. Evaluation of 1025 fetal deaths: proposed diagnostic workup. Am J Obstet Gynecol. 2012;206(1):53 e51–12.

# 13

# Histopathological characterization of corrosion product associated adverse local tissue reaction in hip implants

Benjamin F. Ricciardi[1], Allina A. Nocon[2], Seth A. Jerabek[1], Gabrielle Wilner[3], Elianna Kaplowitz[3], Steven R. Goldring[3], P. Edward Purdue[3] and Giorgio Perino[4*]

## Abstract

**Background:** Adverse local tissue reaction (ALTR), characterized by a heterogeneous cellular inflammatory infiltrate and the presence of corrosion products in the periprosthetic soft tissues, has been recognized as a mechanism of failure in total hip replacement (THA). Different histological subtypes may have unique needs for longitudinal clinical follow-up and complication rates after revision arthroplasty. The purpose of this study was to describe the histological patterns observed in the periprosthetic tissue of failed THA in three different implant classes due to ALTR and their association with clinical features of implant failure.

**Methods:** Consecutive patients presenting with ALTR from three major hip implant classes ($N = 285$ cases) were identified from our prospective Osteolysis Tissue Database and Repository. Clinical characteristics including age, sex, BMI, length of implantation, and serum metal ion levels were recorded. Retrieved synovial tissue morphology was graded using light microscopy. Clinical characteristics and features of synovial tissue analysis were compared between the three implant classes. Histological patterns of ALTR identified from our observations and the literature were used to classify each case. The association between implant class and histological patterns was compared.

**Results:** Our histological analysis demonstrates that ALTR encompasses three main histological patterns: 1) macrophage predominant, 2) mixed lymphocytic and macrophagic with or without features of associated with hypersensitivity/allergy or response to particle toxicity (eosinophils/mast cells and/or lymphocytic germinal centers), and 3) predominant sarcoid-like granulomas. Implant classification was associated with histological pattern of failure, and the macrophagic predominant pattern was more common in implants with metal-on-metal bearing surfaces (MoM HRA and MoM LHTHA groups). Duration of implantation and composition of periprosthetic cellular infiltrates was significantly different amongst the three implant types examined suggesting that histopathological features of ALTR may explain the variability of clinical implant performance in these cases.

**Conclusions:** ALTR encompasses a diverse range of histological patterns, which are reflective of both the implant configuration independent of manufacturer and clinical features such as duration of implantation. The macrophagic predominant pattern and its mechanism of implant failure represent an important subgroup of ALTR which could become more prominent with increased length of implantation.

**Keywords:** Adverse local tissue reaction, Corrosion products, Revision arthroplasty, Synovial inflammation, Metal-on-metal total hip replacement, Hip resurfacing

* Correspondence: perinog@hss.edu
[4]Department of Pathology and Laboratory Medicine, Hospital for Special Surgery, 535 East 70th Street, New York, NY 10021, USA
Full list of author information is available at the end of the article

# Background

The introduction over the past two decades of alternative bearing surfaces, in particular a new generation of metal-on-metal (MoM) bearing, and increased modularity at the head-neck and neck-stem tapers has attempted to reduce wear debris formation at the bearing surface, risk of dislocation, and improve accurate reproduction of leg length, offset, and version [1–3]. These modifications have had unintended consequences, although clinical concerns regarding formation of corrosion products were raised; in particular, increased rates of adverse periprosthetic soft tissue reactions reported across a diverse spectrum of implant configurations [4–9]. These failures have resulted in extensive soft tissue necrosis, injury to the hip abductors, increased revision complications, and significant patient morbidity [8, 10–12].

Early studies described an unusual pattern of periprosthetic soft tissue inflammation with mixed macrophagic and lymphocytic infiltrates, variable tissue necrosis, vascular wall changes, and cytoplasmic inclusions of uncertain composition in the macrophages, which was collectively described as aseptic lymphocyte dominated vasculitis associated lesion (ALVAL) [13–15]. The formation of corrosion products at modular junctions and/or bearing surface and subsequent penetration into the periprosthetic soft tissue have been a common feature associated with the reaction [5, 16–18]. More recent studies have focused on characterizing the lymphocytic infiltrate, noting mixed interstitial and perivascular B- and T-cell populations with formation of germinal centers or sarcoid-like granulomas in subsets of patients [17, 19, 20].

Unlike the early reports that focused primarily on aspects of lymphocytic infiltrate and necrosis, subsequent studies suggested that the histological spectrum of these reactions, named adverse local tissue reaction (ALTR) or adverse reaction to implant debris (ARMD) is more diverse than originally appreciated, and lymphocyte rich infiltrate with significant necrosis represents only a subset of these cases [17, 20, 21]. In particular, a subgroup of patients with neo-synovial florid macrophagic infiltrate containing wear debris with no or minimal lymphocytic component in their periprosthetic tissue has been described in these studies, although its contribution to implant failure has not been well characterized. It is critical to identify the full spectrum of ALTR failures because different histological subtypes may have unique needs for longitudinal clinical follow-up and complication rates after revision arthroplasty.

In the present study, we report the histological features of 285 cases of ALTR from a large, diverse group of hip implants that includes three major classes: metal-on-metal (MoM) hip resurfacing arthroplasty (HRA), MoM large head total hip arthroplasty (THA), and non-MoM THA with cobalt/chrome (CoCr) dual modular neck. Histopathological analysis of the periprosthetic tissue across the three classes of implants was performed to answer the following research questions: 1. What are the histopathological patterns of soft tissue failure in ALTR; 2. What is the association between implant class and different histopathological features of ALTR; 3. What is the association of histopathological findings with clinical features of implant failure.

# Methods

## Patients

All patients who underwent revision hip arthroplasty between June 2011 and December 2014 implanted with a prosthetic device of the above mentioned classes of implants at risk of ALTR were identified retrospectively from the prospective Osteolysis/Adverse Local Reaction Tissue Database and Repository at our institution (Fig. 1). These patients were all eligible for inclusion in the current study [N = 303]. Exclusion criteria included infection diagnosed in compliance with the criteria reported by the International Consensus Meeting on periprosthetic joint infection and accepted by the Centers for Disease Control [22] [N = 3] with 5 out of 5, 6 out of 6, and 5 out of 5 intraoperative positive cultures, insufficient tissue retrieval for comparative pathologic examination (less than 5 tissue sections and more than 75 % tissue necrosis at light microscopy examination on all slides examined) [N = 13], and two cases for non-ALTR related post-operative complications with histological examination: periprosthetic fracture [N = 1] and recurrent dislocation [N = 1]. The exclusion of these patients left a total of 285 cases for inclusion in this study. In addition, 18 cases were identified with a post-operative unexpected diagnosis of ALTR in conventional MoP implants without dual modular neck that were not consented for inclusion in our registry prospectively and were not eligible for enrollment in the current study.

Patients were divided into three groups based on the design of their implant. Previous work has shown that implant design influences both clinical and pathologic manifestations of ALTR [17]. The three major implant classes examined were: 1. MoM HRA group; 2. MoM large head (≥36 mm) THA with or without cobalt chromium (CoCr) metallic adapter sleeve (MoM LHTHA group); and 3. Metal-on-polyethylene (MoP), ceramic-on-polyethylene (CoP), or ceramic-on-ceramic (CoC) bearing surface with femoral heads <36 mm and (CoCr) dual modular neck (Non-MoM DMNTHA). These represent the most common implant classes that have resulted in ALTR in case reports and case series [5, 23–27]. Demographic data (age, sex, body mass index, duration of implantation, duration of symptoms, implant type) were recorded for each patient when available. The onset of

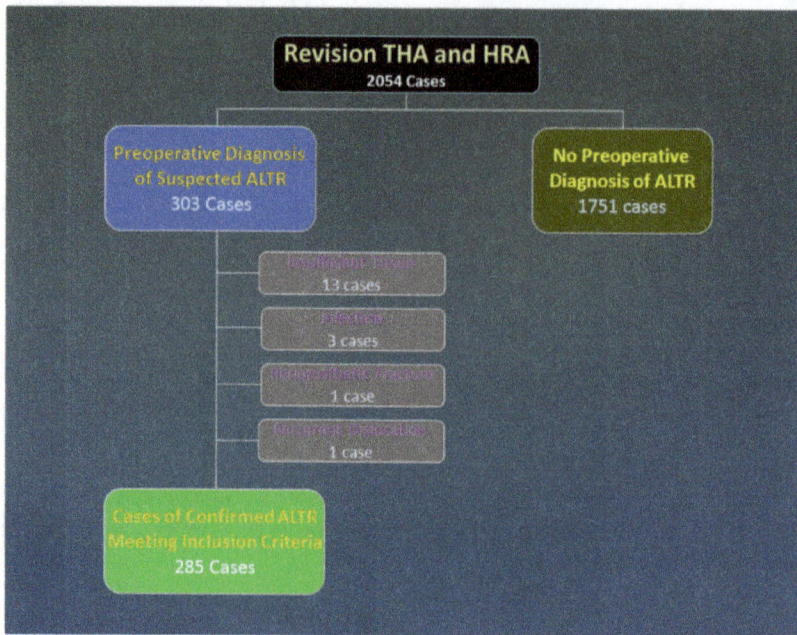

**Fig. 1** Flowchart of case study selection. The flowchart summarizes the process for inclusion and exclusion criteria for the study during the time period June 2011-December 2014, starting with the total number of THA and HRA revisions performed during the study period and ending with the final number of cases examined

symptoms was assessed via questionnaire at the time of revision surgery. Symptoms included increasing pain around the hip and mechanical symptoms such as "grinding sensation". Other symptoms such as discomfort around the hip, although frequent in the Non-MoM DMNTHA group were not considered positive unless progression to pain was recorded before revision. Preoperative serum cobalt and chromium levels were obtained by quantitative inductively coupled plasma-mass spectrometry at the operating surgeons' discretion (ARUP Laboratories, Salt Lake City, Utah). Ethical committee approval was obtained prior to this study and all patients had an informed consent obtained in writing for inclusion in the registry (Institutional Review Board, Hospital for Special Surgery, Protocol Number 26085).

**Tissue collection and sampling**

Tissue collection and sampling for all patients was performed as previously described [17]. Briefly, patients suspected of having ALTR underwent magnetic resonance imaging (MRI) with multi-acquisition variable-resonance image combination (MAVRIC) scan to further reduce susceptibility artifact. Areas of inflammation were identified preoperatively on MRI when available, and used as guidance for tissue sampling by the operating surgeon.

Samples were taken from multiple regions around the hip joint including the periprosthetic pseudocapsule, bursal synovium, and adjacent skeletal muscle when necessary and labeled accordingly. Acetabular and femoral bone samples, core biopsies of osteolytic areas, and/or reamings were collected at the discretion of the operating surgeon to evaluate possible bone marrow involvement when suitable. Extensive sampling was performed at macroscopic examination with care to the orientation of the specimens, including necrotic areas and/or friable, loose material. Femoral heads from resurfacing specimens were separated from the metallic cup at surgery when possible and extensively sampled or subject to multiple biopsies when retrieved in situ. The mean number of individual surgical specimens between the groups was not different [DMN cohort was 4.3 (SD 1.5), for the MoM THA cohort was 3.5 (1.6), and for the resurfacing cohort 3.5 (1.3); $p > 0.05$]. Extensive samples between 5 and 15 tissue blocks containing one or two histological sections were taken depending on the available tissue for each specimen.

**Histological analysis**

Histological analysis was performed as previously described [17]. Briefly, all sections were processed and embedded with standard procedures, stained routinely with hematoxylin-eosin. Cases were scored for this study by an experienced musculoskeletal pathologist (GP) and a surgeon trained in examining periprosthetic tissue from revision hip arthroplasty (BFR). Investigators were blinded from clinical patient characteristics. All cases were examined by both observers. Disagreement was handled by consensus between the two observers. This method of grading and assessment has been reported in previous publication [17] and also validated for intraobserver variability [28]. The ALVAL scoring system proposed by Campbell et al, which was previously used as correlative index with MRI imaging analysis, was recorded for each case [13, 28].

Histological sections were examined for synovial structure, cellularity, macrophage particle content, and bone marrow involvement using a previously described scoring system [17] and summarized in Table 1. Results were expressed as the percentage of samples containing the selected feature. All patients enrolled in our registry over the same time period with a diagnosis of aseptic loosening due to osteolysis with conventional MoP implants without dual modular neck (MoP OLTHA) were subject to the same tissue collection, histological analysis, and scored to serve as non-ALTR controls for pathological data [$N = 31$].

### Histological patterns

Several histological patterns have been observed in ALTR in previous studies [13, 17, 20, 21, 29, 30]. We divided these into four broad groups based on these previous studies: 1) predominantly macrophagic pattern with absent or minimal lymphocytic response, 2) mixed inflammatory pattern, macrophagic and lymphocytic with variable presence of plasma cells, eosinophils, and mast cells, and 3) granulomatous pattern, predominant or associated with the mixed inflammatory pattern; and 4) predominantly lymphocytic pattern with absence of macrophagic component [Table 2]. The macrophagic pattern represents a group of patients with an adverse

soft tissue reaction resulting in implant failure with minimal lymphocytic infiltration [20, 30, 31]. The mixed inflammatory group is divided into two subsets: (A) with and (B) without lymphocytic germinal centers usually associated with tall endothelial cell venules and/or mast cell/eosinophilic infiltrate because the A subset may identify patients with distinct immunologic response [13, 15, 19, 29]. The third group has prominent formation of sarcoid-like granulomas, defined as a nodular collection of epithelioid macrophages with multinucleated giant cells and lymphocytic cuffing associated with large aggregates of corrosion products particles and a mixed macrophagic/lymphocytic infiltrate, possibly representing a subset of patients with distinctive macrophagic features [20, 29]. The fourth group shows perivascular/interstitial lymphocytic infiltrate without macrophagic component [21]. Patients in each implant class were classified based on the predominant histological pattern seen at light microscopy. The rate of appearance of each pattern was compared between the different implant classes.

### Statistics

All demographic and histological variables were compared across the three implant classes. Descriptive statistics are presented as medians and ranges for continuous variables and as frequencies and percentages for categorical variables. Continuous variables were assessed using the Kruskall-Wallis test. Histological patterns amongst the different implant classes were compared using the Fischer's exact test. A multinomial logistic regression was performed in order to identify possible predictive factors for the development of the scale of ALTR severity as described in the Campbell's score. Bonferroni correction was used for pairwise comparisons of histological data adjusted for multiple comparisons.

### Results
#### Demographic results
Implant designs that resulted in cases of ALTR in this study are shown in Table 3. Patients in the HRA group

---

**Table 1** Histological grading system used for all cases of ALTR

| Synovial Structure | Cellularity | Macrophage Content | Bone and Bone Marrow Involvement |
|---|---|---|---|
| Synovial Layer Loss (Present, Absent) | Macrophages (Grade 0–3) | Polyethylene Particles (Present, Absent) | Necrosis (Present, Absent) |
| Cell Exfoliation (Present, Absent) | Lymphocytes (Grade 0–4) | Metal Particles (Present, Absent) | Macrophages (Present, Absent) |
| Soft Tissue Necrosis (Present, Absent) | Stromal Cells (Grade 1–3) | Corrosion Products (None, Intracellular, Extracellular) | Reactive Lymphocytic Aggregates (Present, Absent) |
| Vascular Wall Changes (Present, Absent) | Neutrophils (Present, Absent) | | Germinal Centers (Present, Absent) |
| Granulomas (Present, Absent) | Plasma Cells (Grade 0–2) | | |
| | Eosinophils (Present, Absent) | | |

**Table 2** Histological patterns analyzed in hip replacement failures due to ALTR

| Histological Pattern | Characteristics |
| --- | --- |
| Macrophagic Pattern | Macrophagic infiltrate (grade ≥ 1) without or with minimal evidence of interstitial and/or perivascular lymphocytic infiltrate (<grade 1) |
| Mixed Macrophagic and Lymphocytic Pattern w/wo Plasmacytic Component | Macrophagic (grade ≥ 1) and lymphocytic (grade ≥ 1) infiltrate |
|   Without Presence of Germinal Centers or Eosinophils | |
|   With Presence of Germinal Centers or Eosinophils | |
| Granulomatous Pattern | Any pattern with predominant presence of sarcoid-like granulomas |
| Lymphocytic Pattern | Interstitial and/or perivascular lymphocytic infiltrate without evidence of macrophagic infiltrate |

were younger in age at time of revision relative to the other implant classes (Table 4). Total implantation time was shortest in the Non-MoM DMNTHA group [median 28 months (range 6–65)], and these patients had a significantly shorter duration of implantation relative to the MoM HRA group [median 48 months (range 5–120); $p < 0.001$] and the MoM LHTHA groups [median 60 months (range 23–132); $p < 0.001$] (Table 4). Duration of symptoms prior to revision did not differ between the different implant classes (Table 4). Preoperative serum cobalt and chromium ion levels were increased in the MoM

**Table 3** Retrieved implants with failure due to ALTR

| Non-MoM DMNTHA | Number of Hips |
| --- | --- |
| Rejuvenate (Stryker, Kalamazoo, MI) | 111 |
| ABG II (Stryker, Kalamazoo, MI) | 5 |
| SMF (Smith and Nephew, London, UK) | 3 |
| Redapt (Smith and Nephew, London, UK) | 2 |
| OTI/Encore R-120 (DJO Surgical, Austin, TX) | 1 |
| Aesculap Hip Replacement (Aesculap, Hazelwood, MO) | 1 |
| MoM HRA | |
| Birmingham Hip Resurfacing (Smith and Nephew, London, UK) | 36 |
| Cormet Hip Resurfacing (Corin Group, Cirencester, UK) | 5 |
| Conserve Hip Resurfacing (Wright Medical Technology, Arlington, TN) | 2 |
| ASR Hip Resurfacing (Depuy/Synthes, Warsaw, IN) | 1 |
| MoM LHTHA | |
| Birmingham Hip Replacement (Smith and Nephew, London, UK) | 44 |
| ASR Hip Replacement (Depuy/Synthes, Warsaw, IN) | 22 |
| Pinnacle Ultramet (Depuy/Synthes, Warsaw, IN) | 19 |
| Durom/Metasul (Zimmer, Warsaw, IN) | 10 |
| M2a Magnum (Biomet, Warsaw, IN) | 8 |
| Profemur (Wright Medical Technology, Arlington, TX) | 6 |
| Metal on Metal Bearing S-ROM (Depuy/Synthes, Warsaw, IN) | 4 |
| Conserve Hip Replacement (Wright Medical Technology, Arlington, TN) | 4 |
| Cormet Hip Replacement (Corin Group, Cirencester, UK) | 1 |

HRA and MoM LHTHA groups relative to the Non-MoM DMNTHA group (Table 4). Head sizes were larger in the MoM bearing surface groups (HRA and LHTHA) relative to the Non-MoM DMNTHA group.

### Histological patterns

A summary of the histological patterns seen in each of the three implant classes is shown in Table 5.

The macrophagic pattern is characterized by flat to papillary hypertrophic neo-synovium with a variable amount of macrophagic infiltrate and exfoliation of necrotic forms with absence or presence of giant cells containing fine globular and/or irregular aggregates of greenish corrosion products of variable dimension with or without particles of needle-shaped and/or irregular conventional black metallic debris and absent or minimal interstitial and/or perivascular lymphocytic infiltrate (Fig. 2a and b). A thick layer of necrosis is usually not present, although infarction of the neo-synovial papillae or a thin layer of superficial necrosis/infarction can be focally present along with variable foci of foamy macrophages. This pattern was seen in 41 % of cases of MoM HRA failures, but was less common in the other two implant classes (MoM LHTHA, 11 % of cases; Non-MoM DMNTHA, 6 % of cases) (Table 5).

The mixed macrophagic and lymphocytic pattern is characterized by a superficial layer of macrophages with or without an interstitial lymphocytic component, a layer of tissue necrosis/infarction of variable thickness or a band of desmoplastic fibrosis, a variable deep perivascular lymphocytic infiltrate, and macrophages containing fine globular and/or irregular aggregates of greenish corrosion products with or without particles of needle-shaped and/or irregular conventional black metallic debris (Fig. 2c and d). A subset of the mixed macrophagic and lymphocytic pattern shows features usually associated with hypersensitivity/allergy reactions, such as focal or diffuse eosinophilic infiltrate and presence of a large number of mast cells in association with particle-laden macrophages and/or perivascular lymphocytic infiltrate with formation of germinal centers (Fig. 2e and f). Implants with non-MoM bearing surfaces had increased mixed pattern

**Table 4** Demographic characteristics from all three major implant classes

|  | Non-MoM DMNTHA (N = 120 patients) | MoM HRA (N = 44 patients) | MoM LHTHA (N = 113 patients) |
|---|---|---|---|
| Age (years) | 66 (47–87)* | 56 (43–75)* | 60 (31–84)* |
| Sex (% female) | 64 % | 58 % | 54 % |
| Body Mass Index | 28 (17–43)^ | 25 (18–36)^ | 26 (19–59) |
| Implantation Time (months) | 28 (6–65)° | 48 (5–120)° | 60 (23–132)° |
| Symptom Duration (months) | 9 (0–60) | 12 (0–63) | 18 (0–60) |
| Serum Cobalt | 7 (0–169)# | 16 (1–115)# | 13 (4–16)# |
| Serum Chromium | 1 (0–64)§ | 14 (1–160)§ | 60 (23–132)§ |
| Head Size | 28 (22–52)¶ | 46 (38–52)¶ | 46 (36–64)¶ |
| Cup Size | 52 (38–64) | 52 (46–58) | 52 (48–64) |

All values are given as median (range)
*$p < 0.005$ for the MoM HRA group compared to the other two groups
^$p < 0.05$ for the MoM HRA group compared to the non-MoM DMNTHA group ($p = 0.005$)
°$p < 0.05$ for the non-MoM-DMN THA group compared to the MoM HRA group ($p < 0.001$) and the MoM LHTHA group ($p < 0.001$)
#$p < 0.05$ for the non-MoM DMNTHA group compared to the MoM HRA group ($p = 0.042$)
§$p < 0.05$ for the MoM HRA and the MoM LHTHA groups compared to the non-MoM DMNTHA group ($p < 0.001$) and the MoM HRA group compared to the MoM LHTHA group ($p = 0.026$)
¶$p < 0.05$ for the MoM HRA ($p < 0.001$) and the MoM LHTHA ($p < 0.001$) groups compared to the non-MoM DMNTHA group

with hypersensitivity features as a percent of total failures (Non-MoM DMNTHA 32 %) versus implant classes with a MoM bearing surface (HRA 11 % of cases and LHTHA 22 % of cases) (Table 5).

The granulomatous pattern is characterized by predominant isolated or confluent granulomas composed of centrally located large aggregates of particulate corrosion products lined or contained by multinucleated giant cells surrounded by a nodular infiltrate of epithelioid macrophages lined by lymphocytic cuff of variable thickness with or without presence of a plasmacytic component (Fig. 2g and h). A granulomatous pattern was most commonly seen in the Non-MoM DMNTHA (16 % of cases) versus the other two implant classes (Table 5).

A significant association ($p < 0.001$) was found with length of implantation and histological classification on univariate analysis, with longer durations of implantation associated with a macrophagic pattern of failure and shorter durations of implantation associated with granulomatous or a mixed pattern with eosinophils and/or germinal centers. Duration of patient symptoms was not associated with histological classification in univariate analysis ($p = 0.16$).

**Morphology results**

A summary of morphologic findings among the three classes of implants and the control group is shown in Table 6.

Macrophage distributions were significantly different between the three implant classes, and the MoM HRA group had the highest percentage of cases of grade 3 macrophage distribution (95 % of cases) versus MoM LHTHA (65 % of cases; $p = 0.007$) and the Non-MoM DMNTHA (42 % of cases; $p = 0.007$) (Table 6). Compared with the MoP OLTHA group, the MoM HRA and MoM LHTHA had similar macrophage distributions ($p = 0.14$) (Table 6). Non-MoM DMNTHA had decreased macrophage distributions relative to the MoP OLTHA group ($p = 0.007$) (Table 6). Soft tissue necrosis was more common in the Non-MoM DMNTHA (53 % of cases) relative to the other implant classes (32 % in the MoM LHTHA [$p = 0.0048$], 11 % in the MoM HRA group; $p = 0.007$) (Table 6).

Focal or diffuse macrophagic involvement of the bone marrow was observed in the MoM HRA, MoM LHTHA, and the Non-MoM DMNTHA implants (Table 6). More cases of osteolysis/massive particle laden macrophagic infiltration within retrieved periprosthetic bone samples were seen in the MoM HRA relative to the other implant classes (Table 6). Examination of some of the femoral heads retrieved from failed hip resurfacing implants showed florid particle-laden macrophagic infiltrate in the neo-synovium and massive infiltration of the bone marrow with formation of macroscopically evident,

**Table 5** Distribution of the histological patterns in the three implant classes

| Implant class | Macrophagic pattern | Mixed Pattern w/o hypersensitivity features | Mixed Pattern w/Hypersensitivity Features | Granulomatous pattern | Lymphocytic pattern |
|---|---|---|---|---|---|
| Non-MoM DMNTHA | 6 | 46 | 32 | 16 | 0 |
| MoM HRA | 41 | 48 | 11 | 0 | 0 |
| MoM LHTHA | 11 | 62 | 22 | 5 | 0 |

All values are expressed as a percentage of total cases of each histological pattern for a specific implant class

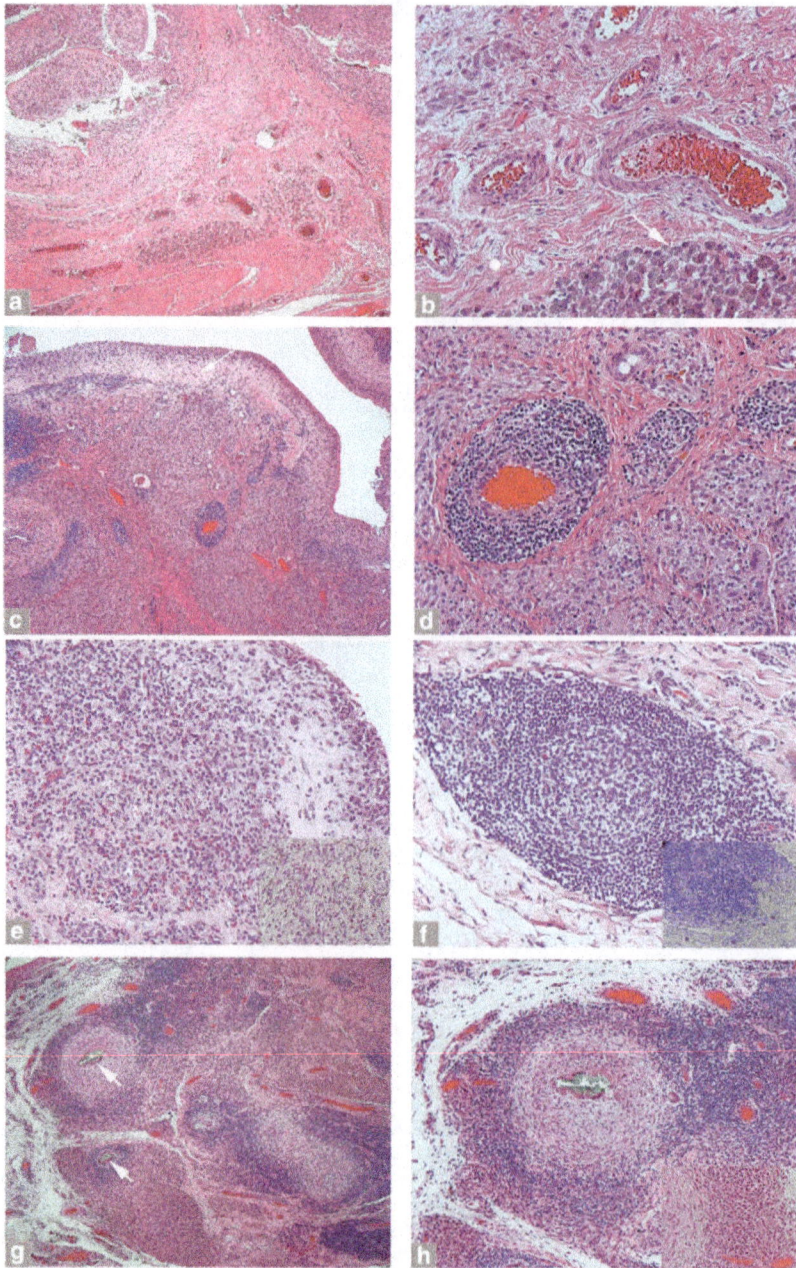

**Fig. 2** Histological patterns of ALTR. *Macrophagic pattern*: **a** Papillary neo-synovium with macrophagic infiltrate and underlying vascular layer (H-E x50). **b** Vascular layer without lymphocytic infiltrate and cluster of particle laden macrophages, white arrow (H-E x400). *Mixed macrophagic and lymphocytic pattern*: **c** Neo-synovium with superficial macrophagic layer and desmoplastic band, white arrow, and perivascular lyphocytic infiltrate (H-E x50). **d** Perivascular lymphocytic infiltrate associated with large clusters of particle laden macrophages (H-E x200). *Subset of the mixed pattern with heightened immunological features*: **e** Neo-synovium with florid interstitial lymphocytic and eosinophilic infiltrate (H-E x200) and association of eosinophils with particle laden macrophages (inset, H-E x400). **f** Perivascular lymphocytic infiltrate with germinal center (H-E x200) associated with numerous mast cells (inset, Toluidine Blue x400). *Granulomatous pattern*: **g** Multiple sarcoid-like granulomas with central aggregate of corrosion products, white arrow (H-E x100). **h** Granuloma at higher power with central collection of epithelioid macrophages and occasional giant cells (H-E x200) and plasmacytic component with binucleated forms admixed with particle laden macrophages (inset, H-E x400)

**Table 6** Significant differences in histological findings from all three implant classes and the control group

| | Non-MoM DMNTHA (N = 123 hips) | MoM HRA (N = 44 hips) | MoM LHTHA (N = 118 hips) | MoP OLTHA (N = 31 hips) |
|---|---|---|---|---|
| Synovial Structure | | | | |
| Synovial Layer Loss (%) | 99 | 89 | 99 | 16.1 |
| Soft Tissue Necrosis (%) | 53‡ | 11‡ | 32‡ | 0‡ |
| Sarcoid-like Granulomas (%) | 16* | 0* | 5* | 0 |
| Campbell Score (median) | 8§ | 5§ | 6§ | - |
| Cellularity | | | | |
| Macrophages (% Grade 1, Grade 2, Grade 3) | 7, 51, 42^ | 0, 5, 95^ | 1, 34, 65^ | 3, 16, 81^ |
| Lymphocytes (% Grade 1, Grade 2, Grade 3, Grade 4) | 7, 29, 34, 24° | 25, 18, 11, 7 ° | 25, 31, 23, 10° | 10, 0, 0, 0° |
| Plasma Cells (% Grade 1, Grade 2) | 26, 18 | 11, 9 | 29, 18 | 0, 0 |
| Eosinophils (%) | 20 | 9 | 17 | 0 |
| Macrophage Content | | | | |
| Polyethylene Particles (%) | 2 | 0 | 0 | 80 |
| Metallic Particles (%) | 8# | 39# | 30# | 65# |
| Corrosion Products (%) | 95 | 100 | 99 | 0 |
| Large Aggregates | 74¶ | 11¶ | 63¶ | 0¶ |
| Bone and Bone Marrow | N = 58 | N = 44 | N = 36 | N = 0 |
| Necrosis (%) | 47 | 11 | 23 | - |
| Macrophage Infiltration (%) | 57 | 67 | 73 | - |
| Germinal Centers (%) | 12 | 2 | 3 | - |
| Osteolysis (# cases) | 4 | 9 | 4 | - |

All values for synovial structure, macrophage content, eosinophils, cell distributions, and bone and bone marrow content expressed as percentage of cases with each morphologic feature
*$p = 0.013$ for Non-MoM DMNTHA versus MoM LHTHA and MoM HRA
^$p = 0.007$ for OL versus Non-MoM DMNTHA; $p = 0.007$ for MoM HRA versus MoM LHTHA; MoM HRA versus Non-MoM DMNTHA, and Non-MoM DMNTHA versus MoM LHTHA
°$p = 0.007$ for significant difference in distributions of lymphocyte grade between all implant classes except MoM LHTHA versus MoM HRA ($p = 0.0023$)
#$p = 0.007$ for OL versus MoM LHTA and Non-MoM DMNTHA; $p = 0.007$ for Non-MoM DMNTHA versus MoM HRA and MoM LHTHA
§$p < 0.001$ for significant difference in Campbell score between ALTR implant classes
‡$p = 0.007$ for OL versus Non-MoM DMNTHA, MoM LHTHA; $p = 0.007$ for MoM HRA versus Non-MoM DMNTHA; $p = 0.009$ MoM HRA versus MoM LHTHA; $p = 0.0048$ MoM LHTHA versus Non-MoM DMNTHA
¶$p = 0.011$ for OL versus MoM HRA; $p = 0.007$ OL versus Non-MoM DMNTHA and MoM LHTHA; $p = 0.007$ for MoM HRA versus MoM LHTHA and Non-MoM DMNTHA; $p = 0.026$ MoM LHTHA versus Non-MoM DMNTHA

macrophage-lined pseudocystic cavities (Fig. 3a, arrow) with marked exfoliation of necrotic forms (Fig. 3b). Macrophages containing greenish particles of corrosion products (Fig. 3b, inset and 3c) sometimes in association with black particles of conventional metallic debris (Fig. 3e and 3f) were observed streaming from the adjacent neo-synovium and infiltrating the bone marrow forming massive aggregates (Fig. 3f) or small clusters and single forms in the fatty marrow (Fig. 3g) or pushing underneath the orthopedic cement border lined by giant cells (Fig. 3c). In some cases, these were associated with large lymphocytic aggregates (Fig. 3h) or without lymphocytic reaction (Fig. 3d). The presence or absence of lymphocytic infiltrate in the bone marrow usually corresponded to the response seen in the neo-synovial membrane.

In the MoM LHTHA, a significant amount of necrotic debris containing macrophagic forms was observed in the metallic femoral head groove of a range of implant manufacturers (Fig. 4a and 4e), deposited from exfoliation of macrophagic viable/necrotic forms containing particles of corrosion products with or without conventional metallic debris (Fig. 4g) from thickened neo-synovial membrane with or without papillary features (Fig. 4b and 4f). Free aggregates of irregular green particles of corrosion products were found in synovial fluid (Fig. 4h, arrow) and in larger aggregates entrapped in necrotic cellular debris (Fig. 4d, arrow).

Lymphocyte distributions were significantly different between the three implant classes, and the MoM HRA group had the lowest percentage of cases of grade 3 and 4 lymphocyte distributions (18 % of cases) relative to the Non-MoM DMNTHA (58 % of cases; $p = 0.0007$), the MoM LHTHA (33 % of cases; $p = 0.0027$) (Table 6). All three ALTR groups had increased lymphocyte distributions relative to the MoP OLTHA group ($p = 0.007$; Table 6). Eosinophils were least common in the MoM HRA (9 % of cases) relative to the Non-MoM DMNTHA

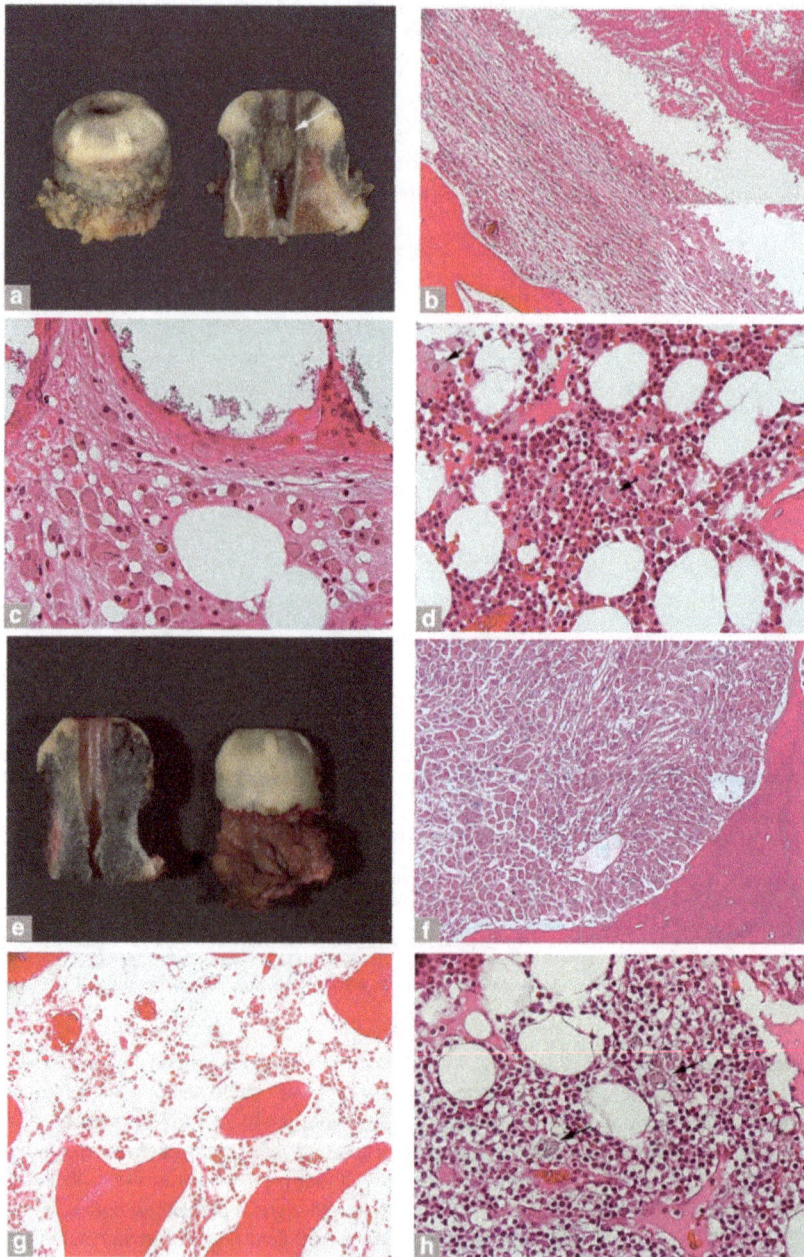

**Fig. 3** Osteolysis features in the MoM RHA group. **a** Femoral head with orthopedic cement cap lined by papillary neo-synovium and showing osteolytic cavity involving the central groove of the metallic stem, white arrow (Smith and Nephew Birmingham, implantation time 48 months). **b** Content of the osteolytic cavity composed of particle laden macrophages with central exfoliation of necrotic forms in the right upper corner (H-E x100) and detail of the cavity lining cell layer containing greenish corrosion products in inset (x400). **c** Particle laden macrophagic infiltrate under the orthopedic cement cap lined by multinucleated giant cells (H-E x400). **d** Hematopoietic marrow with particle laden macrophages without evidence of lymphocytic reaction (H-E x400). **e** Femoral head with orthopedic cement cap lined by papillary neo-synovium with charcoal grey bone marrow, secondary to diffuse permeation by macrophagic infiltrate with metallic wear content (Smith and Nephew Birmingham, implantation time 78 months). **f** Massive macrophagic infiltrate in bone marrow containing greenish particles of corrosion products and black particles of abrasion metallic wear without evidence of osteoclastic activity (H-E x200). **g** Seeding of particle-laden macrophages in fatty marrow indicative of increased motility (H-E x100). **h** Large aggregate of lymphocytes positive for T-cell (CD3) and B-cell (CD20) marker (not shown) with interspersed particle laden macrophages, black arrows (H-E x 400)

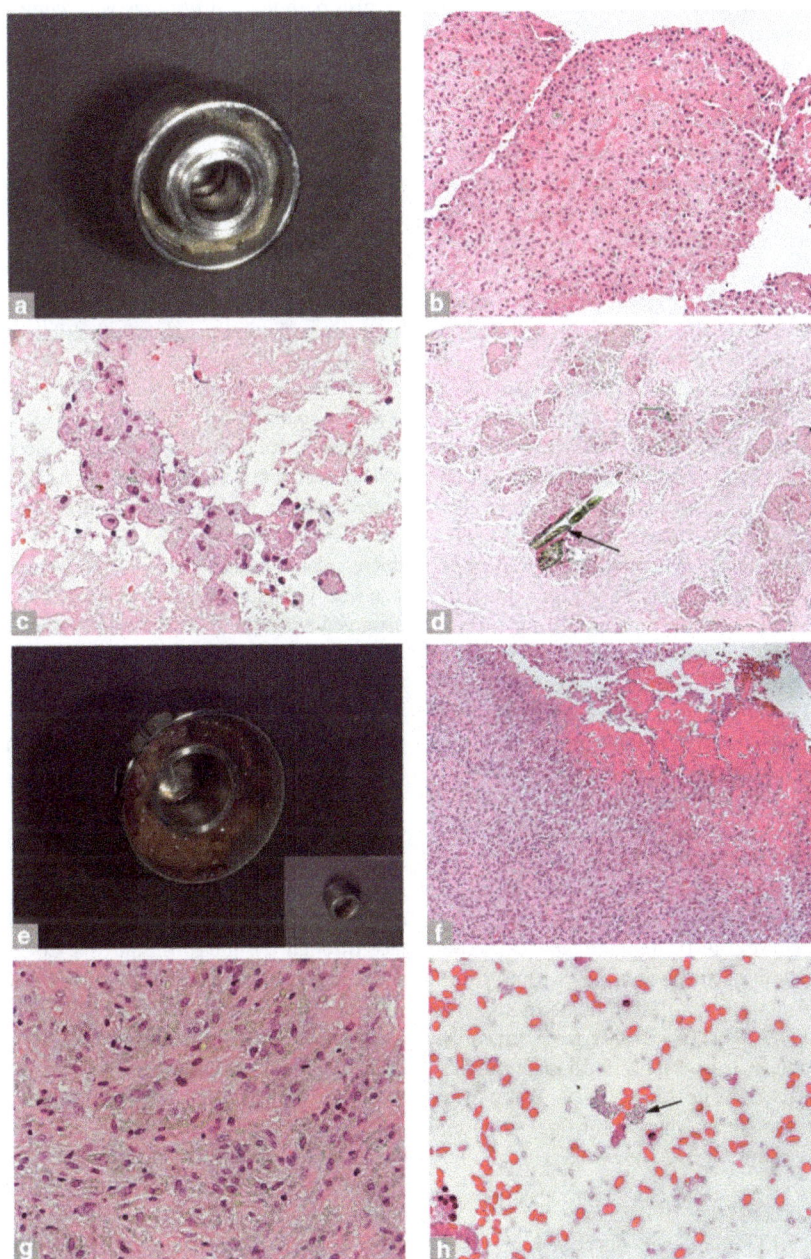

**Fig. 4** Features of macrophagic pattern in the MoM LHTHA group. **a** Metallic femoral head and inserted metallic adapter sleeve (MAS) with groove filled with dense necrotic cellular debris (DePuy ASR, implantation time 61 months). **b** Papillary neo-synovium with florid macrophagic infiltrate and superficial exfoliation of necrotic forms (H-E x200). **c** Mixture of viable and necrotic particle laden macrophages of necrotic cellular debris shown in (A). **d** Necrotic cellular debris with entrapped large aggregates of greenish particulate corrosion products, black arrow (H-E x400). **e** Metallic femoral head and separate MAS (inset) with groove filled with dense necrotic cellular debris (Smith and Nephew Birmingham, implantation time 44 months). **f** Neo-synovium with florid macrophagic infiltrate and marked exfoliation of necrotic cellular debris (H-E x100). **g** Detail of the macrophgic infiltrate containing globular and irregular aggregates of greenish particulate corrosion products (H-E x400). **h** Cluster of aggregates of pale green corrosion products particles detected in smeared synovial fluid pellet spun at 3,000 rpm x 15 min (H-E x 400)

(20 % of cases) and MoM LHTHA (17 % of cases), however without reaching significance ($p = 0.26$) (Table 6).

The observation of particles of conventional metallic debris was less common in the Non-MoM DMN THA (8 % of cases) relative to the MoM HRA (39 % of cases; $p < 0.0001$), the MoM LHTHA (30 % of cases) ($p < 0.0001$). Corrosion products were seen in either intracellular and/or extracellular locations in almost all cases in each group (Table 6). Extracellular aggregates of these corrosion products were less common in the MoM HRA group (11 % of cases) relative to the Non-MoM DMNTHA (74 % of cases; $p = 0.007$) and the MoM LHTHA (63 % of cases; $p = 0.007$) (Table 6). Examples of large aggregates are shown in two Non-MoM DMNTHAs (Fig. 5a and 5e) with similar histological appearance in the neo-synovial membrane (Fig. 5b and 5f). The large aggregates of particles of corrosion products with plate-like, stratified configuration were present on implant components (Fig. 5a, inset and 5e, lower inset), detachable from the surface (Fig. 5h), or embedded in periprosthetic tissue with breakdown in multinucleated giant cells (Fig. 5c and 5d) with or without a granulomatous histological pattern irrespective of implant bearing surface (Fig. 5g and 5d). Sarcoid-like granulomas were more likely to be present in the Non-MoM DMNTHA (16 % of cases) than in the MoM LHTHA (5 % of cases; $p = 0.013$) and MoM HRA (0 % of cases; $p = 0.013$) (Table 6).

Median Campbell (ALVAL) score was lower in implants with MoM bearing surfaces (MoM HRA, median score 5 and LHTHA, median score 6 relative to the Non-MoM DMNTHA, median score 8 ($p < 0.001$). A multinomial logistic regression was performed in order to examine the association between preoperative demographic variables (age, sex, BMI, implant type, duration of symptoms, duration of implantation) with Campbell's ALVAL score at revision. After adjustment, age ($p = 0.010$) and implant type ($p = 0.002$) were the only variables independently associated with Campbell's ALVAL score at revision. The MoM HRA group was an independent factor for a lower score at revision, using MoM bearing surfaces as a reference.

## Discussion

The occurrence of ALTR has been described in cases series for all three classes of implants analyzed in our study [4, 5, 13–15, 24, 27, 30, 32–46]. Recent reports have shown that the histological patterns of ALTR are more diverse than the original description of ALVAL and this complexity may result in different mechanisms of failure, which can have clinical implications for patient surveillance and outcomes after revision arthroplasty [13, 17, 20, 21, 29, 46]. The purposes of this study were to describe the frequency of different histopathological patterns of soft tissue failure in ALTR, their association with different implant class, and the association

of histopathological findings with clinical features of implant failure.

Our histological analysis demonstrates that ALTR encompasses a range of histological patterns ranging from purely macrophagic to mixed lymphocytic and macrophagic with or without features of associated with hypersensitivity (eosinophils/mast cells and/or lymphocytic germinal centers), and predominant sarcoid-like granulomas as previously described [13, 17, 19–21, 29, 46]. This is the largest study to the best of our knowledge to classify the histological patterns of ALTR across a diverse range of implants and its association to their clinical performance.

### Macrophagic pattern

Our results confirm that a macrophage predominant pattern of soft tissue failure exists in ALTR as previously reported, and it occurs more commonly in implants with MoM bearing surfaces [20, 21, 29]. We hypothesize that this is related to surface corrosion generating nanoparticle size wear debris unique to this bearing surface, as originally observed and later characterized by transmission and scanning microscopy [15, 18]. Phagocytosis/pinocytosis of metallic nanoparticle debris into cytoplasmic phagosomes with subsequent release of metallic ions has been shown to produce high level of oxidative stress in macrophages, resulting in a marked increase in reactive oxygen species promoting protein carbonylation, a well-known consequence of cellular oxidative stress, leading to a loss of biological function and ultimately cell death [47]. This process may be accelerated and enhanced by the addition of corrosion wear particles generated at the head-neck taper surface through the interposition of a CoCr metallic adapter sleeve. A proposed mechanism of implant failure of ALTR with the macrophagic pattern due to soft tissue and bone involvement exemplified for a MoM LHTHA is illustrated in Fig. 6. We hypothesize that massive corrosion product-associated macrophage apoptosis, exfoliation of necrotic cellular debris and phagocytized secondary wear particles into the joint fluid alters the bearing surface lubrication in implants with a MoM bearing surface. This failure mechanism would be difficult to replicate in any in-vitro tribology system or constructed tribocorrosion test apparatus [48, 49]. These alterations of the tribological film may lead to accelerated corrosion of the bearing surface and formation of abrasion-induced metallic wear. Clinically, this process may manifest as patient-reported mechanical symptoms that develop years after implantation along with increased serum metallic ion levels as the bearing surface is no longer properly lubricated. Previous studies have also shown that elevated metal ion levels occur due to implant misalignment; however, implant positioning does not account for many clinical failures, and this mechanism could provide an alternative explanation [50].

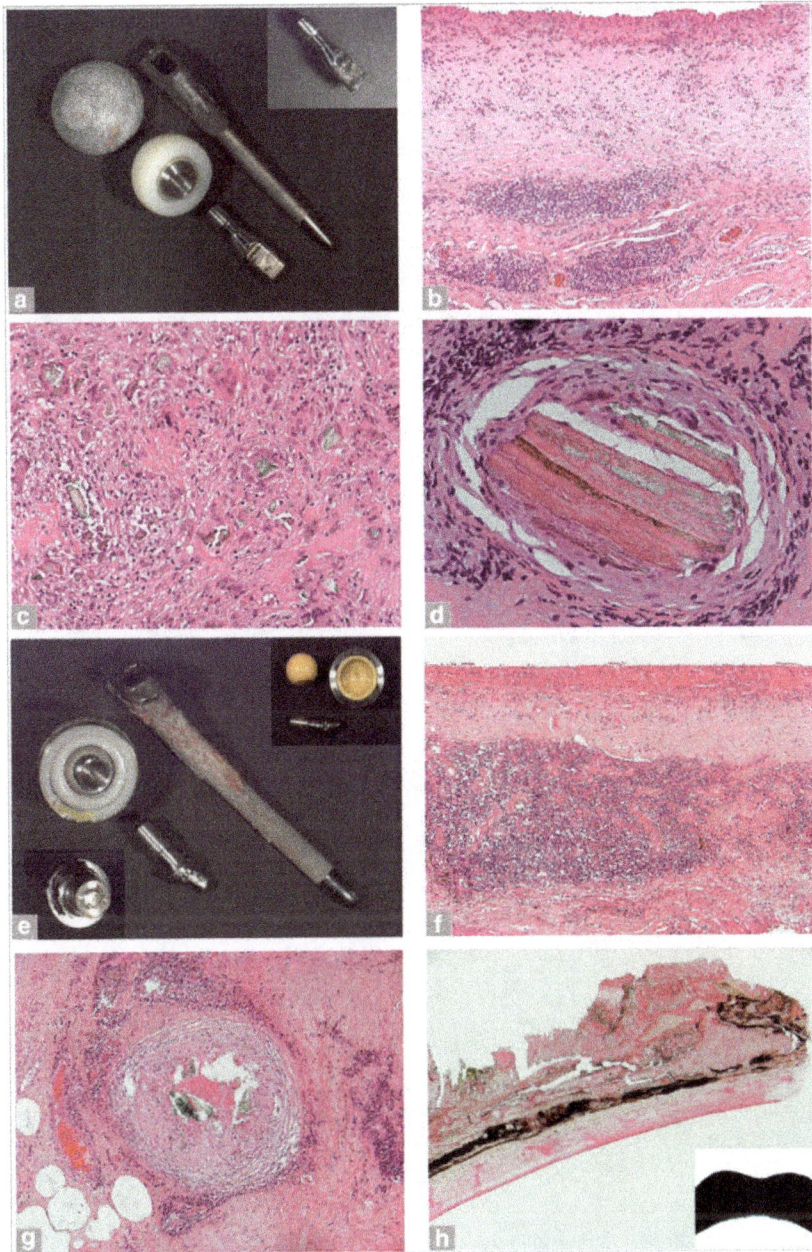

**Fig. 5** Features of corrosion products in the Non-MoM DMNTHA group. **a** MoP THA with CoCr dual exchangeable neck (inset) with corrosion on distal male taper (Stryker Rejuvenate, implantation time 20 months). **b** Neo-synovium showing superficial layer of macrophagic infiltrate and deep lymphocytic infiltrate (H-E x100). **c** Giant cell reaction without formation of granulomas to large aggregates of greenish and corrosion products (H-E x200). **d** Large aggregate of corrosion products with plate-like structure suggestive of layering of corrosion (greenish) and blood (reddish) products (H-E x400). **e** MoP THA with CoCr dual exchangeable neck with original CoC bearing surface and neck (inset, right upper corner) and second revision neck (inset, lower corner) with corrosion products on the male geared surface (OTI Encore, implantation time at first revision 36 months and at second revision 44 months from first revision). **f** Neo-synovium of first revision showing superficial layer of macrophagic infiltrate and dense layer of lymphocytic infiltrate (H-E x100). **g** Sarcoid-like granulomatous reaction with central green aggregates of corrosion products of second revision (H-E x100). **h** Large aggregate of layered corrosion products detached from the dual exchangeable neck (H-E x100) with scalloped shape of the gearing surface (inset)

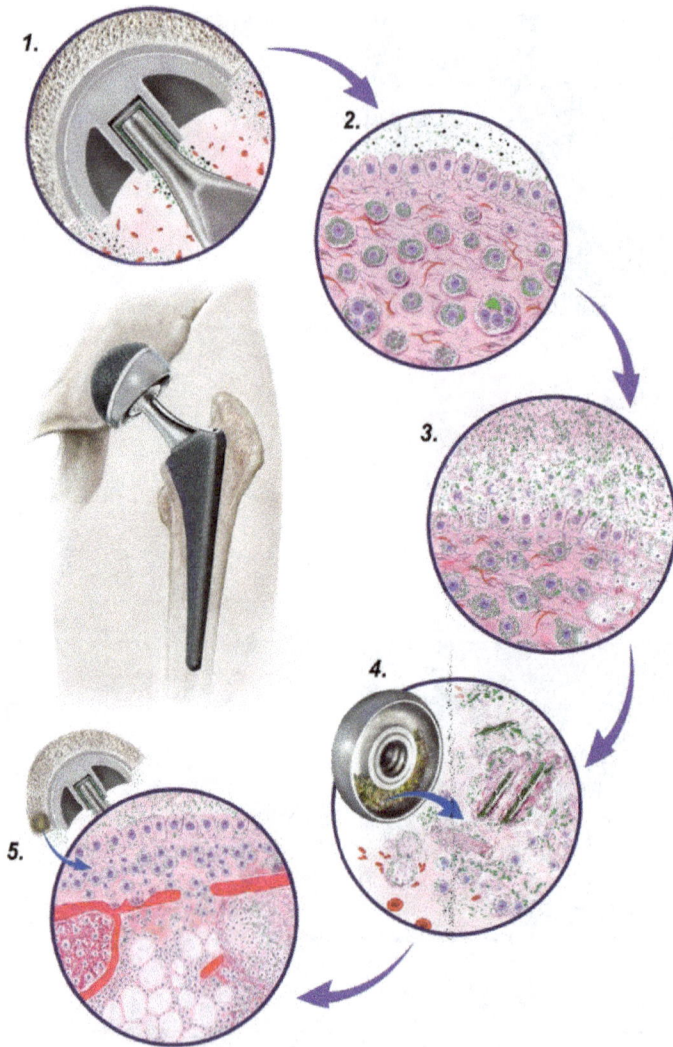

**Fig. 6** Phases of macrophagic pattern of ALTR in MoM LHTHA prosthesis. *Circle 1:* Nano-scale particles generated at the bearing surface by sliding tribocorrosion and nano and micron-scale at the metallic adapter sleeve-femoral neck surface by fretting/crevice corrosion where larger aggregates are formed. Conventional abrasion metallic wear can also be generated at the bearing surface by edge loading and/or neck junction at any time of implantation. *Circle 2:* Phagocytosis/pinocytosis of particulate material by neo-synovial superficial and deep layer macrophages with multinucleated giant cells containing large particulate aggregates. *Circle 3:* Massive apoptosis of neo-synovial particle-laden macrophages through oxidative stress with formation of degenerated foamy forms (right side) and release of necrotic cellular debris and secondary particles of corrosion products/abrasion metallic particles with disruption of cytoplasmic phagosomes. *Circle 4:* Accumulation of viable macrophages, necrotic cellular debris, red blood cells, and entrapped small and large aggregates of primary and secondary particles of corrosion products in the femoral head groove with substantial increase in thickness of the synovial fluid and subsequent modification of its lubrication properties. *Circle 5:* Bone marrow involvement by neo-synovial particle-laden macrophagic infiltrate through resorptive osteoblastic activity and direct invasion through cortical gaps with formation of osteolytic cavity (right side), diffuse seeding of the fatty marrow (middle area), and involvement of the hematopoietic marrow (left side)

The occurrence of macrophagic bone marrow infiltrate with or without associated histological evidence of osteolysis in the MoM HRA class may be explained by three different mechanisms: 1. The well- studied osteoclastic activation; 2. Increased macrophagic motility with mass burden necrosis and formation of pseudocystic cavities in the acetabular and/or femoral bones; 3. Penetration of corrosion particles and viable macrophages pushed by lubrication fluid pressure during motion. This component of the ALTR has been overlooked, but could become clinically significant with extended time of implantation and corrosion wear particle generation, especially for MoM HRA and MoM LHTHA groups [51, 52].

## Mixed macrophagic/lymphocytic pattern

Similar to previous studies, we found a mixed lymphocytic and macrophagic pattern to be common in ALTR however, within this group, the range of cellular infiltrates and tissue morphology suggests that individual variation exists within this pattern. Specifically, we have found the presence of mast cells/eosinophils and/or formation of lymphocytic germinal centers usually associated with tall endothelial cell venules in a subset of patients within this group. Mast cells are difficult to be identified in a crowded inflammatory background with conventional histology, although their presence has been previously demonstrated by immunohistochemistry [17]. The increased presence of mast cells, eosinophilic infiltrate, and lymphocytic germinal centers may be an expression of hypersensitivity/allergy to particulate conventional metallic or corrosion debris in certain subsets of patients. Previous authors have noted a weak correlation between wear characteristics and soft tissue response in a subgroup of patients with ALTR [29, 39]. Subsets of patients with evidence of neo-synovial tertiary lymphoid organs or sarcoid-like granulomas have been noted by previous authors, and these all may represent patient-specific variable immune responses to particulate corrosion debris [17, 19, 20]. Identification of patients with hypersensitivity to metal debris in joint replacement remains controversial because skin patch testing and lymphocyte transformation testing does not reliably predict patient-specific implant performance [53–55]. Systemic toxicity such as cardiomyopathy, neuropathy, and dermatological manifestations has been reported in limited case series, and these findings are typically associated with very high serum ion levels, particularly cobalt [56]. Recent work has shown a prominent up-regulation of interferon gamma associated chemokine expression in ALTR with a mixed lymphocytic and macrophagic pattern [57]. Activation of hypoxia-inducible factor secondary to cellular oxidative stress has also been implicated in this process [47, 58, 59]. Further studies on the molecular signaling pathways involved in ALTR are critical.

Similar to other non-specific foreign body responses, a pure lymphocytic pattern was not observed in our study, and macrophagic phagocytosis of wear particles is a key initial event. This activation of the innate immune system may or may not be associated with subsequent involvement of an adaptive immune response, which may in turn lead to further macrophagic recruitment [29]. We believe that the absence of particle laden macrophages in some reported cases may be related to tissue sampling rather than true absence of such cells from the affected tissues [21].

## Granulomatous pattern

The granulomatous pattern was observed in both THA groups with variable frequency and not in the MoM HRA group. We hypothesize that it requires the presence of large aggregates of particulate corrosion products, which is seldom present in the MoM HRA group. This pattern represents a distinctive patient-dependent macrophagic response which might be similar to the granulomatous reaction observed in sarcoidosis and triggered by exposure to various microbial agents.

## Use of Campbell's ALVAL scoring system

Currently, the Campbell's ALVAL score has been the primary method to assess ALTR in the periprosthetic soft tissue, showing good correlation with MRI studies [28, 60]. Using multinomial logistic regression, we found that implant configuration was associated with the Campbell's ALVAL score. In particular, hip resurfacing was associated with a lower score at revision for ALTR. In our experience the use of the score has limitations in ALTR because it is focused primarily on necrosis, scored twice in the synovial lining and tissue organization sections with a maximum of 3 points each, and the lymphocytic infiltrate, which is given a maximum of 4 points in a total maximum score of 10 [13]. The predominantly macrophagic pattern of soft tissue failure would produce low Campbell's ALVAL scores due to no or minimal lymphocytic infiltrate and no necrosis, but can still result in soft tissue arthroplasty failure. There is no grading of the macrophagic exfoliation and no consideration for macrophagic involvement with or without associated osteolysis in the femoral/acetabular bone marrow, which may have significant clinical implications for implant performance.

## Public health implications

Our study suggests that the histological analysis of periprosthetic tissue in cases of ALTR can provide information that may be useful for longitudinal monitoring of implants. For example, we found that mixed lymphocytic and granulomatous subtypes were associated with shorter durations of implantation and were more common in the MoM LHTHA and Non-MoM DMNTHA with a known occurrence of taper corrosion [5, 7–9, 27, 61, 62]. In contrast, the predominantly macrophagic pattern is more common in the MoM HRA group which generates nano-size corrosion/conventional metallic debris particles only at bearing surface.

The association between histological classification and time to revision may have clinical implications because implants with high number of patients with mixed macrophagic/lymphocytic pattern may fail earlier due to formation of pseudotumors with soft tissue necrosis, and this has resulted in implant recalls, such as the Stryker Rejuvenate and ABGII models. Implants with predominant macrophagic pattern, may fail at medium-long implantation time at an undetermined rate due to changes in the tribological lubrication process and/or macrophagic driven osteolysis. This unpredictable risk at the present time would call for a follow-up program with a frequency and modalities to be determined coupled with studies aiming at identifying biological and cellular factors associated with this type of adverse reaction [52, 63].

Our analysis showed that similar patterns of ALTR were present in implant classes of similar configuration and material composition independent of the manufacturer. This suggests the need for prompt observation and monitoring of any class of implants exhibiting a pattern of early failure with immediate reporting of sentinel cases to regulatory agencies/implant registries with the aim of avoiding high rates of complications for a large number of patients. Additionally, our results have made a case for the inclusion of the pathology report of revision cases in hospital based, regional, and national implant registries as an important and valuable tool in assessing modalities of implant failures along with the implementation of an international consensus classification, as the one recently reported for the periprosthetic soft tissue [64].

### Study limitations

We acknowledge several limitations with the current study. The first and most important is that our analysis is based on our hospital osteolysis/adverse local reaction tissue and repository database, which depends on the patient population admitted to the hospital and histological examination at surgical implant revision end-point. Our hospital serves as a tertiary referral center for revision arthroplasty cases; therefore, we cannot determine the overall class or device-specific implant performance from our data. The second is the attempt to reconstruct the natural history of the adverse reaction based on a single observation at the time of implant revision, although partially compensated for by the extensive tissue sampling. The third is the absence of the following sets of clinical data: a. physical activity pre and post-operative, although it has shown a weak correlation to elevated serum metal ion levels, suggesting that activity-related bearing surface wear plays only a minor role in elevated serum cobalt or chromium levels [65, 66]; b. pre and post-operative bone density, which may influence the occurrence/rate of implant mechanical loosening/osteolysis especially in the female population which requires a sophisticated method for proper assessment, such as high-spatial-resolution bone densitometry with dual-energy X-ray absorptiometric region-free analysis [67], which is not currently performed as standard of care at our institution; c. wear analysis by biomechanics examination of the metal-on-metal implants for surface roughness, although retrieval analysis and blood metal

measurements contribution to the understanding of ALTR has been previously addressed in a comprehensive review and no clear dose–response relationship between wear and ALTR could be established [68].

### Conclusions

ALTR encompasses a diverse range of histological patterns, which are reflective of both the implant configuration independent of manufacturer and clinical features such as duration of implantation. The predominant macrophagic pattern and its mechanism of implant failure represent an important subgroup of ALTR which could become more prominent with increased length of implantation. Further studies should characterize the physical and chemical characteristics of wear particles and the molecular characteristics of the generation and development of these different histological patterns of ALTR and relevant mechanisms of failure in different implant classes and/or specific devices.

### Abbreviations

THA: Total hip arthroplasty; ALVAL: Aseptic lymphocyte dominated vasculitis associated lesion; ALTR: Adverse local tissue reaction; ARMD: Adverse reaction to metallic debris; MoP: Metal-on-polyethylene; CoP: Ceramic-on-polyethylene; DMN: Dual modular neck; MoM: Metal-on-metal; LHTHA: Large head THA; HRA: Hip resurfacing arthroplasty.

### Competing interests

The authors declare they have no competing interests.

### Authors' contributions

BFR – data collection, pathological analysis, data interpretation, manuscript preparation. AAN – statistical analysis, manuscript preparation. SAJ – assist with data interpretation, manuscript preparation. GW – patient enrollment, data collection. EK – patient enrollment, data collection. SRG – assist with data interpretation and study conception, manuscript preparation. PEP – assist with data interpretation and study conception, manuscript preparation. GP – study conception, patient enrollment, pathological analysis, data interpretation, manuscript preparation. All authors read and approved the final manuscript.

### Acknowledgements

We would like to acknowledge the surgeons of the Adult Reconstruction and Joint Replacement Service at the Hospital for Special Surgery for providing periprosthetic tissue for this study; Irina Shuleshko and Yana Bronfman for technical assistance in histology preparation; Philip Rusli for technical assistance for preparation of the manuscript; and Randal McKenzie of McKenzie Illustrations for preparation of the medical illustration.

### Author details

[1]Department of Orthopedic Surgery, Hospital for Special Surgery, New York, NY, USA. [2]Healthcare Research Institute, Hospital for Special Surgery, New York, NY, USA. [3]Division of Research, Hospital for Special Surgery, New York, NY, USA. [4]Department of Pathology and Laboratory Medicine, Hospital for Special Surgery, 535 East 70th Street, New York, NY 10021, USA.

### References

1. Amstutz HC, Grigoris P. Metal on metal bearings in hip arthroplasty. Clin Orthop Relat Res. 1996;329(Suppl):S11–34.
2. Srinivasan A, Jung E, Levine BR. Modularity of the femoral component in total hip arthroplasty. J Am Acad Orthop Surg. 2012;20(4):214–22.

3. Werner PH, Ettema HB, Witt F, Morlock MM, Verheyen CC. Basic principles and uniform terminology for the head-neck junction in hip replacement. Hip Int. 2015;25(2):115–9.

4. Jacobs JJ, Gilbert JL, Urban RM. Corrosion of metal orthopaedic implants. J Bone Joint Surg Am. 1998;80(2):268–82.

5. Cooper HJ, Urban RM, Wixson RL, Meneghini RM, Jacobs JJ. Adverse local tissue reaction arising from corrosion at the femoral neck-body junction in a dual-taper stem with a cobalt-chromium modular neck. J Bone Joint Surg Am. 2013;95(10):865–72.

6. Khair MM, Nam D, DiCarlo E, Su E. Aseptic lymphocyte dominated vasculitis-associated lesion resulting from trunnion corrosion in a cobalt-chrome unipolar hemiarthroplasty. J Arthroplasty. 2013;28(1):196.e11–4.

7. Mao X, Tay GH, Godbolt DB, Crawford RW. Pseudotumor in a well-fixed metal-on-polyethylene uncemented hip arthroplasty. J Arthroplasty. 2012; 27(3):493.e13–7.

8. Munro JT, Masri BA, Duncan CP, Garbuz DS. High complication rate after revision of large-head metal-on-metal total hip arthroplasty. Clin Orthop Relat Res. 2014;472(2):523–8.

9. Witt F, Bosker BH, Bishop NE, Ettema HB, Verheyen CC, Morlock MM. The relation between titanium taper corrosion and cobalt-chromium bearing wear in large-head metal-on-metal total hip prostheses: a retrieval study. J Bone Joint Surg Am. 2014;96(18):e157.

10. Beaver Jr WB, Fehring TK. Abductor dysfunction and related sciatic nerve palsy, a new complication of metal-on-metal arthroplasty. J Arthroplasty. 2012;27(7):1414.e13–5.

11. Kayani B, Rahman J, Hanna SA, Cannon SR, Aston WJ, Miles J. Delayed sciatic nerve palsy following resurfacing hip arthroplasty caused by metal debris. BMJ Case Rep. 2012;2012.

12. Wyles CC, Van Demark 3rd RE, Sierra RJ, Trousdale RT. High rate of infection after aseptic revision of failed metal-on-metal total hip arthroplasty. Clin Orthop Relat Res. 2014;472(2):509–16.

13. Campbell P, Ebramzadeh E, Nelson S, Takamura K, De Smet K, Amstutz HC. Histological features of pseudotumor-like tissues from metal-on-metal hips. Clin Orthop Relat Res. 2010;468(9):2321–7.

14. Davies AP, Willert HG, Campbell PA, Learmonth ID, Case CP. An unusual lymphocytic perivascular infiltration in tissues around contemporary metal-on-metal joint replacements. J Bone Joint Surg Am. 2005;87:18–27.

15. Willert HG, Buchhorn GH, Fayyazi A, Flury R, Windler M, Köster G, et al. Metal-on-metal bearings and hypersensitivity in patients with artificial hip joints. A clinical and histomorphological study. J Bone Joint Surg Am. 2005;87:28–36.

16. Huber M, Reinisch G, Trettenhahn G, Zweymüller K, Lintner F. Presence of corrosion products and hypersensitivity-associated reactions in periprosthetic tissue after aseptic loosening of total hip replacements with metal bearing surfaces. Acta Biomater. 2009;5(1):172–80.

17. Perino G, Ricciardi BF, Jerabek SA, Martignoni G, Wilner G, Maass D, Goldring SR, Purdue PE. Implant based differences in adverse local tissue reaction in failed total hip arthroplasties: a morphological and immunohistochemical study. BMC Clin Pathol. 2014;14:39.

18. Xia Z, Kwon YM, Mehmood S, Downing C, Jurkschat K, Murray DW. Characterization of metal-wear nanoparticles in pseudotumor following metal-on-metal hip resurfacing. Nanomedicine. 2011;7(6):674–81.

19. Mittal S, Revell M, Barone F, Hardie DL, Matharu GS, Davenport AJ, et al. Lymphoid aggregates that resemble tertiary lymphoid organs define a specific pathological subset in metal-on-metal hip replacements. PLoS One. 2013;8(5):e63470.

20. Natu S, Sidaginamale RP, Gandhi J, Langton DJ, Nargol AV. Adverse reactions to metal debris: histopathological features of periprosthetic soft tissue reactions seen in association with failed metal on metal hip arthroplasties. J Clin Pathol. 2012;65(5):409–18.

21. Berstock JR, Baker RP, Bannister GC, Case CP. Histology of failed metal-on-metal hip arthroplasty; three distinct sub-types. Hip Int. 2014;24(3):243–8.

22. Enayatollahi MA, Parvizi J. Diagnosis of infected total hip arthroplasty. Hip Int. 2015;25(4):294–300.

23. Fehring TK, Odum S, Sproul R, Weathersbee J. High frequency of adverse local tissue reactions in asymptomatic patients with metal-on-metal THA. Clin Orthop Relat Res. 2014;472(2):517–22.

24. Junnila M, Seppänen M, Mokka J, Virolainen P, Pölönen T, Vahlberg T, et al. Adverse reaction to metal debris after Birmingham hip resurfacing arthroplasty. Acta Orthop. 2015;86(3):345–50.

25. Kiran M, Boscainos PJ. Adverse reactions to metal debris in metal-on-polyethylene total hip arthroplasty using a titanium-molybdenum-zirconium-iron alloy stem. J Arthroplasty. 2015;30(2):277–81.

26. Meyer H, Mueller T, Goldau G, Chamaon K, Ruetschi M, Lohmann CH. Corrosion at the cone/taper interface leads to failure of large-diameter metal-on-metal total hip arthroplasties. Clin Orthop Relat Res. 2012;470(11):3101–8.

27. Mokka J, Junnila M, Seppänen M, Virolainen P, Pölönen T, Vahlberg T, et al. Adverse reaction to metal debris after ReCap-M2A-Magnum large-diameter-head metal-on-metal total hip arthroplasty. Acta Orthop. 2013;84(6):549–54.

28. Nawabi DH, Gold S, Lyman S, Fields K, Padgett DE, Potter HG. MRI predicts ALVAL and tissue damage in metal-on-metal hip arthroplasty. Clin Orthop Relat Res. 2014;472(2):471–81.

29. Grammatopoulos G, Pandit H, Kamali A, Maggiani F, Glyn-Jones S, Gill HS, Murray DW, Athanasou N. The correlation of wear with histological features after failed hip resurfacing arthroplasty. J Bone Joint Surg Am. 2013;95:e81.

30. Mahendra G, Pandit H, Kliskey K, Murray D, Gill HS, Athanasou N. Necrotic and inflammatory changes in metal-on-metal resurfacing hip arthroplasties. Acta Orthop. 2009;80:653–9.

31. Jacobs JJ, Urban RM, Gilbert JL, Skipor AK, Black J, Jasty M, et al. Local and distant products from modularity. Clin Orthop Relat Res. 1995;319:94–105.

32. Barrett WP, Kindsfater KA, Lesko JP. Large-diameter modular metal-on-metal total hip arthroplasty: incidence of revision for adverse reaction to metallic debris. J Arthroplasty. 2012;27(6):976–83.e1.

33. Fabi D, Levine B, Paprosky W, Della Valle C, Sporer S, Klein G, et al. Metal-on-metal total hip arthroplasty: causes and high incidence of early failure. Orthopedics. 2012;35(7):e1009–16.

34. Gill IP, Webb J, Sloan K, Beaver RJ. Corrosion at the neck-stem junction as a cause of metal ion release and pseudotumour formation. J Bone Joint Surg Br. 2012;94(7):895–900.

35. Hasegawa M, Yoshida K, Wakabayashi H, Sudo A. Prevalence of adverse reactions to metal debris following metal-on-metal THA. Orthopedics. 2013; 36(5):e606–12.

36. Hinsch A, Vettorazzi E, Morlock MM, Rüther W, Amling M, Zustin J. Sex differences in the morphological failure patterns following hip resurfacing arthroplasty. BMC Med. 2011;9:113.

37. Langton DJ, Joyce TJ, Jameson SS, Lord J, Van Orsouw M, Holland JP, et al. Adverse reaction to metal debris following hip resurfacing: the influence of component type, orientation and volumetric wear. J Bone Joint Surg Br. 2011;93(2):164–71.

38. Langton DJ, Sidaginamale R, Lord JK, Nargol AV, Joyce TJ. Taper junction failure in large-diameter metal-on-metal bearings. Bone Joint Res. 2012;1(4): 56–63.

39. Matthies A, Underwood R, Cann P, Ilo K, Nawaz Z, Skinner J, et al. Retrieval analysis of 240 metal-on-metal hip components, comparing modular total hip replacement with hip resurfacing. J Bone Joint Surg Br. 2011;93(3):307–14.

40. Meftah M, Haleem AM, Burn MB, Smith KM, Incavo SJ. Early corrosion-related failure of the rejuvenate modular total hip replacement. J Bone Joint Surg Am. 2014;96(6):481–7.

41. Molloy DO, Munir S, Jack CM, Cross MB, Walter WL, Walter Sr WK. Fretting and corrosion in modular-neck total hip arthroplasty femoral stems. J Bone Joint Surg Am. 2014;96(6):488–93.

42. Nassif NA, Nawabi DH, Stoner K, Elpers M, Wright T, Padgett DE. Taper design affects failure of large-head metal-on-metal total hip replacements. Clin Orthop Relat Res. 2014;472(2):564–71.

43. Pandit H, Glyn-Jones S, McLardy-Smith P, Gundle R, Whitwell D, Gibbons CL, et al. Pseudotumours associated with metal-on-metal hip resurfacings. J Bone Joint Surg Br. 2008;90(7):847–51.

44. Silverton CD, Jacobs JJ, Devitt JW, Cooper HJ. Midterm results of a femoral stem with a modular neck design: clinical outcomes and metal ion analysis. J Arthroplasty. 2014;29(9):1768–73.

45. Vundelinckx BJ, Verhelst LA, De Schepper J. Taper corrosion in modular hip prostheses: analysis of serum metal ions in 19 patients. J Arthroplasty. 2013; 28(7):1218–23.

46. Phillips EA, Klein GR, Cates HE, Kurtz SM, Steinbeck M. Histological characterization of periprosthetic tissue responses for metal-on-metal hip replacement. J Long Term Eff Med Implants. 2014;24(1):13–23.

47. Scharf B, Clement CC, Zolla V, Perino G, Yan B, Elci SG, et al. Molecular analysis of chromium and cobalt-related toxicity. Sci Rep. 2014;4:5729.

48. Rieker CB, Schön R, Konrad R, Liebentritt G, Gnepf P, Shen M, et al. Influence of the clearance on in-vitro tribology of large diameter metal-on-metal articulations pertaining to resurfacing hip implants. Orthop Clin North Am. 2005;36(2):135–42. vii.

49. Mathew MT, Runa MJ, Laurent M, Jacobs JJ, Rocha LA, Wimmer MA. Tribocorrosion behavior of CoCrMo alloy for hip prosthesis as a function of

loads: a comparison between two testing systems. Wear. 2011;271(9–10): 1210–9.

50. Hart AJ, Skinner JA, Henckel J, Sampson B, Gordon F. Insufficient acetabular version increases blood metal ion levels after metal-on-metal hip resurfacing. Clin Orthop Relat Res. 2011;469(9):2590–7.

51. Asaad A, Hart A, Khoo MM, Ilo K, Schaller G, Black JD, Muirhead-Allwood S. Frequent femoral neck osteolysis with Birmingham mid-head resection resurfacing arthroplasty in young patients. Clin Orthop Relat Res. 2015; 473(12):3770–8.

52. Mont MA, Cherian JJ. CORR insights(®): frequent femoral neck osteolysis with Birmingham mid-head resection resurfacing arthroplasty in young patients. Clin Orthop Relat Res. 2015;473(12):3779–80.

53. Hallab NJ, Anderson S, Stafford T, Glant T, Jacobs JJ. Lymphocyte responses in patients with total hip arthroplasty. J Orthop Res. 2005;23(2):384–91.

54. Kwon YM, Thomas P, Summer B, Pandit H, Taylor A, Beard D, et al. Lymphocyte proliferation responses in patients with pseudotumors following metal-on-metal hip resurfacing arthroplasty. J Orthop Res. 2010; 28(4):444–50.

55. Thyssen JP, Menné T. Metal allergy–a review on exposures, penetration, genetics, prevalence, and clinical implications. Chem Res Toxicol. 2010;23(2): 309–18.

56. Bradberry SM, Wilkinson JM, Ferner RE. Systemic toxicity related to metal hip prostheses. Clin Toxicol (Phila). 2014;52(8):837–47.

57. Kolatat K, Perino G, Wilner G, Kaplowitz E, Ricciardi BF, Boettner F, et al. Adverse local tissue reaction (ALTR)associated with corrosion products in metal-on-metal and dual modular neck total hip replacements is associated with upregulation of interferon gamma-mediated chemokine signaling. J Orthop Res. 2015;33(10):1487–97.

58. Nyga A, Hart A, Tetley TD. Importance of the HIF pathway in cobalt nanoparticle-induced cytotoxicity and inflammation in human macrophages. Nanotoxicology. 2015;13:1–13.

59. Vanlangenakker N, Vanden Berghe T, Vandenabeele P. Many stimuli pull the necrotic trigger, an overview. Cell Death Differ. 2012;19(1):75–86. Epub 2011 Nov 11. Review.

60. Burge AJ, Gold SL, Lurie B, Nawabi DH, Fields KG, Koff MF, et al. MR imaging of adverse local tissue reactions around rejuvenate modular dual-taper stems. Radiology. 2015;1:141967.

61. Barry J, Lavigne M, Vendittoli PA. Evaluation of the method for analyzing chromium, cobalt and titanium ion levels in the blood following hip replacement with a metal-on-metal prosthesis. J Anal Toxicol. 2013;37(2):90–6.

62. DeMartino I, Assini JB, Elpers ME, Wright TM, Westrich GH. Corrosion and fretting of a modular hip system: a retrieval analysis of 60 rejuvenate stems. J Arthroplasty. 2015;30(8):1470–5.

63. Hart AJ, Sabah SA, Henckel J, Lloyd G, Skinner JA. Lessons learnt from metal-on-metal hip arthroplasties will lead to safer innovation for all medical devices. Hip Int. 2015;25(4):347–54.

64. Krenn V, Morawietz L, Perino G, Kienapfel H, Ascherl R, Hassenpflug GJ, et al. Revised histopathological consensus classification of joint implant related pathology. Pathol Res Pract. 2014;210(12):779–86.

65. Heisel C, Silva M, Skipor AK, Jacobs JJ, Schmalzried TP. The relationship between activity and ions in patients with metal-on-metal bearing hip prostheses. J Bone Joint Surg Am. 2005;87(4):781–7.

66. Khan M, Kuiper JH, Richardson JB. The exercise-related rise in plasma cobalt levels after metal-on-metal hip resurfacing arthroplasty. J Bone Joint Surg Br. 2008;90(9):1152–7.

67. Morris RM, Yang L, Martín-Fernández MA, Pozo JM, Frangi AF, Wilkinson JM. High-spatial-resolution bone densitometry with dual-energy X-ray absorptiometric region-free analysis. Radiology. 2015;274(2):532–9.

68. Campbell PA, Kung MS, Hsu AR, Jacobs JJ. Do retrieval analysis and blood metal measurements contribute to our understanding of adverse local tissue reactions? Clin Orthop Relat Res. 2014;472(12):3718–27.

# 14

# SOD2 immunoexpression predicts lymph node metastasis in penile cancer

Lara Termini[1*], José H Fregnani[2], Enrique Boccardo[3], Walter H da Costa[4], Adhemar Longatto-Filho[5,6,7], Maria A Andreoli[1], Maria C Costa[1], Ademar Lopes[4], Isabela W da Cunha[8], Fernando A Soares[8], Luisa L Villa[1,9] and Gustavo C Guimarães[4]

## Abstract

**Background:** Superoxide dismutase-2 (SOD2) is considered one of the most important antioxidant enzymes that regulate cellular redox state in normal and tumorigenic cells. Overexpression of this enzyme in lung, gastric, colorectal, breast cancer and cervical cancer malignant tumors has been observed. Its relationship with inguinal lymph node metastasis in penile cancer is unknown.

**Methods:** SOD2 protein expression levels were determined by immunohistochemistry in 125 usual type squamous cell carcinomas of the penis from a Brazilian cancer center. The casuistic has been characterized by means of descriptive statistics. An exploratory logistic regression has been proposed to evaluate the independent predictive factors of lymph node metastasis.

**Results:** SOD2 expression in more than 50% of cells was observed in 44.8% of primary penile carcinomas of the usual type. This expression pattern was associated with lymph node metastasis both in the uni and multivariate analysis.

**Conclusions:** Our results indicate that SOD2 expression predicts regional lymph node metastasis. The potential clinical implication of this observation warrants further studies.

**Keywords:** Penile cancer, Superoxide Dismutase-2, Lymph node metastasis

## Background

Malignant penile tumors are rare in developed countries but exhibit relatively high prevalence in some developing countries. Regional lymph node metastasis is one of the most important prognostic factors in patients with penile carcinoma due to its correlation with the advanced pathological stage of the tumor and tumor-related death [1]. Other factors affecting prognosis are histological grade, tumor thickness, perineural invasion, lymphovascular invasion and pattern of invasion [2,3].

About 50% of the cases in which palpable suspicious lymph node were present, subsequent pathologic analysis failed to find any evidence of metastatic disease in the lymph nodes [4,5]. Conversely, 20% of lymph nodes with no clinical signal of disease display micro metastases [6]. Therefore there is a need to identify other markers that may predict the occurrence of inguinal metastasis, perineural and vascular invasion. The use of these markers could be valuable to better define the subset of patients that will benefit from different therapeutic approaches [2-7].

Several studies have shown that superoxide dismutase 2 (SOD2 or manganese superoxide dismutase) protein expression is up-regulated in colorectal, lung, gastric/esophageal, and cervical cancer cells when compared to normal tissues [8-11]. However, the relationship between SOD2 expression and penile cancer has not been addressed, mainly in terms of regional lymph node metastasis. This study aimed to evaluate the association of SOD2 immunoexpression with inguinal lymph node metastasis and its clinical implication.

## Methods
### Tissue samples

Penile samples from 125 patients were obtained from the Department of Anatomic Pathology, Medical and

* Correspondence: terminilara@gmail.com
[1]Santa Casa de São Paulo, INCT-HPV at Santa Casa Research Institute, School of Medicine, Rua Marquês de Itú, 381, 01223-001 São Paulo, Brazil
Full list of author information is available at the end of the article

Research Center, A. C. Camargo Cancer Center, São Paulo, Brazil. No patient had distant metastasis at the diagnosis and all of them underwent tumor resection between 1953 and 2000. Lymphadenectomy has been performed in 50.4% of the cases and no patient received postoperative radiotherapy. Pathologic T stage was classified according to the TNM system of the International Union Against Cancer, 7th edition [12]. Ethical approval for this study was granted by the Hospital A.C. Camargo Institutional Research Ethics Committee (Project Number 1369/10).

Lymph node status has been defined using the pathologic information from the lymphadenectomy performed in 63 men (pN status). Patients who had not undergone lymph node resection had their lymph node status based on a retrospective longitudinal analysis of regional recurrence. Since no patient received inguinal or pelvic radiation as part of the treatment, those cases with no lymphadenectomy and no regional recurrence in a 3-year follow-up period had their lymph node status classified as "negative" (n = 46). Nevertheless, nine men without lymphadenectomy developed lymphonodal metastatic recurrence during follow-up after penectomy (median time to recurrence: 7.1 months; range: 1.4 – 22.1 months) and consequently they were considered as having "positive nodes" (tumor progression not previously detected). It was not possible to clearly define the regional lymph node status in seven cases with no previous lymphadenectomy. Although they did not have regional recurrence, the follow-up period was less than three years (median follow-up: 24.1 months; range: 8.7 – 35.8 months). These samples were not included in the uni and multivariate analyses.

## Immunohistochemical SOD2 detection

After deparaffinization in xylene and rehydration, antigen retrieval was performed by incubation in boiling citrate buffer pH 6.0 for 20 minutes. Endogenous peroxidase activity was inactivated with 3% hydrogen peroxide. Nonspecific avidin-binding was also blocked (DAKO, X0590, Carpinteria, CA, USA). Samples were incubated with an anti-SOD2 polyclonal antibody (Santa Cruz Biotechnology, sc-18504, Santa Cruz, CA, USA), 1:100 in 1% bovine serum albumin-phosphate buffered solution for 30 minutes at 37°C and for 18 hours at 4°C. Slides were then incubated for 30 minutes at 37°C with biotinylated rabbit anti-goat IgG, (Vector, BA5000, Burlingame, CA, USA) diluted 1:500, followed by incubation for 30 minutes at 37°C with the complex streptavidin and peroxidase (StreptABComplex/HRP Duet Mouse/Rabbit, DakoCytomation, K0492, Glostrup, Denmark), diluted 1:200 and developed using 100 mg of 3,3'-diaminobenzidine tetrahydrochloride (Sigma, D-5637, St Louis, MO, USA), 6% $H_2O_2$ in dimethyl sulphoxide

and counterstained with Harris' hematoxylin. Sections derived from an ovarian papillary serous adenocarcinoma were used as a positive control for SOD2 expression.

In order to verify the specimen quality for immunohistochemistry, all samples were also checked using a cytokeratin panel, which was positive in all cases. In addition, positivity rate of SOD2 expression was analyzed according to the year of patient's admission (1950–1959; 1960–1969; 1970–1979; 1980–1989; 1990–2000) and no statistically significant difference was found. Thus, specimen quality was considered adequate for analysis.

## Evaluation of tissue staining

Positive immunohistochemical reactions were evaluated considering the percentage of stained tumoral cells. Only tissue cores with more than 25% of tumor cells were analyzed. The evaluation was performed by examining the tumor core under X200 magnification. For the statistical analysis, reactions were scored as exhibiting less than 50% stained cells or more than 50% stained cells, as previously reported by our group [11]. Immunohistochemical evaluation was performed independently and blindly by two observers (ALF and FAS). The very few discordant results were discussed by both observers and a final score was established.

## Statistical analysis

The casuistic has been characterized by means of descriptive statistics. Fisher's exact test was employed to compare categorical variables in the univariate analysis. Exploratory logistic regression has been proposed to evaluate the independent predictive factors of inguinal lymph node metastasis. Variables with p value less than 0.10 were included in the multivariate model, which was conducted using a stepwise forward technique. The significance level was set at 5% for all tests.

## DNA extraction

For DNA extraction, several 5 μm sections of the paraffin-embedded samples were collected in 1.5-ml microtubes. Samples were treated with xylene and digested with proteinase-K according to standard protocols described previously [13]. The microtome blade was changed after each block was cut and all the surrounding area and apparatus were cleaned with xylene and ethanol after processing each sample to avoid contamination between the samples. DNA quality was checked by amplification of the human β-globin gene using PCO3+/PCO4+ primers [14].

## HPV typing

HPV detection and genotyping using generic primers (GP5+/GP6+) and type specific probes (6, 11, 16, 18, 31,

**Table 1 Characterization of the population study (n = 125)**

| Variable | Category | N | % |
|---|---|---|---|
| Age | <50 yo | 43 | 34.4 |
| | 50 – 59 yo | 41 | 32.8 |
| | ≥60 yo | 41 | 32.8 |
| pT (TNM) | pT1a | 7 | 5.6 |
| | pT1b | 4 | 3.2 |
| | pT2 | 52 | 41.6 |
| | pT3 | 57 | 45.6 |
| | pT4 | 5 | 4.0 |
| Palpable suspicious regional lymph node | No | 64 | 51.2 |
| | Yes | 59 | 47.2 |
| | Unknown | 2 | 1.6 |
| Regional lymph node status | No metastasis | 74 | 59.2 |
| | Metastasis | 44 | 35.2 |
| | Unknown | 7 | 5.6 |
| Pattern of invasion | Pushing | 14 | 11.2 |
| | Infiltrating | 101 | 80.8 |
| | Unknown | 10 | 8.0 |
| Histological grade | Grade 1 | 15 | 12.0 |
| | Grade 2 | 45 | 36.0 |
| | Grade 3 | 65 | 52.0 |
| Perineural invasion | No | 83 | 66.4 |
| | Yes | 35 | 28.0 |
| | Unknown | 7 | 5.6 |
| Vascular invasion | No | 85 | 68.0 |
| | Yes | 33 | 26.4 |
| | Unknown | 7 | 5.6 |
| Invasion of *corpora cavernous* | No | 22 | 17.6 |
| | Yes | 60 | 48.0 |
| | Missing data | 43 | 34.4 |
| Invasion of *corpora spongiosum* | No | 4 | 3.2 |
| | Yes | 88 | 70.4 |
| | Unknown | 33 | 26.4 |
| Invasion of urethra | No | 42 | 33.6 |
| | Yes | 28 | 22.4 |
| | Unknown | 55 | 44.0 |
| Tumor depth | ≤5 mm | 21 | 16.8 |
| | >5 mm | 92 | 73.6 |
| | Unknown | 12 | 9.6 |
| HPV detection | No | 99 | 79.2 |
| | Yes | 26 | 20.8 |
| SOD2 expression | <50% | 69 | 55.2 |
| | >50% | 56 | 44.8 |

33, 35, 39, 42, 45, 51, 52, 53, 54, 55, 56 and 58), respectively, was performed as previously described [15].

## Results

In the present study we have analyzed by immunohistochemistry the association of SOD2 expression pattern with different tumor aggressiveness and progression variables in 125 primary SCC samples of the usual histological type. Characterization of the population studied is depicted in Table 1. A representative immunostaining for SOD2 in different penile tumor samples exhibiting <50% or >50% stained cells is presented in Additional file 1. Most of the cases was classified as pT2 or pT3 (87.2%) and 44 cases had regional lymph node metastasis at diagnosis. No cases with distant metastasis were observed. Fifty six tumors (44.8%) had SOD2 expression greater than 50%. In about 20% of the cases HPV infection was detected [see Additional file 2]. No relationship was observed between presence of HPV DNA and SOD2 expression (Table 2).

Table 3 shows the regional lymph node status according to the clinical and pathological variables. In the bivariate analysis, metastatic node was associated with palpable suspicious lymph node in the clinical exam (P < 0.001), tumor size (P = 0.045), histological grade (P = 0.013), perineural invasion (P < 0.001), vascular invasion (P = 0.010), tumor depth (P = 0.002) and SOD2 expression (P = 0.002). All these variables were included in the exploratory logistic regression (Table 4), which identified the following independent predictive factors of lymph node metastasis: palpable suspicious nodes (OR = 8.9; 95% CI: 2.7 – 29.2), tumor depth greater than 5 mm (OR = 11.6; 95% CI: 1.4 – 97.1), perineural invasion (OR = 9.6; 95% CI: 2.7 – 33.6) and SOD2 expression greater than 50% (OR = 3.4; 95% CI: 1.1 – 10.1).

**Table 2 Number and percentage of cases according to HPV genotype and SOD2 expression**

| HPV genotype (*) | Category | SOD2 < 50% N | SOD2 < 50% (%) | SOD2 > 50% N | SOD2 > 50% (%) | P value |
|---|---|---|---|---|---|---|
| HPV-16 | No | 59 | (54.6) | 49 | (45.4) | 0.799 |
| | Yes | 10 | (58.8) | 7 | (41.2) | |
| HPV-18 | No | 64 | (54.2) | 54 | (45.8) | 0.458 |
| | Yes | 5 | (71.4) | 2 | (28.6) | |
| HPV non-16/non-18 | No | 67 | (55.8) | 53 | (44.2) | 0.656 |
| | Yes | 2 | (40.0) | 3 | (60.0) | |
| High risk HPV | No | 54 | (53.5) | 47 | (46.5) | 0.497 |
| | Yes | 15 | (62.5) | 9 | (37.5) | |

(*) HPV-16 (n = 17), HPV-18 (n = 7); HPV-11 (n = 3); HPV-6 (n = 3); HPV-35 (n = 1); HPV-39 (n = 1). HPV co-infection has been registered in four cases: HPV-6, 11 (n = 2); HPV 6, 11 and 16 (n = 1); HPV-16, 18 and 39 (n = 1).

**Table 3 Number and percentage of cases with and without regional lymph node metastasis according to clinical and pathological variables**

| Variable | Category | No lymph node metastasis | | Lymph node metastasis | | P value |
|---|---|---|---|---|---|---|
| | | N | (%) | N | (%) | |
| Age | < 50 yo | 26 | (65.0) | 14 | (35.0) | 0.682 |
| | 50 – 59 yo | 27 | (65.9) | 14 | (34.1) | |
| | ≥60 yo | 21 | (56.8) | 16 | (43.2) | |
| Palpable suspicious regional | No | 48 | (84.2) | 9 | (15.8) | <0.001 |
| Lymph node | Yes | 24 | (40.7) | 35 | (59.3) | |
| pT (TNM) | pT1a | 7 | (100.0) | 0 | (0.0) | 0.045 |
| | > pT1a | 67 | (60.4) | 44 | (39.6) | |
| Pattern of invasion | Pushing | 6 | (46.2) | 7 | (53.8) | 0.368 |
| | Infiltrating | 60 | (61.9) | 37 | (38.1) | |
| Histological grade | Grade 1 | 13 | (86.7) | 2 | (13.3) | 0.013 |
| | Grade 2 | 30 | (71.4) | 12 | (28.6) | |
| | Grade 3 | 31 | (50.8) | 30 | (49.2) | |
| Perineural invasion | No | 59 | (75.6) | 19 | (24.4) | <0.001 |
| | Yes | 9 | (26.5) | 25 | (73.5) | |
| Vascular invasion | No | 55 | (68.8) | 25 | (31.2) | 0.010 |
| | Yes | 13 | (40.6) | 19 | (59.4) | |
| Invasion of *corpora cavernous* | No | 14 | (66.7) | 7 | (33.3) | 0.303 |
| | Yes | 28 | (50.9) | 27 | (49.1) | |
| Invasion of *corpora spongiosum* | No | 3 | (75.0) | 1 | (25.0) | 1.000 |
| | Yes | 50 | (60.2) | 33 | (39.8) | |
| Invasion of urethra | No | 26 | (66.7) | 13 | (33.3) | 0.436 |
| | Yes | 14 | (56.0) | 11 | (44.0) | |
| Tumor depth | ≤5 mm | 18 | (90.0) | 2 | (10.0) | 0.002 |
| | >5 mm | 44 | (51.2) | 42 | (48.8) | |
| HPV-16 | No | 64 | (62.1) | 39 | (37.9) | 1.000 |
| | Yes | 10 | (66.7) | 5 | (33.3) | |
| HPV-18 | No | 68 | (61.3) | 43 | (38.7) | 0.255 |
| | Yes | 6 | (85.7) | 1 | (14.3) | |
| SOD2 expression | <50% | 49 | (75.4) | 16 | (24.6) | 0.002 |
| | >50% | 25 | (47.2) | 28 | (52.8) | |

Table 5 summarizes the patient's distribution according to the four predictive factors of inguinal lymph node metastasis found in the multivariate model.

## Discussion

To the best of our knowledge, this is the first study analyzing the expression of SOD2 in a large series of penile carcinoma samples. SOD2 is one of three distinct superoxide dismutases isoforms found in mammals. This protein is found generally in the mitochondrial matrix and is an evolutionary conserved enzyme in a variety of organisms. Superoxide dismutases act as part of the cellular antioxidant system protecting the redox sensitive cellular machinery from damage induced by reactive oxygen species (ROS). This enzyme's activity affects important cellular processes including cell growth, proliferation and differentiation. As a consequence the role of SOD2 in cancer is complex and multifactorial. In fact, the exact role of SOD2 and redox state in cancer onset and progression remains poorly understood. Interestingly, accumulating evidence suggest that reducing oxidative stress levels by increasing SOD2 expression may represent a double-edged sword in tumor development. Reducing oxidative stress may have anti-tumoral effect by preventing DNA damage. This is supported by the observation that SOD2 expression can reduce the

**Table 4 Predictive factors for regional lymph node metastasis according to the exploratory logistic regression**

| Variable | Category | N | Adjusted OR (*) | 95% CI | P value |
|---|---|---|---|---|---|
| Palpable suspicious regional lymph node | No | 49 | 1.0 | Reference | |
| | Yes | 55 | 8.9 | 2.7 – 29.2 | <0.001 |
| Tumor depth | ≤5 mm | 20 | 1.0 | Reference | |
| | >5 mm | 84 | 11.6 | 1.4 – 97.1 | 0.023 |
| Perineural invasion | No | 71 | 1.0 | Reference | |
| | Yes | 33 | 9.6 | 2.7 – 33.6 | <0.001 |
| SOD2 expression | <50% | 57 | 1.0 | Reference | |
| | >50% | 47 | 3.4 | 1.1 – 10.1 | 0.029 |

(*) Number of outcomes included in the analysis: 44 (regional lymph node metastasis).
OR: Odds ratio 95% CI: 95% confidence interval.

**Table 5 Distribution of patients according to the combination of the predictive factors of inguinal lymph node metastasis found in the multivariate model**

| Palpable suspicious lymph node | Tumor depth | Perineural invasion | SOD2 expression (>50%) | Patients at risk n | Patients with inguinal lymph node metastasis | |
|---|---|---|---|---|---|---|
| | | | | | n | (%) |
| No (*1) | ≤5 mm | Absent | - | 9 | 0 | (0.0) |
| | | Absent | + | 4 | 0 | (0.0) |
| | | Present | - | 2 | 0 | (0.0) |
| | | Present | + | 0 | NA | NA |
| | >5 mm | Absent | - | 15 | 2 | (13.3) |
| | | Absent | + | 10 | 2 | (20.0) |
| | | Present | - | 2 | 0 | (0.0) |
| | | Present | + | 7 | 5 | (71.4) |
| Yes (*2) | ≤5 mm | Absent | - | 2 | 0 | (0.0) |
| | | Absent | + | 0 | NA | NA |
| | | Present | - | 1 | 0 | (0.0) |
| | | Present | + | 2 | 2 | (100.0) |
| | >5 mm | Absent | - | 19 | 7 | (36.8) |
| | | Absent | + | 12 | 8 | (66.7) |
| | | Present | - | 7 | 7 | (100.0) |
| | | Present | + | 12 | 11 | (91.7) |
| All cases (*3) | ≤5 mm | Absent | - | 11 | 0 | (0.0) |
| | | Absent | + | 4 | 0 | (0.0) |
| | | Present | - | 3 | 0 | (0.0) |
| | | Present | + | 2 | 2 | (100.0) |
| | >5 mm | Absent | - | 34 | 9 | (26.5) |
| | | Absent | + | 24 | 10 | (41.7) |
| | | Present | - | 9 | 7 | (77.8) |
| | | Present | + | 19 | 16 | (84.2) |

NA: Data not available since any case was observed in this situation.
(*1) Eight cases were not included in this group because they did have either tumor depth or perineural information. SOD2 expression was positive in three of them. All those cases had no lymph node metastasis.
(*2) Four cases were not included in this group because they did have either tumor depth or perineural information. SOD2 expression was positive in one of them. All those cases had no lymph node metastasis.
(*3) Two cases with unknown clinical status of inguinal nodes were included in this group. Both cases had tumor depth > 5 mm, no perineural invasion, positive SOD2 expression and no lymph node metastasis.

malignant potential of several transformed cell lines [10,16]. Conversely, it can be anticipated that SOD2 up-regulation may reduce the level of ROS in tumor cells. This may prevent the accumulation of life incompatible levels of DNA and other macromolecules damage, protecting neoplastic cells from intrinsic cell death mechanisms and favoring their survival and spread [8,9].

Analysis of SOD2 expression conducted in solid tumor samples including colorectal [17,18], gastric and esophageal [19,20], oral [21], lung [22-24], brain [25], cervical [11] and skin [26] carcinomas have often associated its up-regulation with metastasis and poor disease outcome. The molecular mechanisms underlying increased SOD2 and metastasis include the alteration of several cellular pathways. It has been observed that SOD2 overexpression increases matrix metalloproteinases (MMPs)-1, -2, -3, -7, -10, -9 and -11 mRNA levels. In the case of MMP-1 this has been attributed to the activation of the Ras/MAP/extracellular signal-regulated kinase signaling cascade. In the same study SOD2 upregulation was associated with enhanced metastatic potential of fibrosarcoma cells in an animal model [27]. Since MMPs play a critical role in the metastatic process it can be argued that the association between increased SOD2 and poor prognosis observed in certain tumors may be attributed to elevated MMP production/activity. A recent study showed that SOD2 expression was sufficient to overcome ROS mediated growth arrest in prostate carcinoma cells [28]. Besides it was observed that elevated SOD2 levels confer resistance to ROS mediated anoikis in mammary epithelial cells in a process dependent on NFκB activation [29]. Since anoikis resistance is essential for tumor metastasis the anti-anoikis activity of SOD2 implicates this enzyme in the metastatic process. We can, therefore, speculate that increased SOD2 levels may confer an adaptive advantage to tumor cells favoring disease establishment and progression.

We have previously reported that SOD2 is differentially expressed between normal and HPV immortalized keratinocytes [30]. Furthermore, we have recently shown that SOD2 protein expression level is a potential biomarker for the characterization of different stages of cervical neoplasia, which is etiologically linked with infection with high-risk HPV types [11]. A proportion of penile cancers are also associated with HPV, mostly HPV16. In fact, recent evidence suggests that these viruses, particularly HPV16, may be associated with up to 48% of all penile tumors [31].

In the present study no association between SOD2 expression and HPV infection was observed. HPV DNA was detected in 20.8% of the samples analyzed which is below the HPV positivity data reported by others [31,32]. This result is not due to quality of the DNA

recovered from the paraffinized specimens since >98% of them tested positive for globin. The low proportion of HPV-positive specimens detected probably reflects the fact that in our study most of the samples analyzed are of SCC of the usual histological type, which is less frequently associated with HPV infection. Using exploratory logistic regression we observed that SOD2 expression in more than 50% of the cells was an independent predictive factor of lymph node metastasis as were other well documented clinical-pathologic variables such as palpable suspicious nodes, tumor depth >5 mm and perineural invasion [33-36].

Although SOD2 expression was clearly an independent predictive factor of inguinal lymph node metastasis in the multivariate model, its real contribution in clinical practice remains to be determined. Table 5 demonstrates that tumor depth information is able to determine itself the presence of node metastasis, regardless the status of inguinal node in the clinical exam and perineural invasion status. Our results show that SOD2 expression has some value by increasing the risk of metastasis when the tumor depth was greater than 5 mm. All cases of inguinal metastasis, but two, occurred when the tumor depth was greater than 5 mm. Interestingly, the two cases in which lymph node metastasis was observed when tumor depth was less than 5 mm had positive SOD2 immunoexpression. Coincidently, those cases had palpable suspicious lymph nodes in inguinal clinical exam. The implication of SOD2 expression in thin penile tumors is uncertain and should be interpreted with caution because a limited number of cases in this particular setting were observed. However, the potential clinical implications of this observation as well as the contribution of SOD2 assessment in clinical practice warrants further studies.

## Conclusions
SOD2 expression predicts regional lymph node metastasis in usual type squamous cell carcinomas of the penis. Further studies are needed to determine the clinical implication of this factor.

## Additional files

**Additional file 1: Immunohistochemical analysis of SOD2 Expression in penile samples.** Representative immunoreactivity of SOD2 in normal penile epithelium (A) and usual penile squamous cell carcinomas (B-D). Less than 50% of stained cells were observed in (B) while (C) and (D) showed more than 50% of stained cells. Magnification: 200x.

**Additional file 2: Frequency of HPV types in penile SCC samples.** Frequency of HPV types in penile SCC samples.

**Abbreviations**
HPV: Human papillomavirus; ROS: Reactive oxygen species; SOD2: Superoxide dismutase 2 or manganese superoxide dismutase.

## Competing interests

The authors declare that they have no competing interests.

## Authors' contributions

LT conceived the study, participated in its design, was involved in immunohistochemical reactions, manuscript preparation and results discussion. JHF carried out statistical analysis, manuscript drafting and results discussion. EB was involved in co-ordination of the study, in manuscript drafting and results discussion. WHC was involved with statistical analysis and manuscript drafting. AL-F, IWC and FAS performed the revision and classification of all histopathological samples, and gave critical assistance in the Discussion section. MAA and MCC were involved HPV genotyping and immunohistochemical reactions. AL and GCG carried out data bank administration, including patients' clinical follow up data/samples collection. LLV participated in the study design and co-ordination. All authors have read and approved the final version of the manuscript.

## Acknowledgements

We are grateful to Carlos Ferreira do Nascimento, Severino Ferreira, Romulo Akira, Luciane Tsukamoto Kagohara and Suely Nonogaki from the A. C. Camargo Cancer Center, São Paulo, Brazil for technical assistance. Financial support: Dr. Lara Termini (FAPESP 2005/57274-9); Dr. Luisa Lina Villa (FAPESP 2008/57889-1 and CNPq 573799/2008-3).

## Author details

[1]Santa Casa de São Paulo, INCT-HPV at Santa Casa Research Institute, School of Medicine, Rua Marquês de Itú, 381, 01223-001 São Paulo, Brazil. [2]Teaching and Research Institute, Barretos Cancer Hospital, Rua Antenor Duarte Vilela, 1331, 14784-006 Barretos, Brazil. [3]Department of Microbiology, Institute of Biomedical Sciences, University of São Paulo, Av. Prof. Lineu Prestes, 1374 - Ed. Biomédicas II, Cidade Universitária, 05508-900 São Paulo, Brazil. [4]Pelvic Surgery Department, A. C. Camargo Cancer Center, Rua Prof. Antônio Prudente 211, 01509-010 São Paulo, Brazil. [5]Laboratory of Medical Investigation (LIM) 14, Department of Pathology, School of Medicine, University of São Paulo, Av. Dr. Arnaldo 455, 01246-903 São Paulo, Brazil. [6]Life and Health Sciences Research Institute, School of Health Sciences, ICVS/3B's - PT Government Associate Laboratory, University of Minho, Braga, Guimarães, Portugal. [7]Molecular Oncology Research Center, Barretos Cancer Hospital, Pio XII Foundation, Barretos, Rua Antenor Duarte Villela, 1331, 14784-400 Barretos, Brazil. [8]Department of Anatomic Pathology, A. C. Camargo Cancer Center, Rua Prof. Antônio Prudente 109, 01509-900 São Paulo, Brazil. [9]Department of Radiology and Oncology, School of Medicine, University of São Paulo and Cancer Institute of the State of São Paulo, ICESP, Av Dr Arnaldo 250, 01246-000 São Paulo, Brazil.

## References

1. Guimarães GC, Rocha RM, Zequi SC, Cunha IW, Soares FA. Penile cancer: epidemiology and treatment. Curr Oncol Rep. 2011;13(3):231–9.
2. Guimarães GC, Lopes A, Campos RS, Zequi S d C, Leal ML, Carvalho AL, et al. Front pattern of invasion in squamous cell carcinoma of the penis: new prognostic factor for predicting risk of lymph node metastases. Urology. 2006;68(1):148–53.
3. Chaux A, Caballero C, Soares F, Guimarães GC, Cunha IW, Reuter V, et al. The prognostic index: a useful pathologic guide for prediction of nodal metastases and survival in penile squamous cell carcinoma. Am J Surg Pathol. 2009;33(7):1049–57.
4. Guimarães GC, Cunha IW, Soares FA, Lopes A, Torres J, Chaux A, et al. Penile squamous cell carcinoma clinicopathological features, nodal metastasis and outcome in 333 cases. J Urol. 2009;182(2):528–34.
5. Zhu Y, Zhang HL, Yao XD, Zhang SL, Dai B, Shen YJ, et al. Development and evaluation of a nomogram to predict inguinal lymph node metastasis in patients with penile cancer and clinically negative lymph nodes. J Urol. 2010;184(2):539–45.
6. Pompeo AC. Extended lymphadenectomy in penile cancer. Can J Urol. 2005;1:30–6. discussion 97–8.
7. Velazquez EF, Ayala G, Liu H, Chaux A, Zanotti M, Torres J, et al. Histologic grade and perineural invasion are more important than tumor thickness as predictor of nodal metastasis in penile squamous cell carcinoma invading 5 to 10 mm. Am J Surg Pathol. 2008;32(7):974–9.
8. Holley AK, Dhar SK, Xu Y, St Clair DK. Manganese superoxide dismutase: beyond life and death. Amino Acids. 2012;42(1):139–58.
9. Johnson F, Giulivi C. Superoxide dismutases and their impact upon human health. Mol Aspects Med. 2005;26(4–5):340–52.
10. Kinnula VL, Crapo JD. Superoxide dismutases in malignant cells and human tumors. Free Radic Biol Med. 2004;36(6):718–44.
11. Termini L, Filho AL, Maciag PC, Etlinger D, Alves VA, Nonogaki S, et al. Deregulated expression of superoxide dismutase-2 correlates with different stages of cervical neoplasia. Dis Markers. 2011;30(6):275–81.
12. American Joint Committee on Cancer. Penis, in AJCC Cancer Staging Handbook. 7th ed. New York: Springer; 2010. p. 447.
13. Shi SR, Cote RJ, Wu L, Liu C, Datar R, Shi Y, et al. DNA extraction from archival formalin-fixed, paraffin-embedded tissue sections based on the antigen retrieval principle: heating under the influence of pH. J Histochem Cytochem. 2002;50(8):1005–11.
14. Saiki RK, Scharf S, Faloona F, Mullis KB, Horn GT, Erlich HA, et al. Enzymatic amplification of beta-globin genomic sequences and restriction site analysis for diagnosis of sickle cell anemia. Science. 1985;230(4732):1350–4.
15. de Roda Husman AM, Walboomers JM, van den Brule AJ, Meijer CJ, Snijders PJ. The use of general primers GP5 and GP6 elongated at their 3' ends with adjacent highly conserved sequences improves human papillomavirus detection by PCR. J Gen Virol. 1995;76(Pt4):1057–62.
16. Ough M, Lewis A, Zhang Y, Hinkhouse MM, Ritchie JM, Oberley LW, et al. Inhibition of cell growth by overexpression of manganese superoxide dismutase (MnSOD) in human pancreatic carcinoma. Free Radic Res. 2004;38(11):1223–33.
17. Toh Y, Kuninaka S, Oshiro T, Ikeda Y, Nakashima H, Baba H, et al. Overexpression of manganese superoxide dismutase mRNA may correlate with aggressiveness in gastric and colorectal adenocarcinomas. Int J Oncol. 2000;17(1):107–12.
18. Janssen AM, Bosman CB, Kruidenier L, Griffioen G, Lamers CB, van Krieken JH, et al. Superoxide dismutases in the human colorectal cancer sequence. J Cancer Res Clin Oncol. 1999;125(6):327–35.
19. Janssen AM, Bosman CB, van Duijn W, Oostendorp-van de Ruit MM, Kubben FJ, Griffioen G, et al. Superoxide dismutases in gastric and esophageal cancer and the prognostic impact in gastric cancer. Clin Cancer Res. 2000;6(8):3183–92.
20. Hwang TS, Choi HK, Han HS. Differential expression of manganese superoxide dismutase, copper/zinc superoxide dismutase, and catalase in gastric adenocarcinomas and normal gastric mucosa. Eur J Surg Oncol. 2007;33(4):474–9.
21. Liu X, Wang A, Lo Muzio L, Kolokythas A, Sheng S, Rubini C, et al. Deregulation of manganese superoxide dismutase (SOD2) expression and lymph node metastasis in tongue squamous cell carcinoma. BMC Cancer. 2010;10:365.
22. Ho JC-m, Zheng S, Comhair SA, Farver C, Erzurum SC. Differential expression of manganese superoxide dismutase and catalase in lung cancer. Cancer Res. 2001;61(23):8578–85.
23. Kinnula VL, Crapo JD. Superoxide dismutases in the lung and human lung diseases. Am J Respir Crit Care Med. 2003;167(12):1600–19.
24. Svensk AM, Soini Y, Pääkkö P, Hiravikoski P, Kinnula VL. Differential expression of superoxide dismutases in lung cancer. Am J Clin Pathol. 2004;122(3):395–404.
25. Haapasalo H, Kyläniemi M, Paunul N, Kinnula VL, Soini Y. Expression of antioxidant enzymes in astrocytic brain tumors. Brain Pathol. 2003;13(2):155–64.
26. St Clair D, Zhao Y, Chaiswing L, Oberley T. Modulation of skin tumorigenesis by SOD. Biomed Pharmacother. 2005;59(4):209–14.
27. Nelson KK, Ranganathan AC, Mansouri J, Rodriguez AM, Providence KM, Rutter JL, et al. Elevated SOD2 activity augments matrix metalloproteinase expression: evidence for the involvement of endogenous hydrogen peroxide in regulating metastasis. Clin Cancer Res. 2003;9(1):424–32.
28. Das TP, Suman S, Damodaran C. Reactive oxygen species generation inhibits epithelial-mesenchymal transition and promotes growth arrest in prostate cancer cells. Mol Carcinog. 2014;53(7):537–47.
29. Kamarajugadda S, Cai Q, Chen H, Nayak S, Zhu J, He M, et al. Manganese superoxide dismutase promotes anoikis resistance and tumor metastasis. Cell Death Dis. 2013;4:e504.
30. Termini L, Boccardo E, Esteves GH, Hirata Jr R, Martins WK, Colo AE, et al. Characterization of global transcription profile of normal and HPV-immortalized keratinocytes and their response to TNF treatment. BMC Med Genomics. 2008;1:29.

31. Chaux A, Cubilla AL. The role of human papillomavirus infection in the pathogenesis of penile squamous cell carcinomas. Semin Diagn Pathol. 2012;29(2):67–71.
32. Anic GM, Giuliano AR. Genital HPV infection and related lesions in men. Prev Med. 2011;53:36–41.
33. Pizzocaro G, Algaba F, Horenblas S, Solsona E, Tana S, Van Der Poel H, et al. EAU penile cancer guidelines 2009. Eur Urol. 2010;57(6):1002–12.
34. Lopes A, Hidalgo GS, Kowalski LP, Torloni H, Rossi BM, Fonseca FP. Prognostic factors in carcinoma of the penis: multivariate analysis of 145 patients treated with amputation and lymphadenectomy. J Urol. 1996;156(5):1637–42.
35. Ornellas AA, Nóbrega BL, Wei Kin Chin E, Wisnescky A, da Silva PC, de Santos Schwindt AB. Prognostic factors in invasive squamous cell carcinoma of the penis: analysis of 196 patients treated at the Brazilian National Cancer Institute. J Urol. 2008;180(4):1354–9.
36. Cubilla AL. The role of pathologic prognostic factors in squamous cell carcinoma of the penis. World J Urol. 2009;27(2):169–77.

# 15

# Impact of add-on laboratory testing at an academic medical center

Louis S. Nelson[1], Scott R. Davis[1], Robert M. Humble[1], Jeff Kulhavy[1], Dean R. Aman[2] and Matthew D. Krasowski[1*]

## Abstract

**Background:** Clinical laboratories frequently receive orders to perform additional tests on existing specimens ('add-ons'). Previous studies have examined add-on ordering patterns over short periods of time. The objective of this study was to analyze add-on ordering patterns over an extended time period. We also analyzed the impact of a robotic specimen archival/retrieval system on add-on testing procedure and manual effort.

**Methods:** In this retrospective study at an academic medical center, electronic health records from were searched to obtain all add-on orders that were placed in the time period of May 2, 2009 to December 31, 2014.

**Results:** During the time period of retrospective study, 880,359 add-on tests were ordered on 96,244 different patients. Add-on testing comprised 3.3 % of total test volumes. There were 443,411 unique ordering instances, leading to an average of 1.99 add-on tests per instance. Some patients had multiple episodes of add-on test orders at different points in time, leading to an average of 9.15 add-on tests per patient. The majority of add-on orders were for chemistry tests (78.8 % of total add-ons) with the next most frequent being hematology and coagulation tests (11.2 % of total add-ons). Inpatient orders accounted for 66.8 % of total add-on orders, while the emergency department and outpatient clinics had 14.8 % and 18.4 % of total add-on orders, respectively. The majority of add-ons were placed within 8 hours (87.3 %) and nearly all by 24 hours (96.8 %). Nearly 100 % of add-on orders within the emergency department were placed within 8 hours. The introduction of a robotic specimen archival/retrieval unit saved an average of 2.75 minutes of laboratory staff manual time per unique add-on order. This translates to 24.1 hours/day less manual effort in dealing with add-on orders.

**Conclusion:** Our study reflects the previous literature in showing that add-on orders significantly impact the workload of the clinical laboratory. The majority of add-on orders are clinical chemistry tests, and most add-on orders occur within 24 hours of original specimen collection. Robotic specimen archival/retrieval units can reduce manual effort in the clinical laboratory associated with add-on orders.

**Keywords:** Clinical chemistry tests, Clinical laboratory information services, Clinical laboratory services, Hematology, Laboratory automation, Robotics

* Correspondence: mkrasows@healthcare.uiowa.edu
[1]Department of Pathology, University of Iowa Hospitals and Clinics, Iowa City, IA 52242, USA
Full list of author information is available at the end of the article

## Background

Clinical laboratories frequently receive orders to perform additional tests on existing specimens ('add-ons'). Melanson et al. in 2004 was the first published report analyzing the operational impact of add-on testing, demonstrating patterns of misutilization (e.g., failure to follow laboratory testing algorithms in institutional chest pain protocols) in a significant fraction of add-on orders [1]. A follow-up study in 2006 compared add-on testing between two academic hospitals, showing similarities in add-on ordering patterns and proposing strategies to improve the process [2]. There have been several other studies on add-on test ordering, each analyzing less than one month of add-on orders [3–5].

In this study at an academic medical center, we retrospectively analyzed add-on testing data over a five and a half year period (May 2009- Dec 2014). This allowed for the analysis of add-on ordering trends over a much longer period of time than in previous studies. Also, during this time period, the core clinical laboratory of the institution introduced a robotic archival specimen retrieval system that changed the add-on testing procedure. We analyzed the impact of this unit on add-on testing procedure and manual workload.

## Methods

### Institutional setting

The study was approved by the University of Iowa Institutional Review Board as a retrospective study covering the time period from May 2, 2009- December 31, 2014. In this large retrospective study, there was waiver of informed consent and authorization approved by the Institutional Review Board for all subjects. The institution in this study is the University of Iowa Hospitals and Clinics (UIHC), a 730 bed academic medical center that includes an emergency department (ED) with level one trauma capability, adult and pediatric inpatient floors, and multiple intensive care units (ICUs; neonatal, pediatric, medical, cardiovascular, and neurologic/surgical). Outpatient services are located at the main medical campus in Iowa City, IA, as well as at a multi-specialty outpatient facility located three miles away. Smaller primary care clinics are located throughout the local region. A core clinical laboratory within the Department of Pathology provides clinical chemistry and hematopathology testing. Two critical care laboratories (one located near the main operating rooms and another embedded within the neonatal ICU) perform blood gas and activated clotting time testing. There are also separate clinical laboratories for anatomic pathology, blood center, and microbiology/molecular pathology located within the main medical campus.

### Hospital and laboratory informatics

The electronic health record (EHR) for UIHC was Epic (Epic Systems, Inc, Madison, WI). Computerized provider order entry (CPOE) is available in Epic to licensed independent providers. Add-on orders can be placed within the EHR by CPOE or by calling the laboratory. Throughout the period of retrospective study, providers were directed, when feasible, to place orders within the EHR and limit the number of verbal orders requiring laboratory-initiated testing orders. In general, chemistry and hematology tests are all orderable individually. However, there are some panels built in Epic: basic metabolic panel with total calcium (BMP; sodium, chloride, carbon dioxide, potassium, blood urea nitrogen, creatinine, glucose, total calcium), electrolyte panel (sodium, chloride, carbon dioxide, potassium), complete blood count (CBC; white blood cell count, hemoglobin, hematocrit, red blood cell count, platelet count), and lipid panel (total cholesterol, high-density lipoprotein, triglycerides, calculated low-density lipoprotein). For the purposes of analysis in this manuscript, panels were broken apart into individual tests except where described otherwise. Categories of testing were also defined (Table 1) to provide better comparison to other published studies on add-on testing [1, 2, 5].

The laboratory information system (LIS) for all UIHC pathology laboratories until August 2, 2014 was Cerner (Kansas City, MO, USA) "Classic", currently version 015. On August 2, 2014, the clinical pathology laboratories switched to Epic Beaker as the LIS, retaining Cerner as the LIS for anatomic pathology, blood center, and some parts of hematopathology and molecular pathology. The switch to Epic Beaker allowed for accurate capture of the timing of add-on orders relative to when the original specimen was received in the laboratory. During this nearly 5 month period (August 2 to December 31, 2014), there were 56,389 add-on orders with complete time data.

### Laboratory instrumentation and add-on testing procedures

The instrumentation and informatics within the core laboratory of UIHC has been described in detail in previous reports [6, 7]. Throughout the time period of retrospective analysis, the main chemistry instrumentation in the core laboratory was from Roche Diagnostics (Indianapolis, IN, USA). Front-end automation was provided by a Modular Pre-Analytic (MPA)-7 unit. In February 2014, the core laboratory went live with a Roche Diagnostics P701 automated archival/retrieval system. This system changed the add-on process (Fig. 1). Originally, specimens were placed into archival racks by the instrument flexible sample sorters. The most recent racks were kept near the instruments. The racks were then archived manually to a set of refrigerators for storage for 3 to 5 days (dependent on available refrigerator space and number of specimens). The P701 automated the sample storage and retrieval process (Fig. 1b), eliminating manual steps.

The manual effort involved from the moment the add-on is printed into the laboratory to the time the sample is

**Table 1** Abbreviations for assay categories

| Abbreviation | Full Name | Test(s) Included |
|---|---|---|
| A1C | Hemoglobin A1C | Hemoglobin A1C |
| ANEMIA | Anemia Testing | Iron, total iron-binding capacity, ferritin, folate, vitamin $B_{12}$ |
| BILD | Bilirubin, Direct | Direct (conjugated) bilirubin |
| BMP | Basic Metabolic Panel | Sodium, potassium, chloride, carbon dioxide, blood urea nitrogen, creatinine, glucose, and calcium |
| CARDIAC | Cardiac Markers | Creatine kinase-MB, troponin T, N-terminal B-type natriuretic peptide |
| CBC | Complete Blood Count | White blood cell count, red blood cell count, hemoglobin, hematocrit, platelet count |
| CRP | C-Reactive Protein | C-Reactive Protein |
| DIFF | Differential | White blood cell differential |
| ENDO | Endocrinology Testing | Thyroid-stimulating hormone, thyroxine ($T_4$) – total and free, triiodothyronine ($T_3$) – total and free, cortisol, testosterone, and 25-hydroxyvitamin D |
| ESR | Erythrocyte Sedimentation Rate | Erythrocyte sedimentation rate |
| GASES | Blood Gas Analyzer Laboratory Studies[a] | Lactic acid, potassium, glucose, hemoglobin, hematocrit, sodium, chloride, ionized calcium, $pO_2$, $pCO_2$, oxygen saturation, methemoglobin, carboxyhemoglobin |
| HAPT | Haptoglobin | Haptoglobin |
| HEPC | Hepatitis C Antibody | Hepatitis C antibody |
| HBSG | Hepatitis B Surface Antigen | Hepatitis B surface antigen |
| LFP | Liver Function Panel | Albumin, alkaline phosphatase, total bilirubin, total protein, alanine aminotransferase, aspartate aminotransferase, and γ-glutamyltranspeptidase |
| LDH | Lactate Dehydrogenase | Lactate dehydrogenase |
| REFERENCE | Reference Laboratory Testing | All testing referred to external reference laboratory |
| OSMO | Osmolality | Serum and urine osmolality |
| PO4MG | Phosphorus and Magnesium | Phosphorus, magnesium |
| PREALB | Prealbumin | Prealbumin |
| PT/INR | Prothrombin Time/INR | Prothrombin time/International normalized ratio |
| PTT | Partial Thromboplastin Time | Partial thromboplastin time |
| RETIC | Reticulocytes | Reticulocytes |
| TAP | Toxic Alcohol Panel | Sodium, glucose, blood urea nitrogen, osmolality, ethanol |
| URIC | Uric Acid | Uric acid |

[a]These are studies using whole blood and not plasma or serum

loaded on the proper analyzer averaged approximately 3.5 minutes prior to introduction of the P701 (composed in large part in retrieving specimens from racks near instruments or in the refrigerators), and 45 seconds once the P701 was implemented. In the prior system of manual archiving and retrieval, instances where samples were archived improperly could significantly delay the process.

## Results
### Timing trends in add-on testing
In the time period of retrospective study (May 2, 2009 to December 31, 2014), there were a total of 880,359 add-on orders at UIHC. This comprised 3.3 % of the total laboratory test volume performed within the clinical laboratories. The total number of add-on orders increased every year from 2009 to 2013 and then

decreased slightly in 2014 (Fig. 2a, b). Fig. 2c shows the variation of add-on orders by month. The inpatient population had the majority of add-on orders (66.8 %), while the ED and outpatient clinics accounted for 14.8 % and 18.4 % of add-on orders, respectively.

Capture of the exact timing of add-on orders relative to initial specimen collect was only possible with the new LIS (August 2, 2014 – December 31, 2014; complete data available on 56,389 add-on orders). Fig. 3a plots the timing of add-on orders, showing the percentage within periods of time. The majority of add-ons were placed within 8 hours (87.3 %) and nearly all by 24 hours (96.8 %). The timing of ordering varied by patient location. Add-on orders placed for patients in the ED were generally closer to original specimen collect time as compared to inpatient units and outpatient clinics. Nearly 100 % of add-on orders within

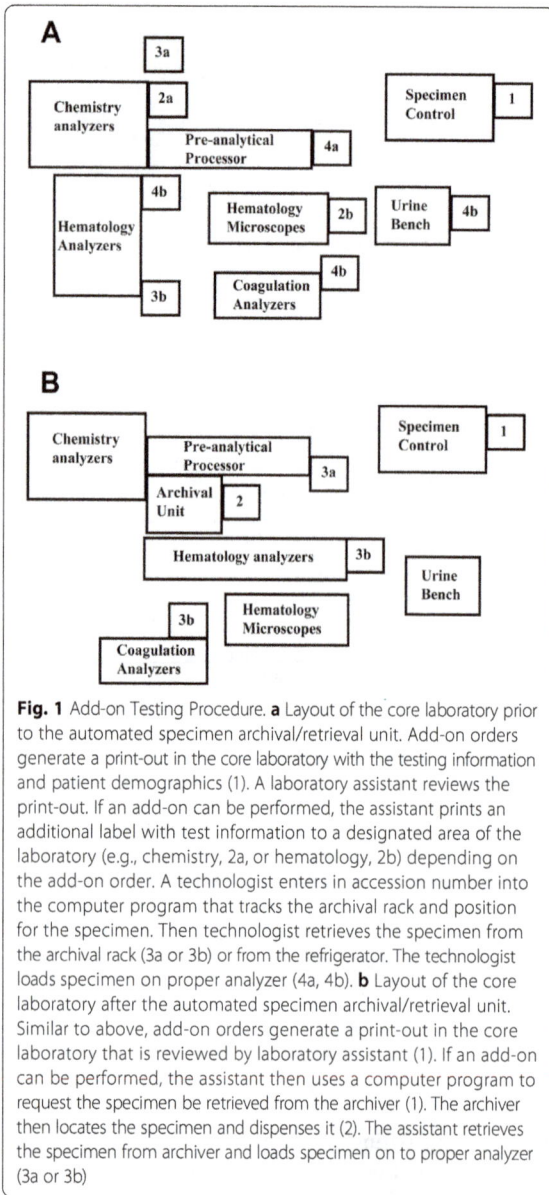

**Fig. 1** Add-on Testing Procedure. **a** Layout of the core laboratory prior to the automated specimen archival/retrieval unit. Add-on orders generate a print-out in the core laboratory with the testing information and patient demographics (1). A laboratory assistant reviews the print-out. If an add-on can be performed, the assistant prints an additional label with test information to a designated area of the laboratory (e.g., chemistry, 2a, or hematology, 2b) depending on the add-on order. A technologist enters in accession number into the computer program that tracks the archival rack and position for the specimen. Then technologist retrieves the specimen from the archival rack (3a or 3b) or from the refrigerator. The technologist loads specimen on proper analyzer (4a, 4b). **b** Layout of the core laboratory after the automated specimen archival/retrieval unit. Similar to above, add-on orders generate a print-out in the core laboratory that is reviewed by laboratory assistant (1). If an add-on can be performed, the assistant then uses a computer program to request the specimen be retrieved from the archiver (1). The archiver then locates the specimen and dispenses it (2). The assistant retrieves the specimen from archiver and loads specimen on to proper analyzer (3a or 3b)

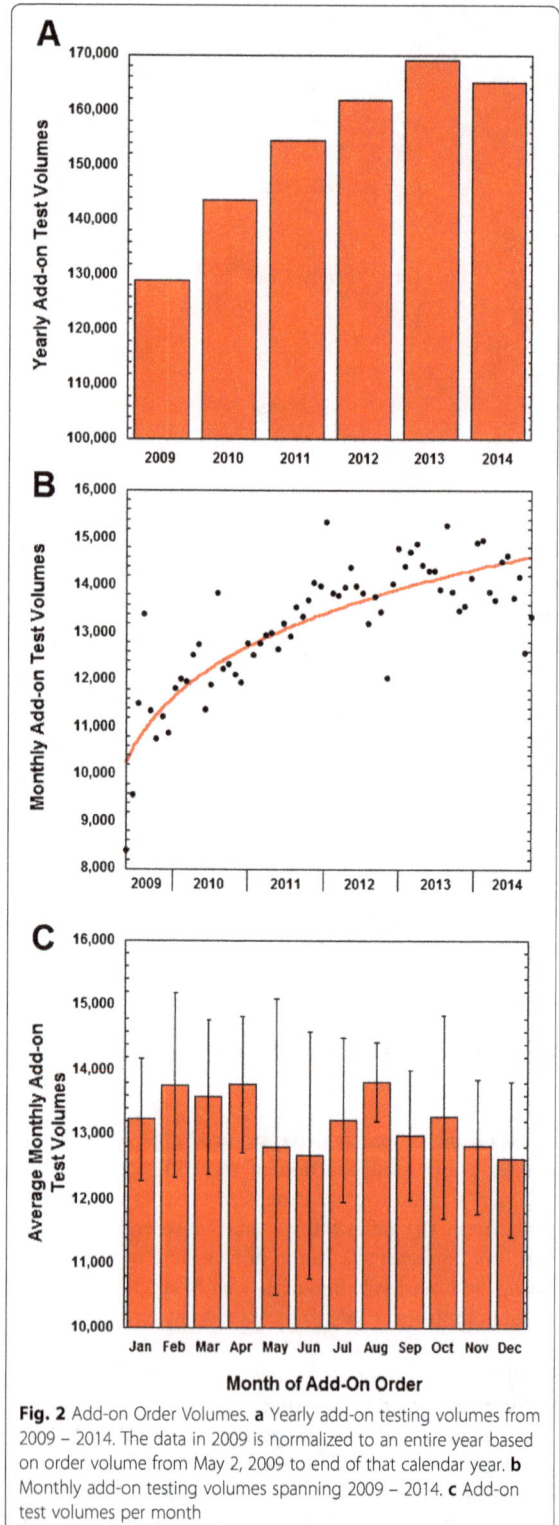

**Fig. 2** Add-on Order Volumes. **a** Yearly add-on testing volumes from 2009 – 2014. The data in 2009 is normalized to an entire year based on order volume from May 2, 2009 to end of that calendar year. **b** Monthly add-on testing volumes spanning 2009 – 2014. **c** Add-on test volumes per month

the ED were placed within 8 hours. Timing of add-on orders for inpatient units and outpatient clinics were similar, except that there was a longer tail of add-on orders placed 24 hours or more later than original specimen collect in the outpatient population (Fig. 3a).

The peak times for add-on order placement were between 08:00 – 12:00, with 47.8 % of add-ons ordered between 07:00 and 13:00 (Fig. 3b). Add-on orders were more frequent during weekdays, with Saturdays and Sundays only accounting for slightly more than 20 % of total add-on volume (Fig. 3c).

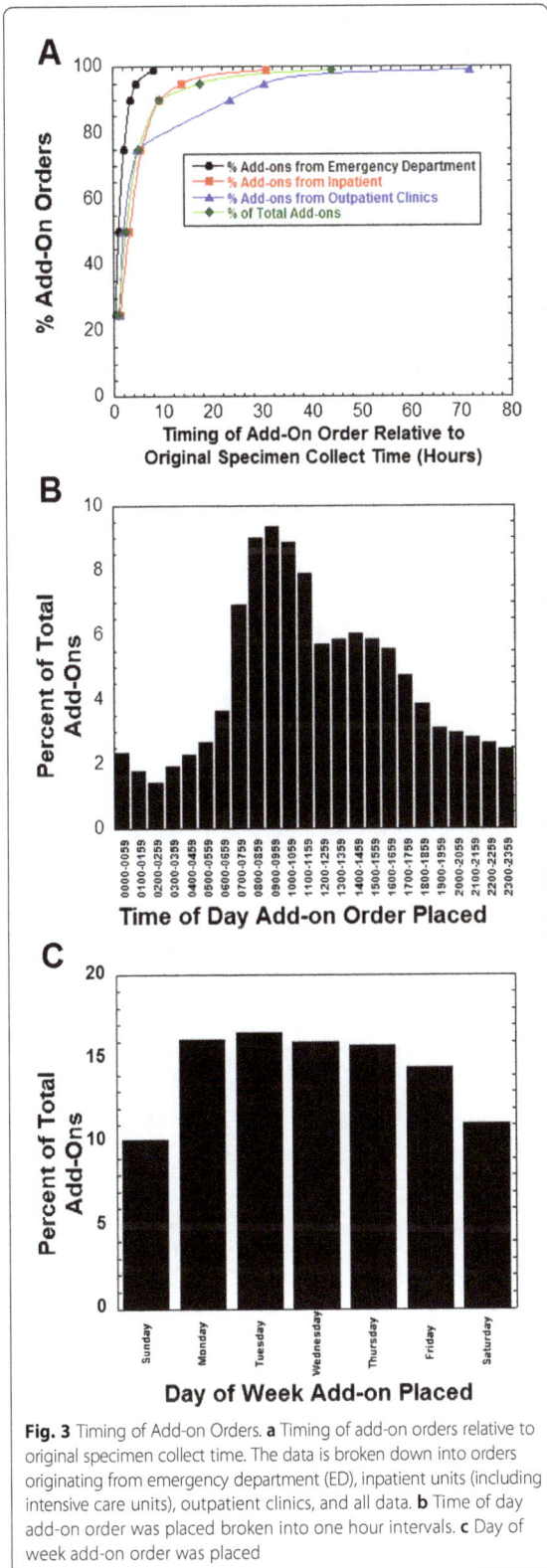

**Fig. 3** Timing of Add-on Orders. **a** Timing of add-on orders relative to original specimen collect time. The data is broken down into orders originating from emergency department (ED), inpatient units (including intensive care units), outpatient clinics, and all data. **b** Time of day add-on order was placed broken into one hour intervals. **c** Day of week add-on order was placed

## Distribution of add-on testing by category of testing

Figure 4 shows a breakdown of add-on testing by category of testing. The majority of the add-on tests were chemistry tests (78.8 % of total add-on orders comprising 3.3 % of overall chemistry test volumes), with the most frequent being within the following categories (all percentages are of the total overall add-on orders): LFP (25.6 %), BMP (11.7 %), MGPO4 (7.0 %), Cardiac (4.6 %), and Anemia (3.2 %). Hematology and coagulation tests were the next most frequent areas of add-on testing. The most frequent hematology and coagulation add-ons were in the following categories (all percentages are of the total overall add-on orders): CBC (2.70 %), Diff (2.19 %), PTT (1.19 %), PT/INR (1.71 %), and ESR (0.85 %). Within the critical care laboratories, the most frequent add-on orders were the following tests performed on blood gas analyzers using whole blood specimens: lactic acid (0.97 %), potassium (0.78 %), glucose (0.62 %), hemoglobin/hematocrit (0.49 %), and sodium (0.49 %). Urinalysis-related tests accounted for less than 1 % of total add-ons. For the critical care laboratory tests, in most cases the parameters had already been determined as part of a cartridge of testing on the blood gas analyzers; results were suppressed from reporting to the LIS if not ordered by the provider. Thus, the add-on order for these tests required only that staff perform the computer steps necessary to release the previously unordered test from the instrument to the LIS.

Table 2 summarizes the most frequent add-on orders broken down into categories of testing. LFP, BMP, MGPO4, ENDO, and CARDIAC ranked in the top ten

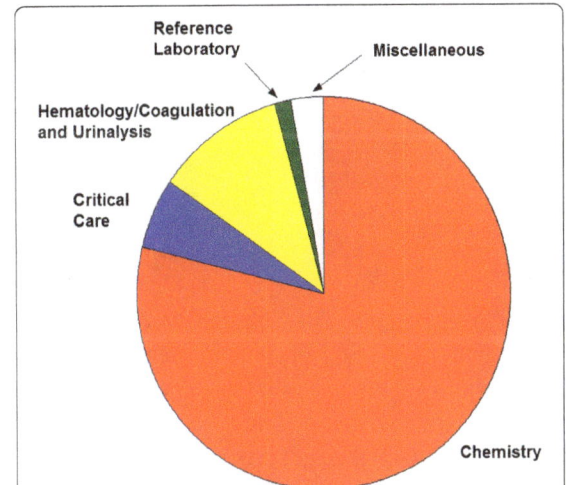

**Fig. 4** Breakdown of Add-on Order Volumes by Category of Testing. The categories of testing are: Clinical Chemistry (performed in core laboratory), Hematology/Coagulation and Urinalysis (performed in core laboratory), Critical Care (blood gases, whole blood electrolytes, and other testing performed in satellite critical care laboratories), Reference Laboratory (testing referred to outside laboratories), and Miscellaneous (all testing not fitting into other categories)

most frequent add-on orders overall and also individually for inpatient units, ED, and outpatient clinics. Not surprisingly, GASES were an infrequent add-on order in the outpatient clinics but were the fourth most common overall add-on order. A1C was more frequently added-on in the outpatient clinics than from the ED or inpatient units. Table 3 lists the most frequent individual tests added-on. The top five most frequent individual add-on tests were magnesium (4.0 %), albumin (3.8 %), alanine aminotransferase (3.8 %), aspartate aminotransferase (3.8 %), and total bilirubin (3.7 %). Table 3 also lists the percentage of times each individual test was ordered as an add-on. For six of the tests (amylase, creatine kinase, hemoglobin A1C, lactate dehydrogenase, lipase, troponin T), over 10 % of orders for that particular test were placed as add-ons.

Reference laboratory testing comprised only 1.4 % of total add-ons, with no single test accounting for more than 0.05 % of total add-ons (Table 4). There were 618 different reference laboratory tests available in the EHR test menu that were ordered at least once as an add-on in the time period of retrospective study. This included 193 orders of "Miscellaneous Test", an order option in the EHR for reference laboratory testing not built in the EHR test menu. Our analysis does not capture attempts

to order reference laboratory testing that could not be completed due to lack of suitable existing specimen.

**Workload impact of add-on testing**

Table 5 summarizes the workload of add-on testing over the period of retrospective study. Of the 880,359 add-on orders, there were 443,411 unique ordering instances, leading to an average of 1.99 add-on tests per instance. Some patients had multiple episodes of add-on test orders at different points in time (e.g., during different days of a multi-day inpatient encounter), leading to an average of 9.15 add-on tests per patient. The introduction of the robotic specimen archival/retrieval unit saved an average of 2.75 mins of laboratory staff manual time per unique ordering instance (Table 5). This translates to 24.1 hr/day less manual effort in dealing with add-on orders.

**Discussion**

Add-on testing can occupy a significant amount of clinical laboratory resources [1, 3–5]. The main challenges are storage of specimens and the labor involved in retrieving specimens for further testing [1, 5]. Add-on testing can theoretically serve a useful purpose in allowing for thoughtful ordering of additional testing based on initial laboratory test results or other clinical data. On the other

**Table 2** Most frequently ordered add-on test categories by ordering location

| Test Category | Inpatient Unit % | Rank | Emergency Department % | Rank | Outpatient Clinics % | Rank | All Locations % | Rank |
|---|---|---|---|---|---|---|---|---|
| LFP | 28.79 % | 1 | 29.86 % | 1 | 16.91 % | 1 | 26.76 % | 1 |
| BMP | 12.00 % | 2 | 10.14 % | 2 | 15.12 % | 2 | 12.30 % | 2 |
| MGPO4 | 7.41 % | 4 | 4.02 % | 4 | 2.87 % | 5 | 6.08 % | 3 |
| GASES | 8.41 % | 3 | 2.51 % | 9 | 0.10 % | 19 | 6.01 % | 4 |
| ENDO | 3.30 % | 6 | 3.09 % | 6 | 8.81 % | 3 | 4.28 % | 5 |
| CARDIAC | 4.19 % | 5 | 7.25 % | 3 | 2.09% | 7 | 4.25 % | 6 |
| ANEMIA | 2.66 % | 7 | 0.78 % | 18 | 6.67 % | 4 | 3.12 % | 7 |
| DIFF | 2.40 % | 8 | 1.73 % | 15 | 1.78 % | 9 | 2.19 % | 8 |
| CBC | 2.24 % | 9 | 1.83 % | 14 | 2.00 % | 8 | 2.14 % | 9 |
| PT/INR | 1.43 % | 12 | 3.57 % | 5 | 0.88 % | 13 | 1.65 % | 10 |
| LIPASE | 1.49 % | 11 | 3.01 % | 8 | 0.77 % | 15 | 1.58 % | 11 |
| A1C | 1.33 % | 14 | 0.95 % | 17 | 2.52 % | 6 | 1.49 % | 12 |
| CRP | 1.29 % | 15 | 2.22 % | 10 | 1.39 % | 11 | 1.45 % | 13 |
| LDH | 1.50 % | 10 | 0.64 % | 19 | 1.43 % | 10 | 1.36 % | 14 |
| AMYLASE | 1.37 % | 13 | 2.02 % | 12 | 0.68 % | 16 | 1.34 % | 15 |
| PTT | 0.97 % | 16 | 3.03 % | 7 | 0.19 % | 17 | 1.13 % | 16 |
| ESR | 0.61 % | 18 | 2.00 % | 13 | 0.78 % | 13 | 0.85 % | 17 |
| BILD | 0.94 % | 17 | 0.59 % | 20 | 0.92 % | 12 | 0.85 % | 18 |
| D-DIMER | 0.24 % | 19 | 2.07 % | 11 | 0.11 % | 18 | 0.48 % | 19 |
| TAP | 0.16 % | 20 | 1.61 % | 16 | 0.03 % | 20 | 0.35 % | 20 |
| Total | 82.7 % | | 82.9 % | | 66.1 % | | 79.7 % | |

**Table 3** Most frequently ordered individual add-on tests

| Test | % of Total Add-on Orders | % of Times Test Ordered as Add-on (vs. Routine) |
|---|---|---|
| Magnesium | 4.0 | 5.9 |
| Albumin | 3.8 | 6.5 |
| Alanine aminotransferase | 3.8 | 5.4 |
| Aspartate aminotransferase | 3.8 | 5.5 |
| Bilirubin, total | 3.7 | 6.4 |
| Alkaline phosphatase | 3.4 | 5.8 |
| Gamma-glutamyltransferase | 3.2 | 4.7 |
| Total protein | 3.1 | 6.3 |
| Phosphorus | 3.0 | 6.9 |
| Troponin T | 2.2 | 14.5 |
| Complete blood count | 2.1 | 1.5 |
| Automated white blood cell differential | 2.1 | 2.3 |
| Creatinine | 1.7 | 1.1 |
| Potassium | 1.6 | 1.1 |
| Thyroid stimulating hormone with reflex to free thyroxine | 1.6 | 9.6 |
| Lipase | 1.6 | 15.9 |
| Hemoglobin A1C | 1.5 | 10.2 |
| Prothrombin time/International normalized ratio | 1.5 | 1.8 |
| Basic metabolic panel with calcium | 1.5 | 1.1 |
| C-Reactive protein | 1.4 | 8.1 |
| Lactic acid dehydrogenase | 1.4 | 10.7 |
| Creatine kinase, total | 1.3 | 22.7 |
| Amylase | 1.3 | 15.3 |
| Blood urea nitrogen | 1.3 | 0.9 |
| Calcium, total | 1.2 | 1.3 |

**Table 4** Most frequently ordered reference laboratory add-on tests

| Test | % of Total Add-on Orders |
|---|---|
| *Helicobacter pylori* antibody, IgG | 0.050 % |
| Mitochondrial M2 antibodies | 0.049 % |
| Hepatitis C virus quantitative PCR | 0.033 % |
| IgG subclasses | 0.022 % |
| Miscellaneous test[a] | 0.019 % |
| Vitamin D, 1,25-dihydroxy | 0.018 % |
| Aldosterone, serum | 0.017 % |
| Alpha-1-antitrypsin, phenotyping | 0.013 % |
| Lyme disease antibodies, IgG and IgM | 0.013 % |
| *Histoplasma* antigen, urine | 0.013 % |

[a]Covers any test ordered that is not on list of laboratory tests built in electronic medical record

**Table 5** Summary of add-on tests

| | |
|---|---|
| Total number of add-ons | 880,359 |
| Unique ordering instances[1] | 443,411 |
| Number of patients | 96,244 |
| Average number of add-on tests per unique ordering instance | 1.99 |
| Average number of add-on tests per patient[2] | 9.15 |
| Estimated hours per day of manual effort for add-on testing prior to introduction of robotic archival storage/retrieval unit | 30.7 |
| Estimated hours per day of manual effort for add-on testing with use of robotic archival storage/retrieval unit | 6.6 |

[1]These are unique add-on orders at a specific time
[2]This includes all add-on tests per each patient, which may span multiple unique ordering instances

hand, add-on testing can also be a result of disorganized ordering practices (e.g., neglecting to order essential laboratory testing upfront) or even misutilization of testing, as has been shown in previous studies [1, 2]. Our analysis does not capture attempts at add-on testing that could not be completed due to lack of existing specimens or add-on testing that was duplicate to previously ordered testing (e.g., hemoglobin/hematocrit placed as add-on when CBC already performed). We have analyzed duplicate testing as an example of misutilization in a previous study [6].

The results of this study are similar to previous studies in showing that the majority of add-ons are clinical chemistry tests [2, 4, 5]. As with previous studies, LFP, BMP, MGPO4, and CARDIAC were in the top tier of ordered add-on tests. Hematology and coagulation testing only accounted for 11.2 % of total add-ons; however, add-ons comprised 5.6 % of the overall hematology/coagulation test volumes. Four common tests (CBC, DIFF, PT/INR, and PT) accounted for over two-thirds of the hematology and coagulation add-on tests.

In the present study, the 5.86 % percent of add-ons for the critical care laboratories posed the least manual effort because in most cases the parameters had already been determined but were suppressed from reporting to the LIS if not ordered by the provider. Therefore, most critical care laboratory add-ons only needed to be sent from instrument to LIS rather than having to locate the sample and analyze it again (assuming specimen would even be viable at that point). Reference laboratory add-ons were only a small fraction of total add-ons but spanned a wide variety of tests. No single reference laboratory test exceeded 0.05 % of total add-ons. These results are comparable to previous studies [2, 5]. Add-on requests for reference laboratory tests not built in the LIS or EHR may entail extra work in first determining the specimen requirements for the requested test and then checking if pre-existing specimens can be used.

Similar to previous studies, our study shows a high fraction of add-ons ordered within eight hours of original specimen collect time [1, 2, 5]. The ED tended to order add-ons more quickly compared to inpatient units and outpatient clinics. Only a small fraction of add-on orders were placed more than 24 hours after original specimen collection. Less than 1 % of total add-ons occurred more than 48 hours after specimen collection. Outpatient clinics accounted for the majority of add-on orders submitted more than 24 hours after original specimen collection, a finding similar to a previous study [5].

Depending on workload, add-on orders can entail substantial manual effort from clinical laboratory staff [1, 2, 4, 5]. In our study, add-ons comprised 3.3 % of overall test volume, a figure that is very close to one previous study [4] and higher than another study [1]. Some laboratories,

including ours, have implemented robotic specimen archival/retrieval units. As we have shown, the estimated impact of this type of unit on manual time can be substantial, with an estimated reduction of 24.1 hrs/day of manual add-on processing time in handling add-on order requests. However, the timing of add-on orders suggests that improvements on this design may include a combination of short-term/rapidly accessible and longer-term/less accessible specimen storage. Storage of specimens in a rapidly accessible buffer (e.g., very close to the chemistry analyzers) for a limited period of time (e.g., between 8 and 24 hours) would capture the majority of add-on orders. After this time period, specimens can be archived for longer-term storage in a space more distant from the instruments. At that point, turnaround time is likely less important.

The main limitations of our study are that the analysis is retrospective and confined to an academic medical center. The results may not generalize to other hospital or clinic settings. Nevertheless, it is hoped that the results described here provide useful to other institutions attempting to manage the challenges of add-on testing.

## Conclusions

Add-on orders significantly impact the workload of the clinical laboratory. In this study at an academic medical center, the majority of add-on orders were clinical chemistry tests, and most add-on orders occur within 24 hours of original specimen collection. Robotic specimen archival/retrieval units can reduce manual effort in the clinical laboratory associated with add-on orders.

### Abbreviations
A1C: Hemoglobin A1C; BILD: Direct bilirubin; BMP: Basic metabolic panel; CBC: Complete blood count; CPOE: Computerized provider order entry; CRP: C-reactive protein; DIFF: White blood count differential; ED: Emergency department; EHR: Electronic health record; ESR: Erythrocyte sedimentation rate; HAPT: Haptoglobin; HBSG: Hepatitis B surface antigen; HEPC: Hepatitis C antibody; ICU: Intensive care unit; LDH: Lactate dehydrogenase; LFP: Liver function panel; LIS: Laboratory information system; OSMO: Serum/plasma osmolality; PO4MG: Phosphorus and magnesium; PREALB: Prealbumin; PT/INR: Prothrombin time/international normalized ratio; PTT: Partial thromboplastin time; TAP: Toxic alcohol panel; UIHC: University of Iowa Hospitals and Clinics; URIC: Uric acid.

### Competing interests
The authors declare that they have no competing interests.

### Authors' contributions
LSN and MDK were involved in the study concept and design, analysis and interpretation of the data, drafting and revisions of the manuscript. SRD, RMH, and JK assisted with data analysis and interpretation. DRA helped with extraction and analysis of data from the laboratory information system. All authors have read and approved the final manuscript.

### Acknowledgements
MDK thanks the Department of Pathology (Dr. Nitin Karandikar, Department Executive Officer) for providing research funding.

### Author details
[1]Department of Pathology, University of Iowa Hospitals and Clinics, Iowa City, IA 52242, USA. [2]Hospital Computing Information Services, University of Iowa Hospitals and Clinics, Iowa City, IA 52242, USA.

**References**
1.  Melanson SF, Hsieh B, Flood JG, Lewandrowski KB. Evaluation of add-on testing in the clinical chemistry laboratory of a large academic medical center: operational considerations. Arch Pathol Lab Med. 2004;128(8):885–9.
2.  Melanson S, Flood J, Lewandrowski K. Add-on testing the clinical laboratory: observations from two large academic medical centers. Lab Med. 2006;37(11):675–8.
3.  Kim JY, Kamis IK, Singh B, Batra S, Dixon RH, Dighe AS. Implementation of computerized add-on testing for hospitalized patients in a large academic medical center. Clin Chem Lab Med. 2011;49(5):845–50.
4.  Loh TP, Saw S, Sethi SK. Clinical value of add-on chemistry in a large tertiary care teaching hospital. Lab Med. 2012;43(3):82–5.
5.  Naumova NN, Schappert J, Kaplan LA. Patterns of add-on tests for hospitalized and for private patient populations. Arch Pathol Lab Med. 2007;131(12):1794–9.
6.  Krasowski MD, Chudzik D, Dolezal A, Steussy B, Gailey MP, Koch B, et al. Promoting improved utilization of laboratory testing through changes in an electronic medical record: experience at an academic medical center. BMC Med Inform Decis Mak. 2015;15:11.
7.  Krasowski MD, Davis SR, Drees D, Morris C, Kulhavy J, Crone C, et al. Autoverification in a core clinical chemistry laboratory at an academic medical center. J Pathol Inform. 2014;5:13.

# 16

# Prevalence and predictors of Pap smear cervical epithelial cell abnormality among HIV-positive and negative women attending gynecological examination in cervical cancer screening center at Debre Markos referral hospital, East Gojjam, Northwest Ethiopia

Melkamu Getinet[1], Baye Gelaw[2], Abinet Sisay[1], Eiman A. Mahmoud[3] and Abate Assefa[2*]

## Abstract

**Background:** Cervical cancer is the leading cause of cancer related death among women in developing countries. Cervical cancer is preceded by cervical surface epithelial cell abnormalities (ECA) which can be detected by Pap smear test. Simultaneous human papillomavirus and human immunodeficiency virus (HIV) infection increases cervical cancer. Data on the prevalence and predictors of ECA among women in Ethiopia is limited. Hence, we aimed to determine the prevalence and associated factors of ECA among women.

**Methods:** A comparative cross-sectional study was conducted among HIV+ and HIV- women attending gynecological examination in cervical cancer screening center at the Debre Markos referral hospital. The study subjects were stratified by HIV status and systematic random sampling method was used to recruit study participants. Cervical smears were collected for Pap smear examination. Logistic regression analysis was employed to examine the possible risk factors of cervical ECA.

**Results:** A total of 197 HIV+ and 194 HIV- women were enrolled in the study. The overall prevalence of cervical ECA was 14.1 % of which the prevalence of atypical squamous cells undetermined significance (ASCUS), low grade squamous intraepithelial lesion (SIL), high grade SIL, squamous cell carcinoma and ASC, cannot exclude high grade SIL (ASCH) were 5.1, 3.8, 4.1 and 1.0 %, 0.0 % respectively. Significantly higher prevalence of ECA (17.8 %) was observed among HIV+ women (COR 1.9, 95 % CI: 1.1 – 3.4, $p = 0.036$) as compared to HIV-women (10.3 %). Multiple sexual partnership (AOR 3.2, 95 % CI: 1.1 – 10.0, $p = 0.04$), early ages of first sexual contact (<15 years) (AOR 5.2, 95 % CI: 1.5 – 17.9, $p = 0.009$), parity greater than three (AOR 10.9, 95 % CI: 4.2 – 16.8, $p < 0.001$) and long term oral contraceptive pills (OCP) use (AOR 11.9, 95 % CI: 2.1 – 16.7, $p = 0.02$) were significant predictors of prevalence of ECA.

**Conclusions:** Cervical ECA is a major problem among HIV-infected women. Lower CD4+ T-cell counts of below 350 cells/μl, HIV infection, multiple sexual partnership, early age at first sexual contact, parity greater than three and long term OCP use were significant predictors of prevalence of ECA. Strengthening screening program in HIV+ women should be considered.

* Correspondence: abezew@gmail.com
[2]Department of Medical Microbiology, School of Biomedical and Laboratory Sciences, College of Medicine and Health Sciences, University of Gondar, Gondar, Ethiopia
Full list of author information is available at the end of the article

# Background

Squamous intraepithelial lesions (SIL) are an abnormal growth of squamous epithelial cells of the ecto-cervix. Cervical epithelial cell abnormalities (ECA) represent a spectrum of SIL that lie along the pathway, from mild-to-severe dysplasia to invasive cancer [1]. Cervical carcinoma develops gradually through well characterized precursor lesions [2]. Greater than 99.7 % cervical cancer is attributed by *human papillomavirus* (HPV) infection. HPV usually causes a variety of benign papillomatous lesions of the skin and mucosal basal epithelium [3, 4]. There are more than100 different HPV genotypes [5]. Based on oncogenic potential, HPV is classified as high-risk (HR) and low-risk (LR) oncogenic types. HR-HPV types, HPV 16, 18, 31, 33, 35, 39, 45, 51, 52, 56, 58, 59, 68 and 82, cause anogenital cancer [6], while infection with LR-HPV types, HPV 6 and 11, is associated with benign genital warts. HR-HPV types are detected in 99 % of cervical cancer, and about 70 % of cervical cancer is due to HPV 16 and 18 [7].

More than half of sexually active people become infected with HPV during their lifetime [8]. It is estimated that in Ethiopia about 33.6 % of women in the general population has HPV infection [9]. Persistent infection with HR-HPV types over time leads to the development and progression of cervical intraepithelial neoplasia (CIN). Not all women who acquire HPV infection do develop CIN. Rather approximately 90 % of HPV infections clear within 2 years [10]. The peak of HPV infection in women occurs in the late teens and early twenties following sexual exposure [11, 12]. Cervical cancer associated with HPV infection also leads to infertility. There is higher incidence of ECA among women complaining of infertility [13].

Cervical ECA can be detected and classified by cytological screening methods. Well organized programmes of regular gynecological screening and treatment of precancerous lesions have been very effective in preventing cervical cancer [14, 15]. Cytological examination of cervical scrapping from clinically suspicious cases by Papanicolaou (Pap) cytological screening test can detect cervical ECA. The Pap smear identifies any changes in cells of the transformation zone of the cervix [16]. The Bethesda System 2001 classifies ECA into atypical squamous cell (ASC), low-grade squamous intraepithelial lesion (LSIL), high-grade squamous intraepithelial lesion (HSIL) and squamous cell carcinoma (SCC). ASC comprises: ASC of undetermined significance (ASCUS) and ASC, cannot exclude HSIL (ASCH); LSIL encompasses: HPV, mild dysplasia, and CIN1; while HSIL includes: moderate and severe dysplasia, carcinoma in situ, CIN 2, and CIN 3. These categories promote specificity in the mode of treatment [17]. For patients with invasive lesions the stage of a cervical cancer is the most important factor in the selection of treatment modality. For women diagnosed with ASCUS and LSIL follow up with HPV-DNA testing, Pap smear or colposcopy within certain time interval is some of the management options. In general, noninvasive SIL identified using Pap smear only, are treated with superficial ablative procedures such as cryotherapy or laser therapy [18].

On a global level, 75 % of women has abnormal cervical cytology at least once in their life time which may progress to cervical cancer. Cervical cancer is the second most common women cancer worldwide of which 80 % occurs in developing countries. The higher prevalence of cervical ECA due to HPV was reported in African countries [19–21]. Current estimates indicates that in Ethiopia 4648 women are diagnosed annually with cervical cancer and 3235 die from the disease [9]. Several factors such as number of sexual partners and age of first sexual activity, smoking, immune-suppression, and presence of other sexually transmitted infection (STI) can increase the risk of developing cervical cancer [22]. Several studies revealed that human immunodeficiency virus (HIV) infection is associated with an increased risk of HPV related cervical ECA [23–25]. Mortality and morbidity due to cervical cancer is higher among HIV patients [26–28]. HIV infection and cervical cancer among women in Ethiopia are major public health problems. More than 534,000 adult women are estimated to be infected with HIV and at risk of developing cervical cancer. However, Ethiopia has invested little in the infrastructure, training, and laboratory capacity required for successful cytological screening [29]. Though studies have shown that the prevalence of ECA is more common among HIV-infected than non HIV-infected women, such data in Ethiopia is limited. For the development of a rational approach to the screening and the subsequent management of precancerous cervical lesion in HIV-infected women, understanding of the specific risk factors associated with ECA occurrence among HIV- positive women is very much important. The aim of this comparative study was to determine the prevalence of ECA and risk factors associated with its occurrence among HIV+ and HIV-women attending the Debre Markos referral hospital.

# Methods

## Study setting and design

A comparative cross-sectional study was conducted among HIV- and HIV + women attending at the Debre Markos referral hospital cervical cancer screening center from the 1st of March to the 30th of May, 2014. Debre Markos referral hospital is located in Debre Markos town in East Gojjam Zone 300 km North of Addis Ababa. According to July 2014 zonal statistical agency report, the town has an estimated population of 100,000. The hospital has cervical cancer screening and treatment center. The screening service is provided for all HIV+ women. All women attending the Debre Markos referral hospital during the study period for any gynecological problem were eligible for the study. Pregnant women, lactating women and women on menstrual cycle were excluded from the study. The sample size was determined using two population proportion formula with the assumption of 95 % confidence interval (CI), 5 % marginal error and 33.6 % prevalence of ECA among HIV-infected women (15) and 10 % nonresponse rate. Since there is no previous study done in Ethiopia among HIV-women, the prevalence of ECA was assumed to be 50 %. Using this assumptions the final sample size becomes 400 (200 HIV+ and 200 HIV- women). During the study period there were a total of 1600 HIV- and 2000 HIV+ women attending gynecological examination in cervical cancer screening center. The study subjects from both groups were selected by systematic random sampling method.

### Socio-demographic and clinical information
Data was collected after obtaining written informed consent from each participant. A pre-tested structured questionnaire was used to collect socio-demographic and clinical information needed for the study. Socio-demographic and clinical information included in this study were age, marital status, age at first sexual intercourse, number of sexual partners, duration of oral contraceptive pills (OCP) use, condom use, alcohol use, smoking, prostitution, history of STI, CD4 + T-cell count and parity.

### Cytopathological examination
The cervical smear specimens were collected by gynecologist. Cervical smears were taken with a wooden applicator stick, smeared on a microscopic slide, fixed immediately with 95 % ethanol and allowed to air dry. The smears were stained with Pap stain, examined and graded according to the criteria of Bethesda classification system [17]. To ensure the quality of Pap smear results, 20 randomly selected patients were evaluated by gynecologist with colposcopic examination and visual inspection. Moreover, representative smears were reexamined by pathologists at the University of Gondar hospital blinded from the first results. In this regard 30 randomly selected positive and negative slides were blindly rechecked by a pathologist.

### HIV test and CD4+ T cell count
HIV counseling and testing based the national guideline was offered to participants unaware of their HIV status. Whole blood sample of 8 ml was collected from each study subject for HIV testing and CD4+ T-cell counts. HIV testing was done based on current national rapid HIV testing algorithms. For all HIV+ women, CD4+ T-cell counts were determined by Fluorescent Activated Cell Sorter (FACS) count (Becton Dickinson) at Debre Markos referral hospital.

### Statistical analysis
Data was initially registered in a registration book and transferred to excel Microsoft spread sheet. Data was cleaned and checked for completeness before analysis using SPSS version 20 computer software. Descriptive statistical analysis was used to determine the socio – demographic and clinical characteristics of study participants and prevalence of cervical ECA. The prevalence of ECA was stratified by study subjects' HIV status. Associations of patient characteristics with ECA were assessed using a series of bivariate logistic regression analysis. Then, to control simultaneously for the possible confounding effects of the different variables; a multivariable model was fitted with stepwise variable selection among variables having p-value $\leq 0.2$ at bivariate analysis. In both bivariate and multivariate analyses, the associations were expressed in odds ratios (OR) and 95 % CI. For all cases p-value $<0.05$ were considered statistically significant.

### Ethical approval
The study was reviewed and approved by ethical review committee of School of Biomedical and Laboratory Sciences, College of Medicine and Health sciences, University of Gondar and official permission was obtained from Debre Markos referral hospital higher management. A written informed consent was obtained from each study participant. All Pap smear positive results were referred to the department of obstetrics and gynecology for immediate treatment. The patients record were made anonymous and any identifying information were removed prior to analysis. Individual records were coded and accessed only by research staff members.

### Results
#### Consistency of microscopy and colposcopic examinations
Pap smear microscopic examination was undertaken initially by trained laboratory technologist. Results obtained were compared with results obtained by a pathologist and gynecologist for consistency. In this regard, ten positive Pap smeared slides were given to three of the readers and examined blindly. There was no discrepancy between the results of the laboratory technologist and the pathologist or the gynecologist results except for one sample that was diagnosed as LSIL by the laboratory technologist but as ASCUS by the pathologist (Table 1).

**Table 1** Consistency of the results of the 3 readers

| Sample No | Reader A | | | Reader B | | | Reader C | | |
|---|---|---|---|---|---|---|---|---|---|
| | Method | Result | Grade | Method | Result | Grade | Method | Result | Grade |
| 20 | Msy | ECA | 1 | Msy | ECA | 1 | Cpy | ECA | - |
| 55 | Msy | ECA | 2 | Msy | ECA | 2 | Cpy | ECA | - |
| 90 | Msy | ECA | 3 | Msy | ECA | 3 | Cpy | ECA | - |
| 111 | Msy | ECA | 1 | Msy | ECA | 1 | Cpy | ECA | - |
| 146 | Msy | ECA | 2 | Msy | ECA | 2 | Cpy | ECA | - |
| 244 | Msy | ECA | 2 | Msy | ECA | 1 | Cpy | ECA | - |
| 281 | Msy | ECA | 1 | Msy | ECA | 1 | Cpy | ECA | - |
| 307 | Msy | ECA | 1 | Msy | ECA | 1 | Cpy | ECA | - |
| 331 | Msy | ECA | 3 | Msy | ECA | 3 | Cpy | ECA | - |
| 343 | Msy | ECA | 1 | Msy | ECA | 1 | Cpy | ECA | - |

*Reader A* trained data collector, *Reader B* pathologist, *Reader C* Gynecologist, *Msy* Microscopy, *Cpy* Colposcopy, *ECA* Epithelial cell abnormality, *Grade 1* atypical squamous cell undetermined significance, *Grade 2* Low grade squamous intraepithelial lesion, *Grade 3* High grade squamous intraepithelial lesion, *Grade 4* squamous cell carcinoma

## Socio-demographic data and clinical characteristics of the patients

A total of 400 women (200 HIV+ and 200 HIV- women) were enrolled in the study, but 9 patients (3 HIV+ and 6 HIV-) were excluded because the smears were not adequate for evaluation. Therefore, further analyses were restricted to 391 study subjects. The mean age of the study subjects was 35.02 years with standard deviation of ±8.41 years. Two hundred and thirty (58.8 %) of the women were married, and only 65 (16.6 %) were employed. Majority of the study participants (59.1 %) were urban dwellers. Hundred and seventy six (45.0 %) of the women had no formal education (Table 2).

The number of life time sexual partners, greater than two, was higher in HIV+ women (66.6 %) as compared to HIV- ones (33.6 %). First sexual contact at early age (<18 years) was also higher among HIV+ women (56.0 %) than HIV- women (44.0 %). About 26.1 % of the study subjects had a history of STI. Two hundred and sixty seven participants (68 %) were accustomed to alcohol intake and 0.8 % was currently smoking. About 5.4 % of women used OCP for greater than 5 years and only 14.8 % of the women used condom. The number of parity greater than two was lower in HIV+ women compared to that of HIV- women (Table 3).

## Clinical examination and Pap smear results

Clinical investigation was also conducted for all study subjects and 16.4 % (64/391) were found to have abnormal clinical findings. Among patients who had abnormal clinical results, 60.9 %( 39/64) were positive for HIV. Abnormal vaginal discharge and contact bleeding were the most common clinical findings. In 56 (14.3 %) of the women abnormal vaginal discharge was observed, whereas 8 (2.0 %) of the women had contact bleeding. Pap smear examination revealed that

55 (14.1 %) patients were positive for cervical ECA. Higher prevalence of ECA (17.8 %) was observed in HIV+ women, of which the prevalence of ASCUS was 5.6 % (n = 11), 0.0 % ASCH, 6.1 % LSIL (n = 12), 5.1 % HSIL (n = 10) and 1.0 % SCC (n = 2). On the other hand, a 10.3 % cervical ECA prevalence was found among HIV- women with a prevalence of 4.6 % (n = 9), 0(0.0 %), 1.5 % (n = 3), 3.1 % (n = 6) and 1.0 % (n = 2) for ASCUS, ASCH, LSIL, HSIL and SCC respectively (Table 4).

The prevalence of cervical ECA was high (51.9 %) among HIV+ women with CD4 + T-cell count <200 cells/μl. The prevalence of ECA among women with CD4 + T-cell counts of 200–349 cells/μl and 350–500 cells/μl were 18.5 % (n = 10) and 12.7 % (n = 7), respectively. On the other hand, relatively low prevalence (6.6 %) of ECA was found among women with CD4 + T-cell count greater than 500/ μl (Fig. 1).

## Risk factor analysis for cervical epithelial cell abnormality

Both bivariate and multivariate logistic regression analyses were employed to determine factors associated with ECA. All variables tested in the bivariate logistic regression analysis were entered into multivariate analyses if they have p-value of ≤0.2. The highest prevalence of cervical ECA (25.0 %) was observed in older age women (>45 years of old). Moreover, bivariate analysis showed that the prevalence of ECA was significantly higher among patients within the age groups of 30–45 years old and above (crude odds ratio (COR) 2.5, 95 % CI: 1.2 – 5.1, $p = 0.012$; COR 4.2, 95 % CI: 1.7 – 10.5, $p = 0.002$ respectively) as compared to younger women. Residence, educational status, condom use, smoking and alcohol consumption were not associated with the development of ECA.

**Table 2** Socio-demographic characteristics of women attending cervical cancer screening center at Debre Markos referral hospital

| Characteristics | HIV status | | Total n % | |
|---|---|---|---|---|
| | Positive n (%) | Negative n (%) | | |
| Age( in year) | | | | |
| <30 | 73(49.0) | 76(51) | 149 | 38.1 |
| 30-45 | 102(51.5) | 96(48.5) | 198 | 50.6 |
| >45 | 22(50.0) | 22(50.0) | 44 | 11.3 |
| Marital status | | | | |
| Married | 92(40.0) | 138(60.0) | 230 | 58.8 |
| Single | 10(32.3) | 21(67.7) | 31 | 7.9 |
| Divorced | 49(69.0) | 22(31.0) | 71 | 18.2 |
| Widowed | 46(78.0) | 13(22.0) | 59 | 15.1 |
| Marital status | | | | |
| Orthodox | 185(52.4) | 168(47.6) | 353 | 90.3 |
| Muslim | 5(31.2) | 11(68.8) | 16 | 4.1 |
| Protestant | 7(31.8) | 15(68.2) | 22 | 5.6 |
| Residence | | | | |
| Rural | 70(43.8) | 90(56.2) | 160 | 40.9 |
| Urban | 127(55.0) | 104(45.0) | 231 | 59.1 |
| Educational status | | | | |
| Illiterate | 96(54.5) | 81(45.5) | 176 | 45.0 |
| Primary school | 59(58.4) | 41(40.6) | 101 | 25.8 |
| Secondary& above | 42(37.2) | 71(62.8) | 113 | 28.9 |
| Occupation | | | | |
| Employed | 24(36.9) | 41(63.1) | 65 | 16.6 |
| House wife/Farmer | 81(41.9) | 112(58.1) | 193 | 49.4 |
| No work | 32(68.1) | 15(31.9) | 47 | 12.0 |
| Daily laborer | 20(90.9) | 2(9.1) | 22 | 5.6 |
| Commercial sex worker | 8(50.0) | 8(50.0) | 16 | 4.1 |
| Others | 32(66.7) | 16(33.3) | 48 | 12.3 |

*HIV* Human immunodeficiency virus

The higher proportion of cervical ECA (63.6 %) was accounted by HIV+ women. Even though HIV infection was not found as an independent risk factor for ECA in multivariate analysis, in the bivariate analysis it was significantly associated with developing ECA (COR 1.9, 95 % CI:1.1 – 3.4, $P = 0.036$). A downward trend of the prevalence of ECA along the increment of CD4+ T-cell counts was observed among HIV+ women. Significantly higher prevalence of ECA were observed in HIV+ women with CD4+ T-cell counts <200 cells/µl (adjusted OR (AOR) 14.1, 95 % CI: 6.7 – 16.4, $p < 0.001$) and between 200 and 349 cells/µl all (AOR 9.6, 95 % CI: 1.8 – 11.5, $p = 0.008$) as compared to patients with CD4+ T-cell counts of above 500 cells/µl.

Women with a previous history of multiple lifetime sexual partners (more than two), were at high risk for developing ECA when compared to their counterparts with one or two sexual partner (AOR 3.2, 95 % CI: 1.0 – 10, $p = 0.048$). Early age at first sexual contact (<15 years) was also identified as a significant risk factor for the development of ECA (AOR 5.2, 95 % CI: 1.5– 17.9, $p = 0.009$). Association of marital status for the development of ECA was analyzed. Widowed (AOR3.2, 95 % CI: 1.2 – 8.8, $p = 0.021$) and divorced (AOR 3.0; 95 % CI: 1.1 – 8.1; $p = 0.029$) women were at higher risk than women who are married. Women with high parity (parity greater than four) were ten folds more likely to develop ECA (AOR10.9, 95 % CI; 4.2 – 16.8, $p < 0.001$) than women with parity lower than three. OCP users for more than five years were found to be at higher risk of developing ECA (AOR11.9, 95 % CI: 2.1 – 16.7, $p = 0.02$) (Table 5).

## Discussion

The study showed that microscopic examination of Pap smear results by a trained laboratory technologist are comparable with the microscopic examination results of the same preparation observed by a pathologist. The current accepted practice is for the Pap smear to be examined by pathologist, while nurse responsibility is collection of the sample of cervical cells, and the technician responsibility is to prepare the slides with the pathologist responsible for slide readings and final reporting of findings. The comparable accuracy of the trained technologist reports of the Pap smear to the pathologist reports may indicate the possible utilization of trained technicians in the interpretations of Pap smears at the peripheral health facility where there is no pathologist.

In this study, 16.4 % of the women had abnormal clinical findings. The most prevalent clinical finding (13.4 %) was abnormal vaginal discharge but only 2.0 % of the women had contact bleeding. Vaginal discharge is often a normal and regular occurrence. There are, however, types of discharge that may suggest underlying infectious etiology. Such abnormal discharge was considered when the vaginal discharge was yellow or green in color, chunky in consistency, and have a foul odor. Most abnormal discharges in the study were caused by yeast or bacterial infection. The prevalence of abnormal gynecological findings such as abnormal vaginal discharge and contact bleeding of the current study was relatively lower than abnormal clinical findings reported from India which was 20 % and 6.7 % respectively [30].

In this study, the overall prevalence of cervical ECA based on Pap smear test was 14.1 % in which the prevalence of ASCUS, ASCH, LSIL, HSIL and SCC were 5.1, 0.0, 3.8, 4.1 and 1.0 % respectively. The prevalence of ECA among HIV+ women was 17.8 % which is quite

**Table 3** Behavioral and clinical characteristics of women attending cervical cancer screening unit at Debre Markos referral hospital

| Variable | | HIV status | | Total | |
|---|---|---|---|---|---|
| | | Positive n (%) | Negative n (%) | N | % |
| No. of life time sexual partner | 1-2 | 106(41.7) | 148(58.3) | 254 | 65.0 |
| | >2 | 91(66.4) | 46(33.6) | 137 | 35.0 |
| Age of 1st sexual contact | <18 | 160(56.0) | 126(44.0) | 286 | 73.1 |
| | 18-20 | 25(32.0) | 53(68.0) | 78 | 19.9 |
| | >20 | 12(44.4) | 15(55.6) | 27 | 6.9 |
| Alcohol use | Yes | 142(53.2) | 125(46.8) | 267 | 68.3 |
| | No | 55(44.4) | 69(55.6) | 124 | 31.7 |
| Smoking | Yes | 2(66.7) | 1(33.3) | 3 | 0.8 |
| | No | 195(50.3) | 193(49.7) | 388 | 99.2 |
| History of STI | Yes | 66(64.7) | 36(35.3) | 102 | 26.1 |
| | No | 131(45.3) | 158(54.7) | 289 | 73.9 |
| Duration of OCP usage | <5 years | 43(55.8) | 34(44.2) | 77 | 19.7 |
| | >5 years | 13(61.9) | 8(38.1) | 21 | 5.4 |
| Condom use | Always | 40(69.0) | 18(31.0) | 58 | 14.8 |
| | Some times | 52(46.8) | 59(53.2) | 111 | 28.4 |
| | Never | 105(47.3) | 117(52.7) | 222 | 56.8 |
| Parity | ≤2 | 122(52.6)) | 110(47.4) | 232 | 59.3 |
| | 3-4 | 39(49.4) | 40(50.6) | 79 | 20.2 |
| | >4 | 36(45.0) | 44(55.0) | 80 | 20.5 |

*HIV* Human immunodeficiency virus, *OCP* Oral contraceptive pills, *STI* Sexually transmitted infection

higher than from that of ECA among HIV- women. Relatively concordant results on the prevalence of ECA among HIV-infected women were reported from Tanzania (17 %) [31] and Thailand (15.4 %) consisting of ASCUS 2.8 %, LSIL 8.5 %, and HSIL 3.5 % [32]. On the other hand, lower prevalence of ECA (2.8 %) was reported among Turkish women of which 2.2 % was ASCUS, 0.5 % LSIL, 0.1 % HSIL and 0.0 % SCC [33]. In different regions of Nigeria, Pap smear screening have shown a lower prevalence of HPV induced cervical ECA (7.6 – 13.2 %) [34, 35]. Similarly, based on Bethesda

System ECA classification, the study conducted in Nigeria among young females indicated that the prevalence of ASCUS was 7 %, LSIL 12.2 %, HSIL 7.7 % and SCC 0.7 % [35]. Another study among Italian women also reported 2.8 % ASCUS, 6.2 % LSIL and 1.7 % HSIL cervical cytological abnormalities [36]. In contrast, higher prevalence of HPV induced cervical ECA was observed in South Africa in which 41.7, 70.2 and 83 % were ASCUS, LSILS and HSIL, respectively [21]. In

**Table 4** The prevalence of epithelial cell abnormality among women attending cervical cancer screening unit at Debre Markos referral hospital

| Cervical cytology result | | HIV status | | Total tested | |
|---|---|---|---|---|---|
| | | Positive | Negative | n | % |
| NIL | | 162(82.2 %) | 174(89.7 %) | 336 | 85.9 |
| ECA | | 35(17.8 %) | 20(10.3 %) | 55 | 14.1 |
| Types of ECA | ASCUS | 11(5.6 %) | 9(4.6 %) | 20 | 5.1 |
| | LSIL | 12(6.1 %) | 3(1.5 %) | 15 | 3.8 |
| | HSIL | 10(5.1 %) | 6(3.1 %) | 16 | 4.1 |
| | SCC | 2(1.0 %) | 2(1.0 %) | 4 | 1.1 |

*NIL* Negative for intraepithelial lesion, *ECA* Cervical epithelial cell abnormality, *ASCUS* atypical squamous cell undetermined significance, *LSIL* Low grade squamous intraepithelial lesion, *HSIL* High grade squamous intraepithelial lesion, *SCC* squamous cell carcinoma, *HIV* Human immunodeficiency virus

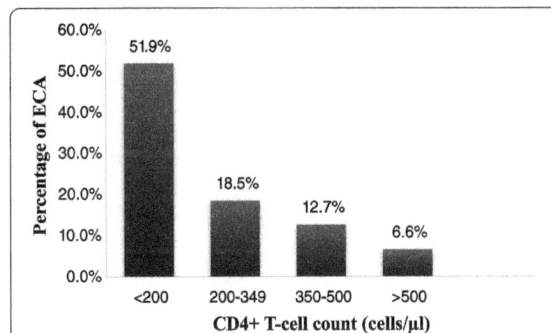

**Fig. 1** Proportion of cervical epithelial cell abnormality (ECA) compared with the CD4 + T-cell count level of HIV+ women. Increasing prevalence of cervical ECA was observed along with the concomitant decreasing of CD4 + T-cell count which indicates a direct relationship between the occurrence of cervical ECA and CD4 + T-cell count level

**Table 5** Bivariate and multivariate analysis of risk factors for cervical ECA among women attending cervical cancer screening unit at Debre Markos referral hospital

| Variables | | Cervical ECA | | COR (95 % CI) | P | AOR (95 % CI) | P |
|---|---|---|---|---|---|---|---|
| | | Yes | No | | | | |
| | | No (%) | No (%) | | | | |
| Age (in year) | <30 | 11(7.4) | 138(92.6) | 1 | | 1 | |
| | 30-45 | 33(16.7) | 165(83.3) | 2.5(1.22, 5.11) | 0.012 | 0.8(0.30, 2.09) | 0.648 |
| | >45 | 11(25.0) | 33(75.0) | 4.2(1.67, 10.47) | 0.002 | 0.6(0.18, 2.25) | 0.493 |
| Marital status | Married | 21(9.1) | 209(90.9) | 1 | | 1 | |
| | Single | 1(3.2) | 30(96.8) | 0.3(0.04, 2.55) | 0.290 | 1.2(0.11,12.43) | 0.869 |
| | Divorced | 15(21.1) | 56(78.9) | 2.7(1.29, 5.50) | 0.008 | 3.2(1.19, 8.77) | 0.021 |
| | Widowed | 18(30.5) | 41(69.5) | 4.4(2.14, 8.91) | 0.000 | 3.0(1.12, 8.09) | 0.029 |
| Education | NFE | 35(19.8) | 142(80.2) | 2.6(0.87, 7.69) | 0.087 | 2.2(0.69, 6.67) | 0.181 |
| | Primary | 16(9.5) | 152(90.5) | 1 | | 1 | |
| Occupation | Employed | 6(9.2) | 59(90.8) | 1 | | 1 | |
| | HW | 28(18.3) | 165(81.7) | 1.8(0.29, 10.76) | 0.275 | 0.4(0.10, 1.88) | 0.536 |
| | DL | 10(16.7) | 50(83.3) | 2.9(0.64, 12.86) | 0.167 | 0.3(0.05, 1.86) | 0.205 |
| | CSW | 4(18.2) | 18(81.8) | 1.6(0.27,9.93) | 0.004 | 0.1(0.01, 0.95) | 0.046 |
| | Others | 7(14.6) | 41(85.4) | 2.6(0.80, 8.25) | 0.081 | 0.8(0.17, 1.16) | 0.112 |
| Age of 1st sex (in year) | <15 | 42(23.5) | 137(76.5) | 7.7(2.68, 22.28) | <0.001 | 5.2(1.49, 17.95) | 0.009 |
| | 15-18 | 9(8.4) | 98(91.6) | 2.3(069, 7.77) | 0.173 | 2.4(0.61, 9.49) | 0.208 |
| | >18 | 4(3.8) | 101(96.2) | 1 | | 1 | |
| No. of sexual partner | 1-2 | 21(8.3) | 233(91.7) | 1 | | 1 | |
| | 3-4 | 34(24.8) | 103(75.2) | 3.6(1.84, 6.96) | <0.001 | 3.2(1.00, 10.03) | 0.048 |
| History of STI | Yes | 21(20.6) | 81(79.4) | 1.9(1.06, 3.53) | 0.029 | 1.5(0.67, 3.42) | 0.314 |
| | No | 34(11.8) | 255(88.2) | 1 | | 1 | |
| OCP user (in year) | <5 | 7(9.1) | 70(90.9) | 1 | | 1 | |
| | ≥5 | 16(76.2) | 5(23.8) | 30.0(7.6, 118.37) | <0.001 | 11.9(2.11, 16.69) | 0.020 |
| | No | 14(11.3) | 110(88.7) | 1 | | 1 | |
| Parity | ≤2 | 13(5.6) | 219(94.4) | 1 | | 1 | |
| | 3-4 | 6(10.7) | 50(89.3) | 3.2(1.36, 7.30) | 0.007 | 1.7(0.53, 5.44) | 0.362 |
| | >4 | 36(35.0) | 67(65.0) | 7.9(3.67, 16.92) | <0.001 | 10.9(4.16, 16.75) | <0.001 |
| HIV status | Negative | 20(10.3) | 174(89.7) | 1 | | 1 | |
| | Positive | 35(17.8) | 162(82.2) | 1.9(1.04, 3.38) | 0.036 | 1.4(0.62, 3.16) | 0.410 |
| CD4 + T-cell count (cells/ µl) | <200 | 14(51.9) | 13(48.1) | 15.3(4.33, 54.31) | <0.001 | 14.1(6.69, 16.4) | <0.001 |
| | 200-349 | 10(18.5) | 44(81.5) | 3.2(0.95, 11.01) | 0.060 | 9.6(1.79, 11.54) | 0.008 |
| | 350-500 | 7(12.7) | 48(87.3) | 2.1(0.57, 7.52) | 0.265 | 5.8(0.98,31.62) | 0.052 |
| | >500 | 4(6.6) | 57(93.4) | 1 | | 1 | |

*HIV* Human immunodeficiency virus, *COR* crude odds ratio, *AOR* adjusted odds ratio, *CI* confidence interval, *P* p- value, *OCP* Oral contraceptive pills, *STI* Sexually transmitted infection, *NFE* No formal education, *CSW* Commercial sex worker, *HW* House wife, *DL* Daily laborer

another study carried among Turkish women, higher prevalence of ECA (54.8 %) was observed. The prevalence of ASCUS was 36.7 %, LSIL 16.8 %, HSIL 1.3 % [37]. The discrepancy in the prevalence of ECA between these studies may be due to differences in the study population. Higher prevalence of ECA observed from our finding and the report from South Africa may be due to the inclusion of high number of HIV-infected women. HIV is reported as one of the independent risk factor for development of cervical ECA and cervical cancer.

Women in the age groups of 30 years and older were at greater risk of developing ECA in the present study. There are also some other study findings which indicate that older age women had greater risk for the development of ECA. Cervical cancer mortality, usually occurring among unscreened women, increases with age, with the maximum mortality rate reported for white women between age 45 years and 70 years, and for black women in their 70s [38, 39]. Mortality among women with negative Pap smear screening is low at all ages. The prevalence of SCC and ASCUS were 36.4 and 81.8 % respectively among women <30 years of age. ASCUS was found to be highest in the youngest age group women in this study.

The study participants were stratified by their HIV status and data of 197 (50.4 %) HIV+ and 194 (49.6 %) HIV- women were analyzed. We found higher prevalence of cervical ECA (17.8 %) among HIV+ women as compared to HIV- women (10.3 %). This finding was very similar to the study finding reported from Brazil where ECA was more common in the HIV+ group (12.1 %) compared to the HIV- group (5.4 %) [40]. In a study finding reported from India, all cervical ECA (26.35 %) were found among HIV+ women [41]. HIV infection is one of the major risk factor that contributes for the growth of cervical ECA. HIV leads to an increased risk of CIN and cervical cancer [40]. Up to 20 % of HIV co-infected patients develop HPV-induced premalignant lesions of the uterine cervix within three years of HIV diagnosis [42]. Progression of an untreated HPV-induced dysplastic lesion can lead to invasive cervical cancer, an AIDS defining illness [43].

Moreover, the prevalence of ECA in this study was significantly higher among HIV+ women with lower CD4 + T-cell counts of < 350 cells/µl. Statistically significant downward trends of the prevalence of ECA along the increment of CD4+ T-cell counts in HIV+ women was observed in the present study. Similarly, higher prevalence of ECA among HIV+ women with lower CD + T-cell counts of <200 cells/µl was reported [40, 44]. There are study reports that documented the higher risk of cervical ECA when CD4+ T-cell counts fall below < 200 cells/µl [25, 28]. Decreased CD4+ T-cells count and increased HIV-RNA levels are risk factors for CIN. In addition, it has also been shown that with decreasing numbers of CD4+ T-cells, there is an increase in both frequency and severity of cervical dysplasia in HIV-infected women [36, 45]. Significant correlation was reported between low levels of CD4+ T-cells, high HIV-viral load and risk of CIN [46]. A Brazilian study demonstrated that immunosuppressed women had a higher risk of lesion recurrence as compared to women with a CD4+ T-cells count > 200 cells/µl [47].

In our study widowed (30.5 %) and divorced (21.1 %) women were significantly at higher risk for the development of ECA when compared to married (9.1 %) women. This difference might be due to divorced and widowed women may have multiple sexual partners when compared to married women. This finding is supported by the report from Ghana in which higher prevalence of ECA (21.3 %) was observed in polygamous women when compared to monogamous women (13.9 %) [48]. In this study, women with a history of STI were 1.5 times more likely to develop cervical ECA than women with no history of STI. Previous reports also demonstrated that genital infections were risk factors for the acquisition of HPV infection and the progression of cervical cancer [35, 43, 44].

We identified earlier initiation of first sexual contact (<15 years) as a significant risk factor for the development of ECA. Women with previous history of multiple life time sexual partners (more than two) were also at high risk for developing ECA which is supported by the study reported from Tanzania (44). Another most important finding of this study was that women with higher parity (greater than four) were 10.9 times more likely to develop ECA as compared to women with parity less than three. OCP users for more than 5 years had higher risk for the presence of ECA than their counterparts. Similar study supported that the prevalence of cervical cancer associated death in Ghana [48] among OCP users was higher.

### Limitation

The limitation of this study is that the number of study participants is relatively small for an epidemiological study; the results may only be applied to Northwest Ethiopia. Most of the study subjects were patients with gynecological problems which may not represent the general population. The result of this study also may not represent the hospital catchment population for most of women attending the cervical screening center are HIV+. The short duration of the study did not allow the adequate follow up of the disease progression. Moreover, the study didn't further assess the etiology of the ECA.

### Conclusions

Women infected with HIV had a greater risk of developing cervical ECA than HIV- women. There was a downward trend of the prevalence of ECA along the increment of CD4+ T-cell counts among HIV-infected women. Lower CD4+ T-cell counts of below 350 cells/µl, earlier initiation of first sexual contact (at the age of <15 years), parity greater than four, being widowed and divorced, multiple sexual partnership (more than three partners) and long term OCP use were significant predictors of increased risk of cervical ECA. Hence, cytological screening program should be targeting specifically HIV+ women. Awareness creation on risk factors as multiple sexual partnership and sexual initiation at earlier age should be provided.

## Abbreviations

ASCUS: Atypical squamous cell undetermined significance; CIN: Cervical intraepithelial neoplasia; ECA: Cervical epithelial cell abnormality; HIV: Human immunodeficiency virus; HR: High risk; HPV: *Human papillomavirus*; HSIL: High grade squamous intraepithelial lesion; LR: Low risk; LSIL: Low grade squamous intraepithelial lesion; NIL: Negative for intraepithelial lesion; OCP: Oral contraceptive pills; SCC: Squamous cell carcinoma; SIL: Squamous intraepithelial lesion; STI: Sexually transmitted infection.

## Competing interests

The authors declare that they have no competing interests.

## Authors' contributions

MG proposed the initial idea for the study. MG, BG and AA contributed to the study design. MG and AS collected all the data. All authors analyzed and interpreted the data. MG drafted the manuscript. All authors contributed to the writing of the manuscript. AA prepared the manuscript for publication. All authors read and approved the final manuscript.

## Authors' information

MG: MSc in medical microbiology; BG: PhD, associate professor of medical microbiology; AA: MSc, lecturer in clinical microbiology; AS: MD, gynecologist; EM: Professor, MD, MPH, Pathology, Director of Global Health Program.

## Acknowledgements

We would like to thank Debre Markos hospital for all the help and support provided during data collection, cytopathological examination and other laboratory investigation. We also thank the Amhara Regional Health Bureau for financial support. We gratefully acknowledge all study participants for their participation in the study. Lastly we would like to acknowledge University of Gondar department of pathology for examination of Pap smear slides.

## Author details

[1]Debre Markos Referral Hospital, Debre Markos, Ethiopia. [2]Department of Medical Microbiology, School of Biomedical and Laboratory Sciences, College of Medicine and Health Sciences, University of Gondar, Gondar, Ethiopia. [3]Department of Basic Sciences, College of Osteopathic Medicine, Touro University, Vallejo, CA, USA.

## References

1. Tornesello ML, Buonaguro L, Giorgi-Rossi P, Buonaguro FM. Viral and cellular biomarkers in the diagnosis of cervical intraepithelial neoplasia and cancer. Biomed Res Int. 2013;2013:519619.
2. Saslow D, Castle PE, Cox JT, Davey DD, Einstein MH, Ferris DG, et al. American Cancer Society Guideline for human papillomavirus (HPV) vaccine use to prevent cervical cancer and its precursors. CA Cancer J Clin. 2007;57:7–28.
3. Trottier H, Franco EL. The epidemiology of genital human papillomavirus infection. Vaccine. 2006;24 Suppl 1:S1–15.
4. Pande S, Jain N, Prusty BK, Bhambhani S, Gupta S, Sharma R, et al. Human papillomavirus type 16 variant analysis of E6, E7, and L1 genes and long control region in biopsy samples from cervical cancer patients in north India. J Clin Microbiol. 2008;46:1060–6.
5. Gagnon S, Hankins C, Tremblay C, Forest P, Pourreaux K, Coutlée F, et al. Viral polymorphism in human papillomavirus types 33and 35 and persistent and transient infection in the genital tract of women. J Infect Dis. 2004;190:1575–85.
6. Ault KA. Epidemiology and natural history of human papillomavirus infections in the female genital tract [Review]. Infect Dis Obstet Gynecol. 2006;Suppl:40470.
7. Bosch F, Sanjose S. Chapter 1: human papillomavirus and cervical cancer–burden and assessment of causality. J Natl Cancer Inst Monogr. 2003;3–13.

8. Gillison ML, Broutian T, Pickard RK, Tong ZY, Xiao W, Kahle L, et al. Prevalence of oral HPV infection in the United States, 2009–2010. JAMA. 2012;307:693–703.
9. World Health Organization (WHO). Human Papillomavirus and Related Cancers. Summary Report Update. 2010. Available at: http://screening.iarc.fr/doc/Human%20Papillomavirus%20and%20Related%20Cancers.pdf.. Accessed on Dec 23, 2013.
10. Franco EL, Villa LL, Sobrinho JP, Prado JM, Rousseau MC, Désy M, et al. Epidemiology of acquisition and clearance of cervical human papillomavirus infection in women from a high-risk area for cervical cancer. J Infect Dis. 1999;180:1415–23.
11. Kerr DJ, Fiander AN. Towards Prevention of Cervical Cancer in Africa. 2009. Available at: www.afrox.org. Accessed on Dec 15, 2013.
12. Hariri S, Unger ER, Sternberg M, Dunne EF, Swan D, Patel S, et al. Prevalence of genital human papillomavirus among females in the United States, the National Health and Nutrition Examination Survey, 2003–2006. J Infect Dis. 2011;204:566–73.
13. Abdull Gaffar B, Kamal MO, Hasoub A. The prevalence of abnormal cervical cytology in women with infertility. Diagn Cytopathol. 2010;38:791–4.
14. Hailu A, Mariam DH. Patient side cost and its predictors for cervical cancer in Ethiopia: a cross sectional hospital based study. BMC Cancer. 2013;13:69.
15. Cutts FT, Franceschi S, Goldie S, Castellsague X, de Sanjose S, Garnett G, et al. Human papillomavirus and HPV vaccines: a review. Bull. 2007; 85(9):719–26.
16. Luyten A, Buttmann-Schweiger N, Luyten K, Mauritz C, Reinecke-Lüthge A, Pietralla M, et al. Early detection of CIN3 and cervical cancer during long-term follow-up using HPV/Pap smear co-testing and risk-adapted follow-up in locally organized screening programs. Int J Cancer. 2014;135:1408–16.
17. Solomon D, Davey D, Kurman R, Moriarty A, O'Connor D, Prey M, et al. Bethesda 2001 Workshop: The 2001 Bethesda System: terminology for reporting results of cervical cytology. JAMA. 2002;287:2114–9.
18. Mayrand MH, Duarte-Franco E, Rodrigues I, Walter SD, Hanley J, Ferenczy A, et al. Human papillomavirus DNA versus Papanicolaou screening tests for cervical cancer. N Engl J Med. 2007;357:1579–88.
19. Richter K, Becker P, Horton A, Dreyer G. Age-specific prevalence of cervical human papillomavirus infection and cytological abnormalities in women in Gauteng Province, South Africa. S Afr Med J. 2013;103:313–7.
20. Allan B, Marais DJ, Hoffman M, Shapiro S, Williamson AL. Cervical human papillomavirus (HPV) infection in South African women: implications for HPV screening and vaccine strategies. J Clin Microbiol. 2008;46:740–2.
21. Firnhaber C, Van Le H, Pettifor A, Schulze D, Michelow P, Sanne IM, et al. Association between cervical dysplasia and human papillomavirus in HIV seropositive women from Johannesburg South Africa. Cancer Causes Control. 2010;21:433–43.
22. Daniel T, Juana S. Human Papillomavirus infection and cervical cancer: pathogenesis and epidemiology. 2007. Available at: http://www.formatex.org/microbio/pdf/pages680-688.pdf. Accessed on Dec 8, 2013.
23. Kravchenko J, Akushevich I, Sudenga SL, Wilson CM, Levitan EB. ShresthaS: Transitional probability-based model for HPV clearance in HIV-1-positiveadolescent females. PLoS One. 2012;7:e30736.
24. Abraham AG, D'Souza G, Jing Y, Gange SJ, Sterling TR, Silverberg MJ, et al. Invasive cervical cancer risk among HIV-infected women: a North American multi-cohort collaboration prospective study. J Acquir Immune Defic Syndr. 2013;62:405–13.
25. Terry R. Management of patients with atypical squamous cells of undetermined significance (ASCUS) on Papanicolaou smears. J Am Osteopath Assoc. 1996;96(8):465–8.
26. Elfström KM, Herweijer E, Sundström K, Arnheim-Dahlström L. Current cervical cancer prevention strategies including cervical screening and prophylactic human papillomavirus vaccination: a review. Curr Opin Onco. 2014;26:120–9.
27. Palefsky J. HPV infection and HPV-associated neoplasia in immunocompromised women. Int J Gynaecol Obstet. 2006;94:S56–64.
28. Anastos K, Hoover DR, Burk RD, Cajigas A, Shi Q, Singh DK, et al. Risk factors for cervical precancer and cancer in HIV-infected, HPV-positive Rwandan women. PLoS One. 2010;5:e13525.
29. Combating-Cervical-Cancer-in-Ethiopia.pdf. 2010. http://www.pathfinder.org/publications-tools/pdfs/Combating-Cervical-Cancer-in-Ethiopia.pdf. Accessed on Feb 15, 2015.
30. Srivastava S, Gupta S, Roy JK. High prevalence of oncogenic HPV-16 in cervical smears of asymptomatic women of eastern Uttar Pradesh, India: a population-based study. J Biosci. 2012;37:63–72.

31. Obure J, Olola O, Swai B, Mlay P, Masenga G, Walmer D. Prevalence and severity of cervical squamous intraepithelial lesion in a tertiary hospital in northern Tanzania. Tanzan J Health Res. 2009;11:163–9.

32. Chalermchockcharoenkit A, Chayachinda C, Thamkhantho M, Komoltri C. Prevalence and cumulative incidence of abnormal cervical cytology among HIV-infected Thai women: a 5.5-year retrospective cohort study. BMC Infect Dis. 2011;11:8.

33. Açikgöz A, Ergör G. Cervical cancer risk levels in Turkey and compliance to the national cervical cancer screening standard. Asian Pac J Cancer Prev. 2011;12:923–7.

34. Patricia A, Marco T, Suelene B. Cervical Cytopathology in a Population of HIV-Positive and HIV-Negative Women. J Trop Med. 2012;869758.

35. Durowade KA, Osagbemi GK, Salaudeen AG, Musa OI, Akande TM, Babatunde OA, et al. Prevalence and risk factors of cervical cancer among women in an urban community of Kwara State, north central Nigeria. J Prev Med Hyg. 2012;53:213–9.

36. Meloni A, Pilia R, Campagna M, Usai A, Masia G, Caredda V, et al. Prevalence and molecular epidemiology of human papillomavirus infection in Italian women with cervical cytological abnormalities. J Public Health Res. 2014;3:157.

37. Atilgan R, Celik A, Boztosun A, Ilter E, Yalta T, Ozercan R. Evaluation of cervical cytological abnormalities in Turkish population. Indian J Pathol Microbiol. 2012;55:52–5.

38. Saslow D, Runowicz CD, Solomon D, Moscicki AB, Smith RA, Eyre HJ, et al. American Cancer Society guideline for the early detection of cervical neoplasia and cancer. CA Cancer J Clin. 2002;52:342–62.

39. National Institutes of Health Consensus Development Conference Statement: cervical cancer, April 1–3. National Institutes of Health Consensus Development Panel. J Natl Cancer Inst Monogr. 1996;1996:vii–xix.

40. Heard I, Tassie JM, Schmitz V, Mandelbrot L, Kazatchkine MD, Orth G. Increased risk of cervical disease among human immunodeficiency virus-infected women with severe immunosuppression and high human papillomavirus load(1). Obstet Gynecol. 2000;96:403–9.

41. Lima MA, Tafuri A, Araújo AC, Lima LM, Melo VH. Cervical intraepithelial neoplasia recurrence after colonization in HIV-positive and HIV-negative women. IntJ Gynecol Obstet. 2009;104:100–04.

42. Jamieson DJ, Duerr A, Burk R, Klein RS, Paramsothy P, Schuman P, et al. Characterization of genital human papillomavirus infection in women who have or who are at risk of having HIV infection. Am J Obstet Gynecol. 2002;186:21–7.

43. Hatuvedi AK, Madeleine MM, Biggar RJ, Engels EA. Risk of human papillomavirus -associated cancers among persons with AIDS. J Natl Cancer Inst. 2009;101:1120–30.

44. Kafuruki L, Rambau PF, Massinde A, Masalu N. Prevalence and predictors of cervical intraepithelial neoplasia among HIV infected women at Bugando Medical Centre, Mwanza-Tanzania. Infect Agent Cancer. 2013;8(1):45.

45. Harris TG, Burk RD, Palefsky JM, Massad LS, Bang JY, Anastos K, et al. Incidence of cervical squamous intraepithelial lesions associated with HIV sero-status, CD4 cell counts, and human papillomavirus test results. JAMA. 2005;293:1471–6.

46. Hawes SE, Critchlow CW, Sow PS, Touré P, N'Doye I, Diop A, et al. Incident high-grade squamous intraepithelial lesions in Senegales women with and without human immunodeficiency virus type 1 (HIV-1) and HIV-2. J Natl Cancer Inst. 2006;98:100–9.

47. Russomano F, Paz BR, Camargo MJ, Grinstejn BG, Friedman RK, Tristao MA, et al. Recurrence of cervical intraepithelial neoplasia in human immunodeficiency virus-infected women treated by means of electrosurgical excision of the transformation zone (LLETZ) in Rio de Janeiro, Brazil. Sao Paulo Med J. 2013;131(6):405–10.

48. Domfeh A, Wiredu E, Adjei A, Ayeh-Kumi P, Adiku T, Tettey Y, et al. Cervical human papillomavirus infection in Accra, Ghana. Ghana Med J. 2008;42:71–8.

# 17

# A retrospective analysis of breast cancer subtype based on ER/PR and HER2 status in Ghanaian patients at the Korle Bu Teaching Hospital, Ghana

Bernard Seshie[1], Nii Armah Adu-Aryee[2], Florence Dedey[2], Benedict Calys-Tagoe[3] and Joe-Nat Clegg-Lamptey[2*]

## Abstract

**Background:** Breast cancer is a heterogeneous disease composed of multiple subgroups with different molecular alterations, cellular composition, clinical behaviour, and response to treatment. This study evaluates the occurrence of the various subtypes and their clinical and pathological behaviour in the Ghanaian breast cancer population at the Korle Bu Teaching Hospital (KBTH).

**Methods:** Retrospective review of case notes of patients who had completed treatment for breast cancer at the KBTH within the last 5 years was conducted between April 2011 and March 2012. Subtypes were determined by immunohistochemistry classification based on expression of estrogen receptor (ER), progesterone receptor (PR), and human epidermal growth factor receptor-2 (HER-2).

**Result:** A total of 165 cases contributed to this study. The mean age at diagnosis was 52.5 ± 12.1 years. Tumour size ranged from 0.8 cm to 15 cm with a mean of 4.9 ± 2.8 cm and median of 4 cm. Tumour grade was Grade I 8.3 %, Grade II 60.8 % and Grade III 30.8 %. ER, PR and HER2/neu receptor positivity was 32.1, 25.6 and 25.5 % respectively. Almost half (49.4 %) of the study population had triple negative tumours. Luminal A, luminal B and non-luminal HER2 were 25.6, 12.2, and 12.8 % respectively. No statistically significant association was seen between subtype and tumour size, tumour grade, lymph node status and age at diagnosis.

**Conclusion:** Triple negative tumour is the most occurring subtype in the Ghanaian breast cancer population treated at the Korle Bu Teaching Hospital. Lack of association seen between subtypes and their clinical and pathological behaviour could be due to small sample size.

**Keywords:** Breast cancer, Subtype, ER, PR, HER2

## Background

Breast cancer is still the most common cancer in women comprising 16 % of all female cancers worldwide [1]. With increasing improvement in treatment modalities like hormonal and chemotherapy, however, mortality has declined [2]. But this decline is faster in white Americans compared to black Americans in the United States of America, although the incidence of breast cancer is lower in the latter [3]. The poorer prognosis in blacks has been attributed to a number of factors, including the observation that blacks appear to be at higher risk of breast cancer at an early age, and are diagnosed with more aggressive and advanced tumours [4, 5]. In Ghana, where more than 50 % of patients present with locally advanced or metastatic disease, 5-year survival was reported as only 25.3 % in 2001 [6].

It is now clear that breast cancer is a heterogeneous disease of multiple subgroups with different molecular alterations, cellular composition, clinical behaviour, and response to treatment [7–9]. Hence, standard clinical prognostic features such as age, tumour size, nodal status, grade, and hormone receptor status may be inaccurate.

* Correspondence: clegglamptey@chs.edu.gh
[2]Department of Surgery, School of Medicine and Dentistry, University of Ghana, Accra, Ghana
Full list of author information is available at the end of the article

Consequently, many patients are perhaps given treatment they may not need and benefit from. On the other hand, the true risk in some patients is underestimated and some may be given false assurances of favourable prognosis [10].

Several studies have attested to the higher prevalence of triple negative tumours with poorer prognosis in breast cancer patients of African origin [5, 11], although a study from Nigeria reported no difference in the pattern of hormone receptors in the African breast cancer population compared to other populations [12].

This study was undertaken to determine the occurrence of the various subtypes of breast cancer in Ghanaian patients seeking treatment at the Korle Bu Teaching Hospital and to determine the clinical and pathological behaviour of the different subtypes (grade, tumour size, lymph node burden and age at diagnosis).

## Methods

Data for this study was from an ongoing study on upper limb morbidity following treatment of breast cancer in Ghana, which has been approved by the Ethical and Protocol Review Committee, University of Ghana School of Medicine and Dentistry.

### Study population

Korle Bu Teaching Hospital (KBTH) is the largest teaching hospital in Ghana, the leading tertiary hospital and the major referral centre in the country. It also serves as the teaching hospital of the University of Ghana School of Medicine and Dentistry.

Breast Cancer patients who had received and completed treatment for breast cancer at the Korle Bu Teaching Hospital (KBTH) within the last 5 years and were being seen for out-patient review constituted the study population. Data was thus collected between April 2011 and March 2012. During the period 363 consecutive patients who met the above criteria were seen and their case notes reviewed. Immunohistochemistry (IHC) for estrogen receptor (ER), progesterone receptor (PR), and HER-2/neu, which is a prerequisite for this study, was available for 165. They thus constituted the subset for this study. Demographic information (hand dominance and educational level), breast cancer clinico-pathological features (age at diagnosis, tumour size, tumour grade, lymph node status, hormonal receptors status) and treatment modality (type of surgery, chemotherapy) were extracted from the case notes.

Pathology reports from which ER, PR and HER-2/neu, were obtained came from Korle-Bu Teaching Hospital. IHC was performed on formalin-fixed paraffin embedded tissue sections. The ER and PR tests were scored based on an aggregate score of percentage of tumour stained and staining intensity. Aggregate score of more than 2 were considered positive; that is, a minimum of 1–10 % stained associated with minimum intensity. HER-2/neu was considered positive if an IHC 3+ result was found. Flourescence in situ hybridization (FISH) was not available in the institution.

For this study we used Immunohistochemistry (IHC) classification that categorizes tumours according to the expression of estrogen receptor (ER), progesterone receptor (PR), and HER-2/neu. Expression of basal cytokeratin 5/6 and EGFR were not determined in these cases. Hence the triple negative tumours included both core basal phenotype, equivalent to the basal-like by gene expression profiling, and five negative phenotype.
Below is the categorization used:

Luminal A (ER/PR+, HER2-)
- ER+/PR+/HER2-; ER-/PR+/HER2-; or ER+/PR-/HER2-

Luminal B (ER/PR+, HER2+)
- ER+/PR+/HER2+; ER-/PR+/HER2+; or ER+/PR-/HER2+

Non-luminal HER2 (ER-/PR-/HER2+)
- ER-/PR-/HER2+

Triple Negative (ER-/PR-/HER2-)
- ER-/PR-/HER2-

Histological grading was by the Bloom-Richardson grading system that combined scores for nuclear grade, tubule formation and mitotic rate [13].

### Statistical analysis

SPSS 16.0 was used for the descriptive data analysis. To test for association between subtype and tumour grade, and subtype and lymph node burden contingency table was used and Chi Square test done. One-way ANOVA was conducted to compare the differences in tumour size and age at diagnosis between breast cancer subtypes.

### Results

A total of 165 cases contributed to this study. The mean age at diagnosis was $52.5 \pm 12.1$ years. The youngest patient in the study group was 24 years and the oldest person was 77 years at the time of diagnosis. Figure 1 shows the age distribution at the time of diagnosis. The educational level of the study population is as shown in Fig. 2.

In 50.9 % of the study population the tumour was located in the left breast with the remaining 49.1 % in the right breast. Over 90 % of the patients were right handed. There was however, no correlation between hand dominance and tumour site (Spearman's correlation value of 0.034, p-value of 0.666).

Tumour size ranged from 0.8 cm to 15 cm with a mean of $4.9 \pm 2.8$ cm and median of 4. Eight tumours were ≥10 cm. Tumour size (T in TNM classification)

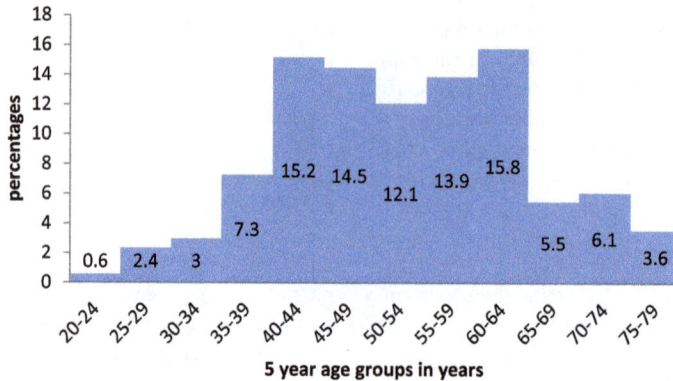

**Fig. 1** Age distribution of study patient

values were available for 155 cases. T1 (maximum diameter 2 cm or less) tumour was present in 17/155 (11 %) and T2 (size more than 2 cm but not more than 5 cm), T3 (bigger than 5 cm) and T4 (spread to chest wall, or skin—including inflammatory cancer) tumours were 71 (45.8 %), 42 (27.1 %), and 25 (15.2 %) respectively.

The majority of tumours were Grade 2. The distribution of tumour grade is shown in Fig. 3.

Mastectomy was done in 97.6 % (161/165) of cases. Only 4 cases (2.4 %) had breast conservation surgery (BCS). Apart from 2 patients who had sentinel node biopsy, all the other patients had axillary clearance. Less than 10 lymph nodes were removed in 52.2 % of cases. Mean lymph node (LN) removal was $9.4 \pm 4.3$ and mean LN involvement was $3.3 \pm 3.6$. Regional LN involvement (TNM) in 137 patients in which data was available was N0 47 (34.3 %), N1 35 (25.5 %), N2 46 (33.6 %) and N3 9 (6.6 %).

ER, PR and HER 2 neu receptor positivity was 32.1 % (53/165), 25.6 % (42/164) and 25.5 % (40/157) respectively. The distribution of the receptor status by tumour size, tumour grade and LN positivity is shown in Table 1.

Data for breast cancer subtype was available for 156 cases. Almost half (49.4 %) of the study population had triple negative tumours. The distribution of various subtypes is as shown in Fig. 4.

The distribution of the subtype by tumour size, tumour grade and LN positivity is shown in Table 2. Luminal A subtype constituted 53.3 % of T1 tumours, whereas triple negative subtype represented 50 % of T2 tumours, 57.1 % of T3 tumours and 50 % of T4 tumours. However, the difference in tumour size among the subtypes was not significant ($F_{3, 113} = 1.26$, $p = 0.262$). Regarding tumour grade, 45.5 % of Grade 2 tumours and 52.8 % of Grade 3 tumours were triple negative subtype. But there was no statistically significant association between tumour grade and subtype ($p$-value = 0.515). Although 51.1 % of N2 and 66.7 % of N3 lymph node status were triple negative subtype, no significant association was seen statistically ($p$-value = 0.547). The same applied to age at diagnosis ($F_{3, 152} = .507$, $p = 0.678$).

In the study population, 43.1 % received between 2 to 6 cycles of neoadjuvant chemotherapy. The commonest combination therapy used as neoadjuvant and adjuvant therapy was Cyclophosphamide—Doxorubicin—5 Fluorouracil (CAF) in 85.5 % of cases. 5-Fluorouracil—Epirubicin—Cyclophosphamide (FEC) 6.2 %, Cyclophosphamide—Methotrexate -5-Fluorouracil (CMF) 6.2 %, and Paclitaxel in only 1.4 %.

**Discussion**

In this study of patients treated for breast cancer we found predominance of hormone receptor negative tumours (49.4 %). This is consistent with a study from Kumasi-Ghana between July 2004 and June 2009, which reported 42.5 % triple negative tumours in 54 breast cancer patients [14]. An earlier from the same centre that compared Ghanaian breast cancer patients with black American and white American reported a higher percentage of hormone negative tumours of 82.2 % in Ghanaian women compared

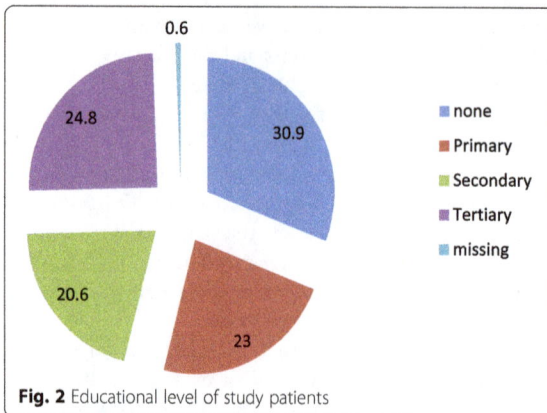

**Fig. 2** Educational level of study patients

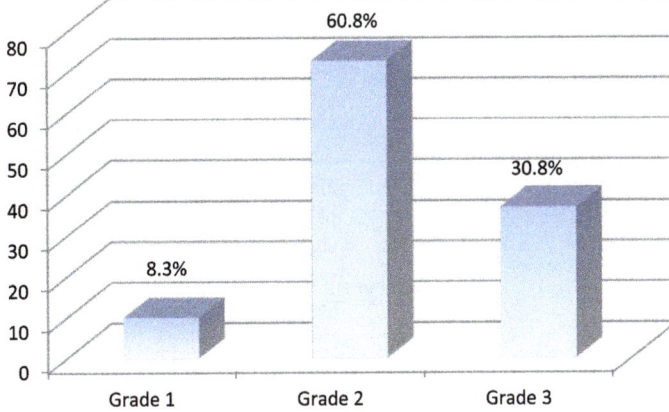

**Fig. 3** Histological grade of tumours

to 26.4 and 16.0 % in black American and white American women respectively [11].

DNA microarray analysis of gene expression has identified five subtypes with different gene expression characteristics and differences in behaviour [15]. The usefulness of gene expression pattern rests in its value as a prognostic maker [16]. Although considered as gold standard it has not been widely used due to expense and difficulty using paraffin-embedded material. Hence, the use of immunohistochemisty (IHC) which is simple, workable, and capable of classifying tumours into subtypes which are surrogates to gene expression pattern [17].

IHC for hormone receptor status, human epidermal growth factor receptor-2 (HER2) status, and at least one basal marker (cytokeratin [CK]5/6 or epidermal growth factor receptor [EGFR]) enable the division of tumours into Luminal 1, Luminal 2, Non-luminal HER2 positive tumours, and triple negative tumours (Fig. 5) and are associated with different behaviour [7].

Using IHC classification based on expression of ER, PR, and HER-2 receptors tumours were grouped in Luminal

**Table 1** Distribution of receptor status by tumour size, grade and LN involvement

| Tumour size | Receptor status | | | | | | | | |
|---|---|---|---|---|---|---|---|---|---|
| | ER+ | ER- | Total | PR+ | PR- | Total | Her2+ | Her2- | Total |
| T1 | 9 (17.6) | 8 (7.7) | 17 (11.0) | 7 (17.5) | 9 (7.9) | 16 (10.4) | 4 (10.8) | 12 (10.8) | 16 (10.0) |
| T2 | 24 (47.1) | 47 (45.2) | 71 (45.8) | 21 (52.3) | 50 (43.9) | 71 (46.1) | 17 (46.9) | 49 (44.1) | 66 (44.6) |
| T3 | 12 (20.6) | 30 (28.8) | 42 (27.1) | 6 (15.0) | 36 (31.6) | 42 (27.3) | 9 (24.3) | 33 (29.7) | 42 (28.4) |
| T4 | 6 (11.8) | 19 (18.3) | 25 (6.1) | 6 (15.0) | 19 (16.7) | 25 (16.2) | 7 (18.9) | 17 (15.3) | 24 (16.2) |
| Total | 51 | 104 | 155 | 40 | 114 | 154 | 37 | 111 | 148 |
| Tumour grade | | | | | | | | | |
| 1 | 5 (50) | 5 (50) | 10 | 4 (40) | 6 (60) | 10 | 3 (33.3) | 6 (66.7) | 9 |
| 2 | 24 (32.9) | 49 (67.1) | 73 | 23 (31.9) | 49 (68.1) | 72 | 21 (30.4) | 48 (69.6) | 69 |
| 3 | 8 (21.6) | 29 (78.4) | 37 | 5 (13.5) | 32 (86.5) | 37 | 8 (22.2) | 28 (77.8) | 36 |
| Total | 37 | 83 | 120 | 32 | 87 | 119 | 32 | 82 | 114 |
| Lymph node positivity | | | | | | | | | |
| N0 | 12 (25.5) | 35 (74.5) | 47 | 8 (17.0) | 39 (83.0) | 47 | 11 (25.0) | 33 (75.0) | 44 |
| N1 | 13 (32.1) | 22 (62.9) | 35 | 12 (34.3) | 23 (65.7) | 35 | 8 (25.0) | 24 (75.0) | 32 |
| N2 | 16 (34.8) | 30 (65.2) | 46 | 10 (22.2) | 35 (77.8) | 45 | 12 (26.1) | 34 (73.9) | 46 |
| N3 | 2 (22.2) | 7 (77.8) | 9 | 0 (0) | 9 (100) | 9 | 3 (33.3) | 6 (66.7) | 9 |
| Total | 43 | 94 | 137 | 30 | 106 | 136 | 34 | 97 | 131 |

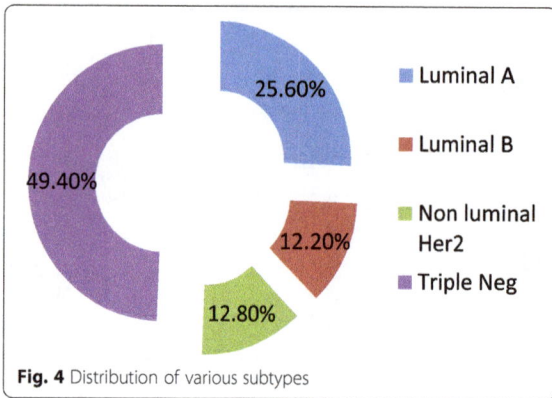

**Fig. 4** Distribution of various subtypes

A, Luminal B, Non-luminal HER-2 and triple negative tumours. We observed a high prevalence of triple negative subtype. Indeed, almost half of the cases were triple negative. This is consistent with some studies from Nigeria and Senegal in which majority of tumours were basal-like 27 % or unclassified 28 % subtype (surrogate for triple negative) [18]. However, this is in contrast to another study from Nigeria in which majority of tumours were Luminal A (77.6 %) [12]. Luminal A, although the second most frequently occurring subtype in our study, was present in only 25.60 % of cases. One limitation to our study was the non availability of retrospective data on basal markers (cytokeratin [CK]5/6 or epidermal growth factor receptor [EGFR]) as they are not routinely done in

**Table 2** Distribution of subtype by tumour size, grade and LN involvement

| Subtype | | | | | |
|---|---|---|---|---|---|
| Tumour size | Luminal A | Luminal B | Non luminal Her2 | Triple Neg | Total |
| T1 | 8 (53.3) | 2 (13.3) | 2 (13.3) | 3 (20.0) | 15 (100) |
| T2 | 17 (25.8) | 10 (15.2) | 6 (9.1) | 33 (50.0) | 66 (100) |
| T3 | 9 (21.4) | 4 (9.5) | 5 (11.9) | 24 (57.1) | 42 (100) |
| T4 | 5 (20.8) | 2 (8.3) | 5 (20.8) | 12 (50.0) | 24 (100) |
| Total | 39 | 18 | 18 | 72 | 147 |
| Tumour grade | | | | | |
| 1 | 3 (33.3) | 2 (22.2) | 1 (11.1) | 3 (33.3) | 9 |
| 2 | 17 (25.0) | 10 (14.7) | 10 (14.7) | 31 (45.5) | 68 |
| 3 | 9 (25.0) | 1 (2.8) | 7 (19.4) | 19 (52.8) | 36 |
| Total | 29 | 13 | 18 | 53 | 113 |
| Lymph node positivity | | | | | |
| N0 | 10 (22.7) | 4 (9.1) | 7 (15.9) | 23 (52.3) | 44 |
| N1 | 12 (37.5) | 4 (12.5) | 4 (12.5) | 12 (37.5) | 32 |
| N2 | 10 (22.2) | 7 (15.6) | 5 (11.1) | 23 (51.1) | 45 |
| N3 | 0(0) | 2 (22.2) | 1 (11.1) | 6 (66.7) | 9 |
| Total | 32 | 17 | 17 | 64 | 130 |

our centre. This would have enabled us stratify the triple negative tumours into 5 negative phenotype (non-basal triple negative) and core basal phenotype which many studies had shown to have different behaviour with the latter being more aggressive [5, 8, 17, 19, 20].

In addition, BRCA 1 and 2 mutations have not been determined in our study population. Hence, we are unable to evaluate their contribution to the high prevalence of triple negative tumours in this study. However, several studies have documented high proportion of triple negative breast cancer in carriers of these germ-line mutations, especial BRCA 1 [21–25]. Future research is needed in this area because of its implications for treatment. Triple negative breast cancer patients with BRCA 1 or BRCA like tumours can benefit from treatment with PARP inhibitors [26].

In this study triple negative tumours appeared to be associated with high mean tumour size and higher proportion of T2, T3 and T4 tumours compared to other subtypes. Indeed, 53.3 % of T1 tumours were luminal A subtype whereas over 50 % T2 to T4 tumours were Triple negative tumours. They also constitute greater proportion of Grade 2 and Grade 3 tumours and N2 and N3 tumours. These are consistent with other studies that have shown that triple negative breast cancer has very unfavourable and aggressive clinicopathological features [5, 11]. However, we failed to find significant statistical association.

Our findings have implication for treatment of breast cancer in Ghana. In the past, patient with breast cancer were treated blindly with tamoxifen. However, approximately 50 % of our patients may not be suitable for hormonal or targeted therapy because they are either negative for ER/PR or do not over express HER2. Hence, they will not benefit from the advantages of these modalities of treatment [27–30]. Currently chemotherapy remains the only systemic treatment for this category of patients. Fortunately, core basal phenotype which is a subset of triple negative breast cancer has the greatest short-term effect from cytotoxics compared to all other subtypes. But this cannot be said about the 5 negative phenotype [31]. Several studies using post treatment American Joint Committee on Cancer tumour-node-metastasis staging for invasive carcinoma have documented higher complete pathological response in the core basal phenotype of triple negative breast cancer compared to all other subtypes [5, 31]. However, they still have poorer prognosis due to higher likelihood of relapse in those with residual disease [9, 31].

Several of these studies demonstrated the importance of neo-adjuvant chemotherapy in triple negative breast cancer patients. This is not for the sole purpose of tumour reduction to facilitate surgery, but also to assess response to cytotoxic drugs and predict the likelihood of

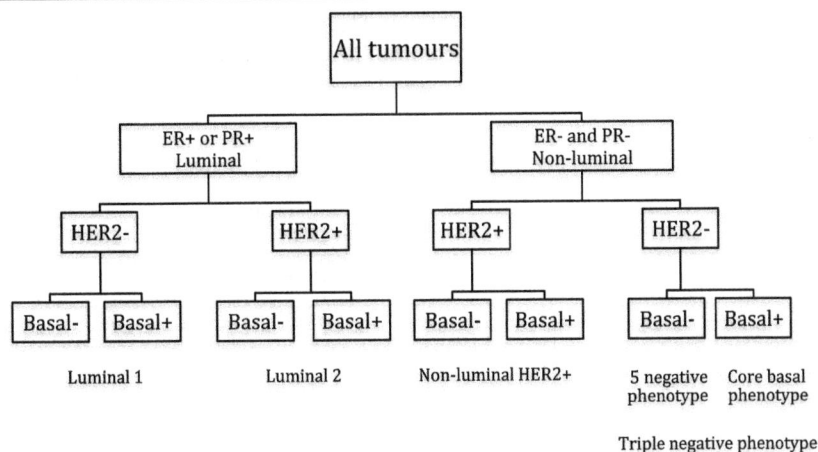

**Fig. 5** Classification of breast cancer subtype according to IHC marker profile [7]

relapse in patients with residual disease. But in our study only 43.1 % received between 2 to 6 cycles of neo-adjuvant chemotherapy. In our study 85.5 % of patient received CAF either as neo-adjuvant, adjuvant or both despite almost half of the patients being triple negative. However, studies have shown that basal-like and HER2+ subtypes are more sensitive to neo-adjuvant chemotherapy with paclitaxel- and doxorubicin-containing regimes compared to the luminal subtype [9]. Also for the triple negative tumours (especially BRCA—mutated disease), platinum based chemotherapy and PARP inhibitors may hold some promise [32, 33]. The neoadjuvant/adjuvant treatment of the patients in our study therefore appears to be suboptimal.

For surgical treatment, 97.6 % of the patients had mastectomy, a rather high rate compared to what is reported in Europe, North America and Japan (between 27.5 to 64 % [34–37]. Breast conserving surgery was only done in 2.4 % of our patients, a rather low rate as compared to rates of 54 % to over 70 % elsewhere [35–39]. As many as 66 % of the patients in this study presented with a T1 or 2 tumours while almost 60 % had N0 or 1 lymph node staging. Breast conservation surgery may have been suitable for many of these patients. However, almost half of the patients had triple negative subtype and about 91 % had grade 2 and 3 tumours. These factors, as well as increasing tumour size, have been found to be independent predictors of mastectomy but are not contraindications to BCS [34, 36, 38, 40],. Although there is no optimal mastectomy rate [41], evidence suggests that our patients may be presenting late and refusing treatment for breast cancer partly because of the fear of mastectomy. Indeed, in a previous study at the KBTH, fear of mastectomy was the reason for delayed

presentation and absconding before and during treatment in 24.2 and 57.2 % of patients respectively [42]. Hence, more breast conservation should be encouraged where indicated.

The limitation of this study was the small sample size. We were thus unable to demonstrate statistically any association between the subtypes and clinical and pathological behaviour. We did not also have information about the menopausal status of the participants to determine the proportions of the various subtypes that were premenopausal.

**Conclusion**

Triple negative tumour is the most commonly occurring subtype in the Ghanaian breast cancer population treated at the Korle Bu Teaching Hospital. Hence, blind hormonal therapy is not justifiable. Lack of significant association between subtypes and their clinical and pathological behaviour could be due to the small sample size. We recommend the inclusion of basal makers in the IHC panel on routine basis.

**Abbreviations**
KBTH: Korle Bu Teaching Hospital; ER: Estrogen receptor; PR: Progesterone receptor; HER2: Human epidermal receptor 2; IHC: Immunohistochemistry; EGFR: Epidermal growth factor receptor; ESBC: Early stage breast cancer; BCS: Breast conservation surgery; CK: Cytokeratin; CAF: Cyclophosphamide–Doxorubicin–5 Fluorouracil; FEC: 5Fluorouracil–Epirubicin-Cyclophosphamide; CMF: Cyclophosphamide- Methotrexate-5 Fluorouracil; LN: Lymph node.

**Competing interests**
The authors declare that they have no competing interests.

**Authors' contribution**
BS, NAA, BCT, FD and JNCL conceptualized the study. BS collected data and all authors analysed the data. BS drafted the manuscript and NAA, BCT, FD and JNCL reviewed and revised the manuscript. All authors read and approved the final manuscript.

## Acknowledgements

We thank the following for their roles in the acquisition of the data:
Desmond Ampaw-Asiedu
Doris Kpogo
Janet Adade

## Author details

[1]Department of Surgery, Tema General Hospital, Tema, Ghana. [2]Department of Surgery, School of Medicine and Dentistry, University of Ghana, Accra, Ghana. [3]Department of Community Health, School of Public Health, University of Ghana, Accra, Ghana.

## References

1. WHO. The Global Burden of Disease: 2004 Update. 2008.
2. Jatoi I, Chen BE, Anderson WF, Rosenberg PS. Breast Cancer Mortality Trends in the United States According to Estrogen Receptor Status and Age at Diagnosis. J Clin Oncol. 2007;25(13):1683–90.
3. Ries LA, Eisner MP, Kosary CL. Cancer Statistics review 1975-2000. In: National Cancer Institute. 2003.
4. Newman LA. Breast Cancer in African American women. Oncologist. 2005;10:1–14.
5. Carey LA, Perou CM, Livasy CA, Dressler LG, Cowan D, Conway K, et al. Race, Breast Cancer Subtypes, and Survival in the Carolina Breast Cancer Study. JAMA. 2006;295:2492–502.
6. Baako BN, Badoe EA. Treatment of Breast Cancer in Accra: 5 year Survival. Ghana Med J. 2001;35:90–5.
7. Blows FM, Driver KE, Schmidt MK, Broeks A, van Leeuwen FE, et al. (2010) Subtyping of Breast Cancer by Immunohistochemistry to Investigate a Relationship between Subtype and Short and Long Term Survival: A Collaborative Analysis of Data for 10,159 Cases from 12 Studies. PLoS Med 7(5): e1000279. doi:10.1371/journal.pmed.1000279.
8. de Ruijter TC, Veeck J, de Hoon JPJ, van Engeland M, Tjan-Heijnen VC. Characteristics of triple-negative breast cancer. J Cancer Res Clin Oncol. 2011;137:183–92.
9. Rouzier R, Perou CM, Fraser Symmans W, Ibrahim N, Cristofanilli M, Anderson K, et al. Breast Cancer Molecular Subtypes Respond Differently to Preoperative Chemotherapy. Clin Cancer Res. 2005;11:5678–85.
10. Bergh J, Holmquist M. Who should not receive adjuvant chemotherapy? International databases. J Natl Cancer Inst Monogr. 2001;30:103–8.
11. Stark A, Kleer CG, Martin I, Awuah B, Nsiah-Asare A, Takyi V, et al. African Ancestry and Higher Prevalence of Triple-Negative Breast Cancer. Cancer. 2010;116:4926–32.
12. Adebamowo AC, Famooto A, Ogundiran OT, Aniagwu T, Nkwodimmah C, Akang EE. Immunohistochemical and molecular subtypes of breast cancer in Nigeria. Breast Cancer Res Treat. 2008;110:183–8.
13. Bloom HJ, Richardson WW. Histological grading and prognosis in breast cancer; a study of 1409 cases of which 359 have been followed for 15 years. Br J Cancer. 1957;11(3):359–77.
14. Ohene-Yeboah M, Adjei E. Breast cancer in Kumasi, Ghana. Ghana Med J. 2012;46(1):8–13.
15. Perou CM, Sùrlie T, Eisen MB, van de Rijn M, Jeffrey SS, Rees CA, et al. Molecular portraits of human breast tumours. Nature. 2000;406.
16. Sørliea T, Perou CM, Tibshiranie R, Aas T, Geisler S, Johnsen H, et al. Gene expression patterns of breast carcinomas distinguish tumor subclasses with clinical implications. Proc Natl Acad Sci U S A. 2001;98(199):10869–74.
17. Nielsen TO, Hsu FD, Jensen K, Cheng M, Karaca G, Hu Z, et al. Immunohistochemical and Clinical Characterization of the Basal-Like Subtype of Invasive Breast Carcinoma. Clin Cancer Res. 2004;10:5367–74.
18. Huo D, Ikpatt F, Khramtsov A, Dangou J-M, Nanda R, Dignam J, et al. Population Differences in Breast Cancer: Survey in Indigenous African Women Reveals Over-Representation of Triple-Negative Breast Cancer. J Clin Oncol. 2009;27:4515–21.
19. Pang J, Toy KA, Griffith KA, Awuah B, Quayson S, Newman LA, et al. Invasive breast carcinomas in Ghana: high frequency of high grade, basal-like histology and high EZH2 expression. Breast Cancer Res Treat. 2012;135(1):59–66.
20. Yang XR, Sherman ME, Rimm DL, Lissowska J, Brinton LA, Peplonska B, et al. Differences in Risk Factors for Breast Cancer Molecular Subtypes

21. Lakhani SR, Van De Vijver MJ, Jacquemier J, Anderson TJ, Osin PP, McGuffog L, et al. The pathology of familial breast cancer: predictive value of immunohistochemical markers estrogen receptor, progesterone receptor, HER-2, and p53 in patients with mutations in BRCA1 and BRCA2. J Clin Oncol. 2002;20(9):2310–8.
22. Foulkes WD, Stefansson IM, Chappuis PO, Begin LR, Goffin JR, Wong N, et al. Germline BRCA1 mutations and a basal epithelial phenotype in breast cancer. J Natl Cancer Inst. 2003;95(19):1482–5.
23. Fostira F, Tsitlaidou M, Papadimitriou C, Pertesi M, Timotheadou E, Stavropoulou AV, et al. Prevalence of BRCA1 mutations among 403 women with triple-negative breast cancer: implications for genetic screening selection criteria: a Hellenic Cooperative Oncology Group Study. Breast Cancer Res Treat. 2012;134(1):353–62.
24. Young SR, Pilarski RT, Donenberg T, Shapiro C, Hammond LS, Miller J, et al. The prevalence of BRCA1 mutations among young women with triple-negative breast cancer. BMC Cancer. 2009;9:86.
25. Villarreal-Garza C, Weitzel JN, Llacuachaqui M, Sifuentes E, Magallanes-Hoyos MC, Gallardo L, et al. The prevalence of BRCA1 and BRCA2 mutations among young Mexican women with triple-negative breast cancer. Breast Cancer Res Treat. 2015;150(2):389–94.
26. McCabe N, Turner NC, Lord CJ, Kluzek K, Bialkowska A, Swift S, et al. Deficiency in the repair of DNA damage by homologous recombination and sensitivity to poly(ADP-ribose) polymerase inhibition. Cancer Res. 2006;66(16):8109–15.
27. Early Breast Cancer Trialists' Collaborative Group (EBCTCG). Effects of chemotherapy and hormonal therapy for early breast cancer on recurrence and 15-year survival: an overview of the randomised trials. Lancet. 2005;365(9472):1687–717.
28. Samphao S, Eremin JM, El-Sheemy M, Eremin O. Treatment of established breast cancer in post-menopausal women: role of aromatase inhibitors. Surgeon. 2009;7(1):42–55.
29. Romond EH, Perez EA, Bryant J, Suman VJ, Geyer Jr CE, Davidson NE, et al. Trastuzumab plus adjuvant chemotherapy for operable HER2-positive breast cancer. N Engl J Med. 2005;353(16):1673–84.
30. Pienkowski T, Zielinski CC. Trastuzumab treatment in patients with breast cancer and metastatic CNS disease. Ann Oncol. 2010;21(5):917–24.
31. Carey LA, Claire DE, Sawyer L, Gatti L, Moore DT, Collichio F, et al. The Triple Negative Paradox: Primary Tumor Chemosensitivity of Breast Cancer Subtypes. Clin Cancer Res. 2007;13:2329–34.
32. Silver DP, Richardson AL, Eklund AC, Wang ZC, Szallasi Z, Li Q, et al. Efficacy of Neoadjuvant Cisplatin in Triple-Negative Breast Cancer. J Clin Oncol. 2010;28(7):1145–53.
33. Rottenberg S, Jaspers JE, Kersbergen A, van der Burg E, Nygren AO, Zander SA, et al. High sensitivity of BRCA1-deficient mammary tumors to the PARP inhibitor AZD2281 alone and in combination with platinum drugs. Proc Natl Acad Sci U S A. 2008;105(44):17079–84.
34. Feigelson HS, James TA, Single RM, Onitilo AA, Aiello Bowles EJ, Barney T, et al. Factors associated with the frequency of initial total mastectomy: results of a multi-institutional study. J Am Coll Surg. 2013;216(5):966–75.
35. Hanagiri T, Nagata Y, Monji S, Shinohara S, Takenaka M, Shigematsu Y, et al. Temporal trends in the surgical outcomes of patients with breast cancer. World J Surg Oncol. 2012;10:108.
36. McGuire KP, Santillan AA, Kaur P, Meade T, Parbhoo J, Mathias M, et al. Are mastectomies on the rise? A 13-year trend analysis of the selection of mastectomy versus breast conservation therapy in 5865 patients. Ann Surg Oncol. 2009;16(10):2682–90.
37. Damle S, Teal CB, Lenert JJ, Marshall EC, Pan Q, McSwain AP. Mastectomy and contralateral prophylactic mastectomy rates: an institutional review. Ann Surg Oncol. 2011;18(5):1356–63.
38. Garcia-Etienne CA, Tomatis M, Heil J, Friedrichs K, Kreienberg R, Denk A, et al. Mastectomy trends for early-stage breast cancer: a report from the EUSOMA multi-institutional European database. Eur J Cancer. 2012;48(13):1947–56.
39. Dragun AE, Huang B, Tucker TC, Spanos WJ. Increasing mastectomy rates among all age groups for early stage breast cancer: a 10-year study of surgical choice. Breast J. 2012;18(4):318–25.
40. Mahmood U, Hanlon AL, Koshy M, Buras R, Chumsri S, Tkaczuk KH, et al. Increasing national mastectomy rates for the treatment of early stage breast cancer. Ann Surg Oncol. 2013;20(5):1436–43.

in a Population-Based Study. Cancer Epidemiol Biomarkers Prev. 2007;16:439–43.

41. Garcia-Etienne CA, Tomatis M, Heil J, Danaei M, Rageth CJ, Marotti L, et al. Fluctuating mastectomy rates across time and geography. Ann Surg Oncol. 2013;20(7):2114–6.

42. Clegg-Lamptey J, Dakubo J, Attobra YN. Why do breast cancer patients report late or abscond during treatment in ghana? A pilot study. Ghana Med J. 2009;43(3):127–31.

# 18

# Uterine myometrial mature teratoma presenting as a uterine mass

Emmanuel Kamgobe[1], Anthony Massinde[1,2†], Dismas Matovelo[1*], Edgar Ndaboine[1,2†], Peter Rambau[3†] and Tito Chaula[1]

## Abstract

**Background:** Teratomas are a germ cell tumors composed of two or more tissues which originate from ectoderm, endoderm or mesoderm. These tumors commonly arise from the ovary although other extragonadal sites can be involved, especially in children.

**Case presentation:** We report a case of a 21-year-old female of Sukuma ethnicity from the northern region of Tanzania who presented with abdominal pain and distension, fever, and abnormal vaginal discharge for the previous three weeks. The patient was also lactating for the previous 8 months following cesarean section delivery. Pelvic ultrasound suggested pelvic abscess but after laparotomy and histological analysis of a bulky uterus removed a diagnosis of mature uterine teratoma was confirmed.

**Conclusion:** Although it is rare, uterine teratoma should be considered in differential diagnosis to any patient with uterine mass even without typical radiological findings.

**Keywords:** Uterine mass, Uterine mature teratoma

## Background

Teratomas are usually composed of two or more embryonic germ layers: ectoderm, endoderm, and mesoderm. Extragonadal teratomas are ectopic to the location in which they are found. Teratomas can be classified as mature or immature on the basis of the presence or absence of immature neuroectodermal tissues in the tumor. Mature tumors have far less tendency to develop into malignancy compared to immature tumors. Teratomas are the most common gonadal tumors. They usually arise in the gonads and often occur in infancy and childhood. Extragonadal teratomas are rare and commonly develop in midline structures [1]. Uterine teratomas, which are part of extra gonadal teratomas of midline structures, account for 1–2 % of all teratomas. Complications during their surgical removal may occur depending on their location or if they are attached to any other structures. There is no documented evidence of metastatic potential [2, 3].

Primary teratomas of the uterus have rarely been reported since Mann's first description of this entity in 1929 [1, 2]. Here we report a case of uterine mature teratoma in a 21-year-old woman with an exceptional presentation of this tumor.

## Case presentation

A 21-year-old female of Sukuma ethnicity from the northern region of Tanzania presented at Bugando Medical Centre (BMC) outpatient clinic in Mwanza city with complaints of abdominal distension and pain, fever and abnormal vaginal discharge for the past 3 weeks. She was apparently lactating for the previous 8 months after cesarean section delivery of her first child. On physical examination, she appeared to be weak, febrile of about 38.5 °C with blood pressure of 110/70 mmHg. She was a blood group 'A' rhesus positive and her hemoglobin level was 6.3 g/dl.

* Correspondence: magonza77@yahoo.co.uk
†Equal contributors
[1]Department of Obstetrics and Gynecology, Catholic University of Health and Allied sciences, P.O.BOX 1464, Mwanza, Tanzania
Full list of author information is available at the end of the article

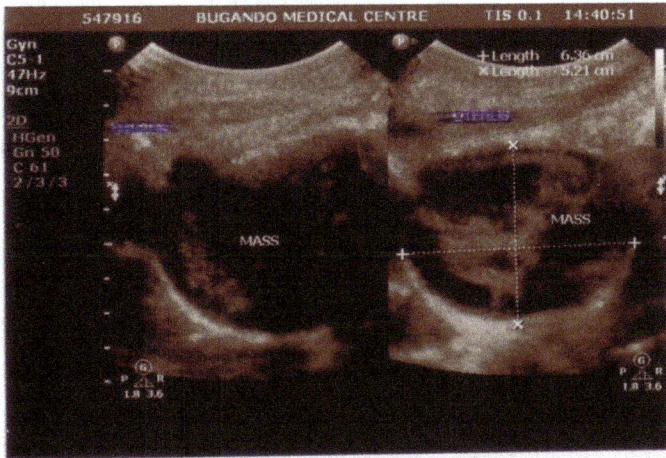

**Fig. 1** An irregular heterogeneous mass with solid echogenic areas surrounded by some fluid with no clear demarcation, measures approximately 5.3*3.4 cm, another hypoechoic mass rounded and capsulated seen posterior to the first mass predominantly cystic with some effective irregular echogenic patches measures 6.3*4.5 cm

On abdominal examination, a sub-umbilical midline scar was seen, and palpable suprapubic mass of about 16 weeks size of the uterus. The mass was soft, tender and mobile. The digital pelvic and vaginal examination elicited a closed cervix with tenderness on mobility and a non-bulging posterior fornix. There was no adnexal mass detected and gloved finger stained with pus-like discharge. Pelvic gynecological ultrasound suggested pelvic abscess (Fig. 1).

Patient was counseled for emergency laparotomy. Intraoperatively, the uterus was found to be bulky with discharging sinus on left fundal position. Both ovaries were healthy-looking and there was no fluid in the pouch of Douglas. The transverse incision was made on the uterus at the level of the discharging sinus. The yellowish mucinous tenacious materials with hairy tissues were observed. The decision to perform a total hysterectomy was reached; in which the removed uterus had hairs and sticky sebaceous matter found freely in the cavity. After surgery, the patient was transfused one unit of blood and intravenous antibiotics ceftriaxone, Gentamycin and Metronidazole were given with an addition of prophylactic Heparin. The patient had an uneventful recovery.

The sample was sent for histological examination. At the pathology department, the bisected uterus of 18 cm × 9 cm × 4 cm with no adnexa was identified. There was a cystic mass of 10 cm on the left fundal position in the myometrium containing hairs, sebaceous material, and pus.

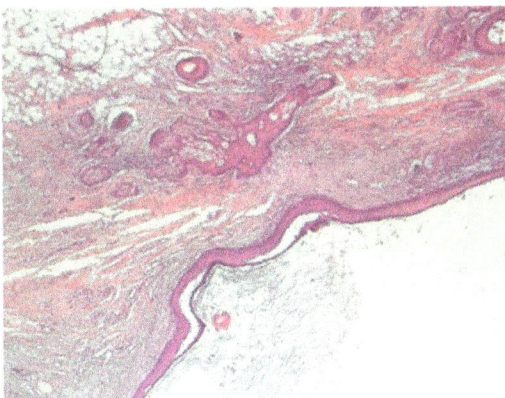

**Fig. 2** H & E histology section showing a cyst lined by squamous epithelium with keratin debris, and dermal appendages (x 10)

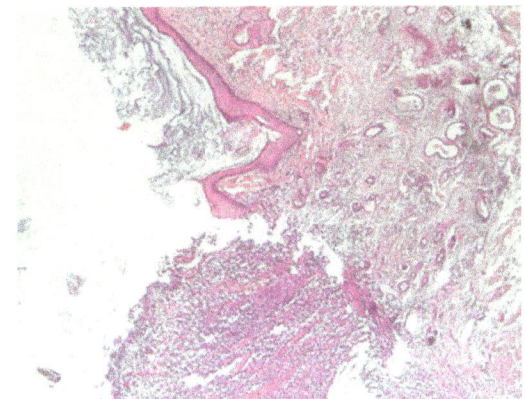

**Fig. 3** The same section showing an area of discontinuous squamous epithelium with inflammatory cells infiltrate (x10)

**Table 1** Clinical and pathological characteristics of patients with primary uterine mature teratoma in the literature

| Author | Age | Symptoms | Site of Tumour | Histology | Treatment | Relapse | Treatment of Relapse |
|---|---|---|---|---|---|---|---|
| Our Case | 21 | Abdominal distension | Uterine corpus | Mature teratoma | Hysterectomy | None | |
| Lim et al., [2011] [6] | 27 | Cervical polyp | Uterine cervix | Mature teratoma with some lymphoid elements | Excision | None | |
| Newsom-Davis et al., [2009] [5] | 82 | Postmenopausal bleeding | Uterine corpus | Mature& Immature Teratoma | Hysterectomy & bilateral salpingooophorectomy | Yes | Taxane, Etoposide & Cisplatin + Surgery |
| Cappelo et al., [2009] [4] | 55 | Asymptomatic (Multiple uterine leiomyomas) | Uterine corpus | Mature teratoma with thyroid differentiation | Hysterectomy | None | |
| Wang et al., [2011] [7] | 46 | Abnormal uterine bleeding | Uterine corpus | Mature cystic teratoma | Hysterectomy | None | |
| Papadia et al., [2007] [8] | 58 | Endometrial polyp/ Abnormal uterine bleeding | Uterine corpus | Mature cystic teratoma | Excision | None | |

The tissue sample was selected and sections were stained by Hematoxylin and Eosin (H&E) and observed by a light microscopy. Histology revealed a cyst in a myometrium contained keratin debris, and it was lined by squamous epithelium with dermal skin appendages with areas of denudation with lymphocyte and neutrophil infiltrate. The myometrium and endometrium was normal. Diagnosis of infected mature teratoma (dermoid cyst) was made (Figs. 2 and 3).

The patient has not shown any sign of disease recurrence for 8 months following hospital discharge.

## Discussion

Mature cystic teratomas of uterus corpus are very rare and thought to originate from displaced germinal cells derived from pluripotential stem cells. The most commonly occurring mature cystic teratomas of the uterus are of the cervical part [2]. The presentation discussed here is unusual because there are only few reported cases of uterine teratomas to date arising from uterine body, and infected teratoma is also a rare event [2]. Extragonadal germ teratomas are very rare, accounting to 1–2 % of all teratomas [4, 5]. Since only few cases have been reported; we report the clinical presentation and pathological characteristics of patients with primary uterine mature teratoma in English literature (Table 1) [4–8].

Our patient was in reproductive age, recently delivered and lactating; the presentation which is likely to develop teratoma due to the possibility of products of conceptus being implanted at any part along the reproductive tract during the process of fertilization according to the Blastomere Theory [8–10]. Although it does not apply to the patient discussed here, it is also possible for teratoma to develop in a newborn by abnormal migratory pathway of primordial germ cells from fetal yolk sac endodermal to the gonadal ridge during early embryogenesis as explained by Parthenogenic theory [3, 5].

Ultrasound images of the patient suggested pelvic abscess, but an explorative laparotomy and histopathological analysis of the excised bulky uterus led to a diagnosis of teratoma. In centers with, CT and MRI, those imaging techniques could have led to a correct diagnosis because of their higher accuracy compared to the ultrasound imaging [5]. Again, our hospital do not have Colour Doppler ultrasound which is superior to other imaging modalities with highest positive predictive value of 9.6 compared to 7.6 for MRI and 3.6 for CT16 [11].

Due to its rarity of occurrence, there is no standard guideline for management of mature uterine teratoma. The few case reports, however, suggest that the best management is complete tumor excision or total abdominal hysterectomy [3, 4, 6–8].

## Conclusion

Although it is rare, uterine teratoma should be considered in differential diagnosis in any patient with uterine mass even without typical radiological findings.

## Consent

"Written informed consent was obtained from the patient for publication of this Case report and any accompanying images. A copy of the written consent is available for review by the Editor of this journal".

### Abbreviations
BMC: Bugando Medical Centre; H&E: Hematoxylin & Eosin.

### Competing interests
We report no conflict of interest and no funding was received for this work.

### Authors' contributions
EK reviewed the patient at emergency unit, did the surgery and drafted the first manuscript. AM reviewed manuscript drafts. DM drafted the first manuscript and reviewed manuscript drafts. EN reviewed manuscript drafts. PR read the histological slides and reviewed manuscript drafts. TC assisted the surgery and reviewed the manuscript which was later approved by all authors.

**Acknowledgment**
The authors would like to thanks all the doctors and nurses at the BMC Emergency unit and Gynecological ward for taking good care of the patient and follow-up.

**Author details**
[1]Department of Obstetrics and Gynecology, Catholic University of Health and Allied sciences, P.O.BOX 1464, Mwanza, Tanzania. [2]Department of Obstetrics and Gynecology, Bugando Medical Centre, P.O.BOX 1370, Mwanza, Tanzania. [3]Department of Pathology, Catholic University of Health and Allied sciences, P.O.BOX 1464, Mwanza, Tanzania.

**References**
1. Cortes J, Llompart M, Rossello J, Rifá J, Más J, Anglada P, et al. Immature teratoma primary of the uterine cervix. First case report. Eur J Gynaecol Oncol. 1989;11(1):37–42.
2. Ben Ameur El Youbi M, Mohtaram A, Kharmoum J, Aaribi I, Kharmoum S, Bouzoubaa A, et al. Primary immature teratoma of the uterus relapsing as malignant neuroepithelioma: case report and review of the literature. Case Rep Oncol Med. 2013;2013:971803.
3. Hamilton CA, Ellison M. Cystic teratoma. Emedicine (http://emedicine.medscape.com.article/281850-overview). 2006.
4. Cappello F, Barbato F, Tomasino RM. Mature teratoma of the uterine corpus with thyroid differentiation. Pathol Int. 2000;50(7):546–8.
5. Newsom-Davis T, Poulter D, Gray R, Ameen M, Lindsay I, Papanikolaou K, et al. Case report: Malignant teratoma of the uterine corpus. BMC Cancer. 2009;9(1):195.
6. Sc L, Ys K, Lee Y, Lee M, Jy L. Mature teratoma of the uterine cervix with lymphoid hyperplasia. Pathol Int. 2003;53(5):327–31.
7. Wang W-C, Lee M-S, Ko J-L, Lai Y-C. Origin of uterine teratoma differs from that of ovarian teratoma: a case of uterine mature cystic teratoma. Int J Gynecol Pathol. 2011;30(6):544–8.
8. Papadia A, Rutigliani M, Gerbaldo D, Fulcheri E, Ragni N. Mature cystic teratoma of the uterus presenting as an endometrial polyp. Ultrasound Obstet Gynecol. 2007;29(4):477–8.
9. NEWTON CW, ABELL MR. Iatrogenic fetal implants. Obstet Gynecol. 1972;40(5):686–91.
10. Tyagi S, Saxena K, Rizvi R, Langley F. Foetal remnants in the uterus and their relation to other uterine heterotopia. Histopathology. 1979;3(4):339–45.
11. Graham L. ACOG releases guidelines on management of adnexal masses. Am Fam Physician. 2008;77(9):1320–3.

# 19

# Primary Burkitt lymphoma of the thyroid gland

Mohamed Allaoui[1*], Ilias Benchafai[2], El Mehdi Mahtat[3], Safae Regragui[3], Adil Boudhas[1], Mustapha Azzakhmam[1], Mohammed Boukhechba[1], Abderrahmane Al Bouzidi[1] and Mohamed Oukabli[1]

## Abstract

**Background:** Primary thyroid lymphoma is an uncommon pathological entity that accounts for only 1 to 5 % of all thyroid malignancies. Primary Burkitt lymphoma of the thyroid gland is very rare. This article presents the first Moroccan case of a primary BL of the thyroid to be reported in the literature to date.

**Case presentation:** We describe here a case of a 70-year-old male who developed a rapidly enlarging thyroid gland with progressive symptoms of compression. Core biopsy confirmed the diagnosis of Burkitt lymphoma. The patient died of septic shock, 2 weeks after the first cycle of appropriate therapeutic chemotherapy.

**Conclusions:** This presentation emphasizes the importance of considering lymphoma when dealing with a thyroid mass, as its management is different from that of other thyroid pathologies, and affords an opportunity to review a very rare type of primary thyroid lymphoma.

**Keywords:** Burkitt lymphoma, Thyroid gland, Chemotherapy

## Background

Primary Burkitt lymphoma (BL) of the thyroid gland is a very uncommon pathological entity with a few isolated case reports in adult patients [1, 2].

This highly aggressive malignancy arises from B-lymphoid cells. It presents usually as a rapidly expanding thyroid mass causing compressive symptoms.

To the best of our knowledge, this article reports the first Moroccan case of a primary BL of the thyroid to be reported in the literature to date.

BL should be promptly recognized because its management is quite different from the treatment of other neoplasms of the thyroid gland. Moreover, this disease is quite curable if diagnosed early and treated appropriately.

## Case presentation

A 70-year-old male presented a rapidly expanding mass of the neck associated with history of airway compression symptoms; progressive dyspnea and dysphonia lasting for 4 weeks, in a context of apyrexia and impairment of general condition. The patient was admitted to the hospital because of increasing dyspnea and urgently received a tracheostomy.

A biopsy of the cervical mass was carried out and the histological examination showed diffuse infiltration of the thyroid gland by a monotonous population of atypical intermediate-sized lymphoid cells (Fig. 1). These last possess scanty amphophilic to basophilic cytoplasm with centrally located nuclei of irregular shape, displaying dispersed basophilic chromatin, and frequent apoptotic figures (Fig. 2). Scattered tingible body type macrophages were also present. Little residual thyroid follicles and some areas of necrosis was observed.

Immunohistochemical staining was then performed and the tumour cells were positive for CD20, CD10 and

* Correspondence: allaoui.m1@gmail.com
[1]Department of Pathology, Military General Hospital Mohammed V, Mohammed V Souissi University - Faculty of Medicine and Pharmacy of Rabat, Hay Riad, Rabat 10000, Morocco
Full list of author information is available at the end of the article

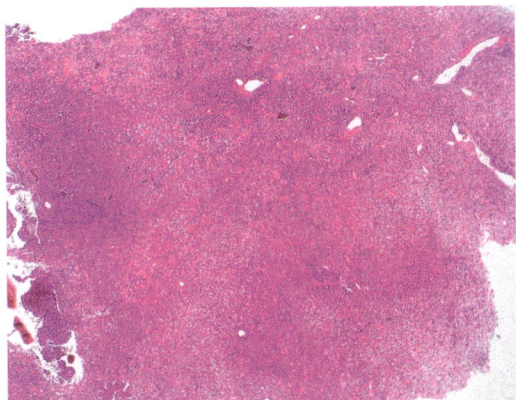

**Fig. 1** Low magnification showing a diffuse infiltration of atypical lymphoid cells in the thyroid gland (haematoxylin & eosin stain, ×50)

BCL6. Ki-67 showed proliferation index approaching 100 %. CD3 and CD5 stained the background T cells (Fig. 3). Immunoreactivity for Epstein-Barr virus (EBV) was negative. The diagnosis of BL was confirmed on fluorescence in situ hybridisation that showed tumour cell positivity for the t (8; 14) translocation. Bone marrow examination was normal.

The patient was transferred to the Clinical Haematology department. On physical examination, he was apyretic and hemodynamically stable with a cervical armouring by a huge mass of hard consistency. Neurological examination shows no sensorimotor deficits.

Other systemic examinations were normal, without any palpable lymphadenopathy or organomegaly.

The computerized tomography (CT) scan showed a heterogeneous process of the thyroid gland measuring $10.5 \times 8.2 \times 6.5$ cm in size, extending up towards the

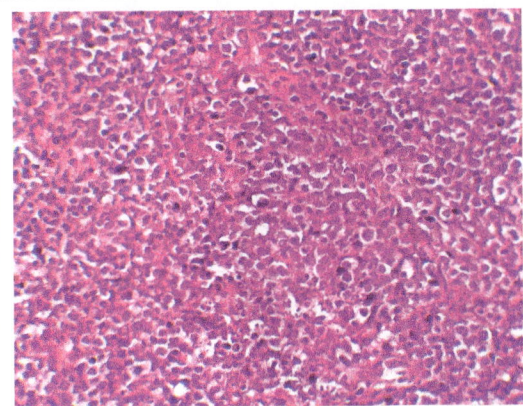

**Fig. 2** Higher magnification showing a monotonous population of intermediate-sized lymphoid cells with scant dark blue cytoplasm, small cytoplasmic vacuoles and tingible-body macrophages (haematoxylin & eosin stain, ×400)

laryngeal region, infiltrating the right vocal cord and reducing the laryngeal lumen (Fig. 4).

The thoraco-abdominal CT scan showed no other localization.

The examination of the cephalorachidian liquid showed no central nervous system involvement. The patient was diagnosed with thyroidal Burkitt lymphoma, stage I of Murphy [3].

After cardiac, renal and liver functions assessment, the patient received chemotherapy according to the LMBA02 protocol [4], group A (Age > 60 years, no CNS nor bone marrow involvement), with a first course of COP (Cyclophosphamide, Vincristine and Prednisone) and intrathecal Methotrexate, followed a week after by a course of R-COPADEM (Rituximab at day 0 and day 6, Cyclophosphamide day 2,3 and 4, Prednisone from day 1 to 5, Doxorubicineat day 2, high dose Methotrexate at day 1 with folic acid rescue from day 2 to day 6 and intrathecal chemotherapy at day 2 and day 6).

At day 15 of chemotherapy, the patient developed febrile neutropenia, refractory to broad-spectrum antibiotics and antifungals. The evolution was marked by the installation of a septic shock with acute respiratory distress syndrome that led to his transfer to intensive care unit where he was intubated and ventilated. The patient died 2 days after.

## Discussion

Primary thyroid lymphoma (PTL) is defined as a lymphoma involving only the thyroid gland or the thyroid gland and adjacent (regional) neck lymph nodes, without contiguous spread or distant metastases from other areas of involvement at diagnosis [5].

PTL is an uncommon pathological entity that accounts for only 1 to 5 % of all thyroid malignancies, comprises approximately 2 % of all malignant extra nodal lymphomas and which predominantly originate from B lymphocytes [5, 6].

The common histological subtypes are diffuse large B-cell lymphoma and mucosa-associated lymphoid tissue (MALT) lymphoma [6–9]. Primary Burkitt lymphoma of the thyroid is very rare with a few isolated case reports (Table 1) [1–3, 10, 11].

Burkitt lymphoma is a highly aggressive disease that is endemic in Africa and sporadic in other parts of the world. The endemic variant is associated with Epstein-Barr virus.

BL was one of the first tumours shown to have a chromosomal translocation that activates an oncogene (c-MYC) [12, 13].

Normally, the thyroid gland does not contain native lymphoid tissue, therefore, the intrathyroid lymphoid tissue that causes thyroid lymphoma comes from the migration of lymphoid tissue into the thyroid during an

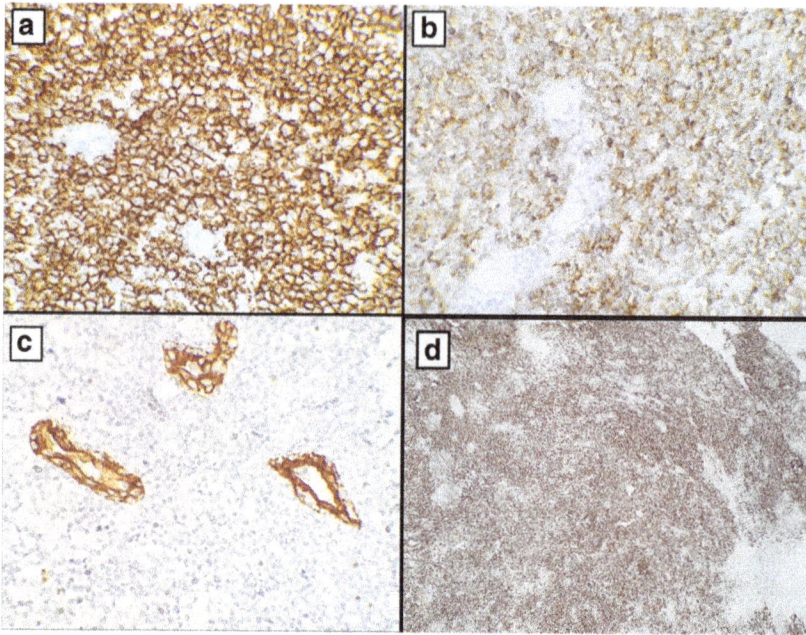

**Fig. 3** Immunohistochemical staining revealed the expression of CD20 (**a**) and CD10 (**b**) by the neoplastic cells. Keratin highlights the lymphoepithelial lesions (**c**). Ki-67 immunostaining showed a high proliferation index (**d**)

inflammatory or immunologic process. The most common condition resulting in lymphoid migration is autoimmune thyroiditis (i.e., Hashimoto's thyroiditis) [14–16]. Large adult population-based as well as retrospective clinicopathological case series suggest that primary thyroid Non-Hodgkin lymphoma NHL typically occur in middle to older-aged persons and have a predilection for females (it have also shown that patients with chronic lymphocytic thyroiditis have a greater risk of subsequently developing thyroid lymphoma when compared to age and gender matched normal individuals) [5, 6, 16–21].

Clinically, lymphomas originating in the thyroid can frequently mimic anaplastic thyroid carcinoma in that both have similar clinical characteristics of rapid growth, which might be associated with compression symptoms dyspnea, dysphagia, pain and hoarseness of voice [2, 22–25].

Ultrasonography is generally the initial diagnostic modality used in the workup of thyroid enlargement and nodules. Although nonspecific, there are certain characteristics that

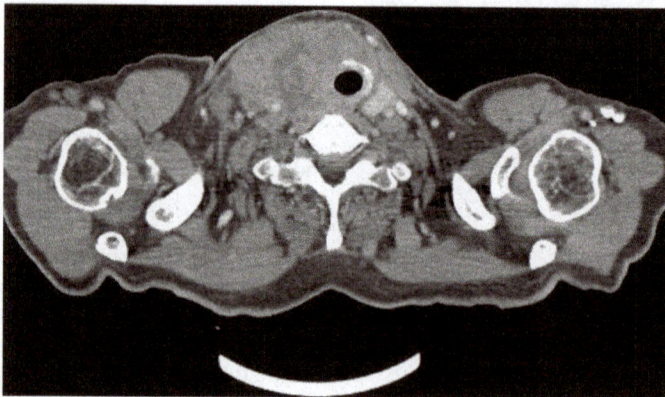

**Fig. 4** CT showing a large heterogeneous mass of the thyroid gland

**Table 1** Clinical and pathological characteristics of patients with primary Burkitt lymphoma of the thyroid gland in the literature

| Author | Age (year) | Sex | Clinical presentation | Size of tumor (cm) | Histology | Translocation type | Treatment | Follow-up time (month) | Evolution |
|---|---|---|---|---|---|---|---|---|---|
| Our case | 70 | M | Rapidly expanding mass of the neck associated with airway compression symptoms | 10.5 | Burkitt lymphoma | t (8; 14) | chemotherapy according to the LMBA02 protocol; with a first course of COP and intrathecal Methotrexate, followed by a course of R-COPADEM. | Patient died | The patient died of septic shock, 2 weeks after the first cycle of chemotherapy |
| Camera et al. [2010] [1] | 56 | M | Incidental discovery of a large left thyroid lobe nodule on CT | 4.9 | Burkitt-like large B–cell lymphoma | | Left lobe thyroidectomy. After diagnosis, The patient was treated with 8 cycles of intensive chemotherapy (cyclophosphamide, vincristine, doxorubicine, and dexamethasone) | 1 | Reduction of all lesions with improvement of symptoms. |
| Kalinyak et al. [2006] [2] | 53 | M | Tracheal compressive symptoms from a rapidly expanding thyroid mass | 6 | Burkitt lymphoma | | Rituxan and CHOP therapy, changed to hyper-CVAD-R chemotherapy. The patient also received a single dose of intrathecal methotrexate | 27 | Patient free of disease after end of treatment |
| Kandil et al. [2012] [10] | 60 | F | Rapidly expanding thyroid mass with airway compression and difficulty in swallowing | 8.7 | Burkitt-like lymphoma (B-cell lymphoma, unclassifiable) | | Rituximab, Cyclophosphamide, Mensa, Vincristine and Doxorubicin | | Successfully treated with 1 cycle of appropriate therapeutic chemotherapy |
| Cooper et al. [2014] [14] | 14 | M | Large predominantly left-sided firm thyroid swelling, with a 3-month history of malaise, lethargy, and weight loss | 6.7 | Burkitt lymphoma | t (8; 14) | COP and prednisolone followed by 2 courses of COPADM, prednisolone and two courses of CYM chemotherapy. This was accompanied by intrathecal chemotherapy | 36 | Disease free 3 years after end of treatment |
| Yildiz et al. [2012] [22] | 31 | M | Rapidly enlarging mass on the fore neck | 4 | Burkitt lymphoma | | R-Hyper-CVAD therapy | 6 | PET-CT scans performed after chemotherapy and at the 6-month follow-up were normal |
| Mweempwa et al. [2013] [24] | 58 | F | Background of benign goiter presented with a rapidly enlarging thyroid mass, causing dysphagia and dyspnea | 8 | Burkitt lymphoma | t (8; 14) | Modified Magrath protocol for Burkitt's lymphoma, low risk disease, which involved having 3 cycles of R-CODOX-M | 4 | Complete resolution of the tumour mass, 4 weeks after end of treatment |
| Liying et al. [2014] [30] | 8 | M | Mass in the right anterior neck with difficulty in swallowing | 4 | Burkitt lymphoma | t (8; 14) | Right lobe thyroidectomy. After diagnosis, the patient underwent alternate R-B-NHL-BFM-90-A and R-B-NHL-BFM-90-B treatment, for 4 cycles each | 48 | After 4 years of follow-up, the patient appears well and remains free of disease |

suggest PTL, based essentially upon ultrasound findings of internal echoes, borders, and posterior echoes. For example, Enhanced posterior echoes help in distinguishing lymphoma from other types of thyroid lesions [26, 27].

Once PTL is suspected based upon clinical presentation and ultrasound findings, the next step in diagnosis is biopsy. Traditionally, open surgical biopsy was felt to be necessary to differentiate thyroid lymphoma from thyroiditis and anaplastic carcinoma. However, with recent advances in immunophenotypic analysis, the accuracy of fine-needle aspiration (FNA) has improved. These advances in diagnosis of PTL mirror those seen with systemic lymphomas with a reported accuracy rate of FNA of 80–100 %. Nevertheless, there are still challenges in

FNA diagnosis of thyroid lymphoma, particularly due to the histological similarities with thyroiditis and the high coincidence of these pathologies within the same gland, which results in increased false-negative rates from sampling error [26].

Histologically, the tumour cells of BL are medium-sized cells (nuclei similar or smaller to those of histiocytes) and show a diffuse monotonous pattern of growth. The cells appear to be cohesive but sometimes exhibit squared-off borders of retracted cytoplasm. The nuclei are round with finely clumped and dispersed chromatin, with multiple basophilic medium-sized, paracentrally situated nucleoli. The cytoplasm is deeply basophilic and usually contains lipid vacuoles. The tumour has an extremely high proliferation fraction (many mitotic figures) as well as a high fraction of apoptosis. A "starry sky" pattern is usually present, which is imparted by numerous benign macrophages that have ingested apoptotic tumour cells [28].

In Burkitt lymphoma, the tumour cells express moderate to strong levels of membrane IgM with light chain restriction and B-cell-associated antigens (CD19, CD20 and CD22), CD10, BCL6, c-MYC and CD38. The neoplastic cells are usually negative or only weakly positive for BCL2 and are uniformly TdT and MUM-1/IRF-4 negative. Nearly 100 % of the cells are positive for Ki67. There are very few admixed T-cells [12, 28–30]. In the present case, the immunophenotype of the atypical lymphoid cells was consistent with these features.

Burkitt lymphoma is characterized at the molecular level by a reciprocal translocation involving the c-MYC proto-oncogene, which normally resides on chromosome 8q24. The most common translocation in Burkitt lymphoma is a t (8;14) (q24;q32), which results in the translocation of c-MYC to the B-cell heavy-chain gene locus on chromosome 14q32. This translocation occurs in approximately 80 % of Burkitt lymphoma cases regardless of the clinical setting. Other variant translocations involve the translocation of c-MYC to the kappa light chain locus on chromosome 2, t (2;8) (p12;q24), which occurs in approximately 15 % of cases, and translocation of c-MYC to the lambda light-chain locus on chromosome 22, t (8;22) (q24;q11), which occurs in approximately 5 % of cases [12, 28, 31].

In addition, it has been confirmed that the occurrence of BL is associated with viral infections, particularly EBV infection. However, the EBV detection rates in different subtypes of BL also vary [32]. EBV infection is detected in the vast majority of endemic BL and ~30 % of sporadic BL [12, 30, 32].

Treatment of Burkitt lymphoma in most centers is guided by the FAB LMB study (cooperative study between the Children's Cancer Group, the Société Francaise d'Oncologie Pediatrique, and the UK Children's Cancer Study Group) [33, 34]. The former consists of initial cytoreduction with cyclophosphamide, prednisolone, and vincristine, followed by more intensive chemotherapy in varying combinations containing doxorubicin, alkylators, vincristine, etoposide and therapy directed to eradicate or to prevent CNS disease such as high dose methotrexate [3, 12].

Aggressive high-dose therapy is needed for adult Burkitt lymphoma. However, interpretation of response is difficult because most studies of this approach have been done with a single protocol in mainly young adults. The regimen generally used in the UK and USA is cyclophosphamide, vincristine, doxorubicin, and highdose methotrexate alternating with ifosfamide, etoposide, and high-dose cytarabine [12].

The use of a less toxic dose adjusted EPOCH (etoposide, prednisone, vincristine, cyclophosphamide, adriamycin) plus rituximab (DA-REPOCH) led to an event free survival of 96 % and an overall survival of 100 % with a median follow up to 86 months in a small studay that included 19 HIV negative patients [35]. The use of rituximab (anti-CD20) in primary therapy has been assessed and a randomized clinical trial including 257 patients demonstrated that the addition of rituximab to the LMB regimen improved the event free survival and the overall survival without adding more toxicities [4].

## Conclusions

In summary, the current study presents a case of sporadic primary BL of the thyroid occurring in a seventy-year-old male, which exhibited the typical morphological features and immunophenotype of BL and which, to the authors' knowledge, is the first case of BL of the thyroid gland to be reported in Morocco. We also emphasize here the importance of considering lymphoma when dealing with a thyroid mass, as its management is different from that of other thyroid pathologies and delaying treatment has an impact on prognosis.

## Consent

Written informed consent was obtained from the patient's family for publication of this case report and any accompanying images. A copy of the written consent is available for review by the Editor of this journal.

## Ethics approval and consent to participate

Not applicable.

**Abbreviations**
BL: Burkitt lymphoma; CT: computerized tomography; EBV: epstein-barr virus; PTL: primary thyroid lymphoma.

**Competing interests**
The authors declare that they have no competing interests.

## Authors' contributions

MA, IB, EMM, SR and MA analyzed and interpreted the patient data, drafted the manuscript and made the figures. MA, AB, MB and MO performed the histological examination and proposed the study. MA, AAB and MO made substantial contributions to conception and design, and revised the manuscript. All authors of this paper have read and given final approval of the version to be published.

## Author details

[1]Department of Pathology, Military General Hospital Mohammed V, Mohammed V Souissi University - Faculty of Medicine and Pharmacy of Rabat, Hay Riad, Rabat 10000, Morocco. [2]Department of Clinical Haematology, Military General Hospital Mohammed V, Mohammed V Souissi University - Faculty of Medicine and Pharmacy of Rabat, Hay Riad, Rabat 10000, Morocco. [3]Department of Otorhinolaryngology, Military General Hospital Mohammed V, Mohammed V Souissi University - Faculty of Medicine and Pharmacy of Rabat, Hay Riad, Rabat 10000, Morocco.

## References

1. Camera A, Magri F, Fonte R, et al. Burkitt-like lymphoma infiltrating a hyperfunctioning thyroid adenoma and presenting as a hot nodule. Thyroid. 2010;20(9):1033–6.

2. Kalinyak JE, Kong CS, McDougall IR. Burkitt's lymphoma presenting as a rapidly growing thyroid mass. Thyroid. 2006;16(10):1053–7.

3. Murphy SB. Classification, staging and end results of treatment of childhood non- Hodgkin's lymphomas: dissimilarities from lymphomas in adults. Semin Oncol. 1980;7:332–9.

4. Ribrag V, Koscielny S, Bouabdallah K, et al. Addition of rituximab improves outcome of HIV negative patients with Burkitt lymphoma treated with the LMBA protocol: results of the randomized intergroup (GRAALL-lysa) LMBA02 protocol [abstract]. Blood. 2012;120(21):Abstract 685.

5. Derringer GA, Thompson LD, Frommelt RA, Bijwaard KE, Heffess CS, Abbondanzo SL. Malignant lymphoma of the thyroid gland: a clinicopathologic study of 108 cases. Am J Surg Pathol. 2000;24:623e39.

6. Pedersen RK, Pedersen NT. Primary non-Hodgkin's lymphoma of the thyroid gland: a population based study. Histopathology. 1996;28(1):25–32.

7. Earnest LM, Cooper DS, Sciubba JJ, Tufano RP. Thyroid MALT lymphoma in patients with a compressive goiter. Head Neck. 2006;28(8):765–70.

8. Yang L, Wang A, Zhang Y, Mu Y. 12 cases of primary thyroid lymphoma in China. J Endocrinol Investig. 2015;38(7):739–44.

9. Alzouebi M, Goepel JR, Horsman JM, et al. Primary thyroid lymphoma: the 40 year experience of a UK lymphoma treatment centre. Int J Oncol. 2012; 40(6):2075–80.

10. Kandil E, Safah H, Noureldine S, et al. Burkitt-like lymphoma arising in the thyroid gland. Am J Med Sci. 2012;343(1):103–5.

11. Ha CS, Shadle KM, Medeiros LJ, Wilder RB, Hess MA, Cabanillas F, et al. Localized non-Hodgkin lymphoma involving the thyroid gland. Cancer. 2001;91:629e35.

12. Molyneux EM, Rochford R, Griffin B, Newton R, Jackson G, Menon G, Harrison CJ, Israels T, Bailey S. Burkitt's lymphoma. Lancet. 2012;379(9822): 1234–44.

13. Jaff ES. The 2008 WHO classification of lymphomas: implications for clinical practice and translational research. Hematology Am Soc Hematol Educ Program. 2009;1:523–31.

14. Cooper K, Gangadharan A, Arora RS, Shukla R, Pizer B. Burkitt lymphoma of thyroid gland in an adolescent. Case Rep Pediatr. 2014;2014(187467):3.

15. Ansell SM, Grant CS, Habermann TM. Primary thyroid lymphoma. Semin Oncol. 1999;26(3):316–23.

16. Widder S, Pasieka JL. Primary thyroid lymphomas. Curr Treat Options Oncol. 2004;5:307e13.

17. Holm LE, Bloomgren H, Lowhagen T. Cancer risks in patients with chronic lymphocytic thyroiditis. N Engl J Med. 1985;312:601–4.

18. Matsuzuka F, Miyauchi A, Katayama S, Narabayashi I, Ikeda H, Kuma K, Sugawara M. Clinical aspects of primary thyroid lymphoma: diagnosis and treatment based on our experience of 119 cases. Thyroid. 1993;3(2):93–9.

19. Isaacson PG. Lymphoma of the thyroid gland. Curr Top Patyhol. 1997;91:1e14.

20. Kossev P, Livolsi V. Lymphoid lesions of the thyroid: review in light of the revised Europeane American lymphoma classification and upcoming World Health Organization classification. Thyroid. 1999;9:1273e80.

21. Saxena A, Alport EC, Moshynska O, Kanthan R, Boctor MA. Clonal B cell populations in a minority of patients with Hashimoto's thyroiditis. J Clin Pathol. 2004;57:1258e63.

22. Yildiz I, Sen F, Toz B, et al. Primary Burkitt's lymphoma presenting as a rapidly growing thyroid mass. Case Rep Oncol. 2012;5(2):388–93.

23. Sarinah B, Hisham AN. Primary lymphoma of the thyroid: diagnosis and therapeutic considerations. Asian J Surg. 2010;33(1):20–4.

24. Mweempwa A, Prasad J, Islam S. A rare neoplasm of the thyroid gland. N Z Med J. 2013;126(1369):75–8.

25. Albert S. Primary Burkitt lymphoma of the thyroid. Ear Nose Throat J. 2013; 92(12):E1–2.

26. Stein SA, Wartofsky L. Primary thyroid lymphoma: a clinical review. J Clin Endocrinol Metab. 2013;98(8):3131–8.

27. Ota H, Ito Y, Matsuzuka F, et al. Usefulness of ultrasonography for diagnosis of malignant lymphoma of the thyroid. Thyroid. 2006;16:983–7.

28. Swerdlow SH, Campo E, Harris NL, et al. WHO classification of tumours of haematopoietic and lymphoid tissues. Lyon: IARC Press; 2008.

29. Chuang SS, Ye H, Du MQ, Lu CL, Dogan A, Hsieh PP, Huang WT, Jung YC. Histopathology and immunohistochemistry in distinguishing Burkitt lymphoma from diffuse large B–cell lymphoma with very high proliferation index and with or without a starry–sky pattern: a comparative study with EBER and FISH. Am J Clin Pathol. 2007;128(4):558–64.

30. Liying Z, Lanxiang G, Guang L, Luping W, Chunwei X, Lin L, Yuwang T, Huiru F, Zhe G. Primary Burkitt's lymphoma of the thyroid without Epstein-Barr virus infection: a case report and literature review. Oncol Lett. 2014;7(5): 1519–24.

31. Hecht JL, Aster JC. Molecular biology of Burkitt's lymphoma. J Clin Oncol. 2000;18(21):3707–21.

32. Queiroga EM, Gualco G, Chioato L, Harrington WJ, Araujo I, Weiss LM, Bacchi CE. Viral studies in Burkitt lymphoma: association with Epstein Barr virus but not HHV 8. Am J Clin Patho. 2008;130:186–92.

33. Patte C, Philip T, Rodary C, et al. High survival rate in advanced-stage B–cell lymphomas and leukemias without CNS involvement with a short intensive polychemotherapy: results from the French pediatric oncology society of a randomized trial of 216 children. J Clin Oncol. 1991;9(1):123–32.

34. Patte C, Auperin A, Michon J, et al. The Societe Francaise d'Oncologie pediatrique LMB89 protocol: highly eff ective multiagent chemotherapy tailored to the tumor burden and initial response in 561 unselected children with B–cell lymphomas and L3 leukemia. Blood. 2001;97:3370–79.

35. Dunleavy K, Pittaluga S, Shovlin M, et al. Low-intensity therapy in adults with Burkitt's lymphoma. N Engl J Med. 2013;369(20):1915–25.

# 20

# Cellular angiofibroma of the vulva: a poorly known entity, a case report and literature review

Mouna Khmou[*], Najat Lamalmi, Abderrahmane Malihy, Lamia Rouas and Zaitouna Alhamany

## Abstract

**Background:** Cellular angiofibroma represents a newly described, site specific tumor. Histologically, CAF is a benign mesenchymal neoplasm characterized by two principal components: bland spindle cells and prominent small to medium-sized vessels with mural hyalinization. The indolent nature of the lesion is underscored by the uniformity of its constituent stromal cells, and their lack of nuclear atypia. Characterization by immunohistochemistry is helpful distinguishing Cellular angiofibroma from other mesenchymal lesions.

**Case presentation:** We report the case of a 37-year-old woman, presenting with a painless nodule involving the vulva. This lesion had gradually increased in size; a simple excision was performed, and follow up was unremarkable. Gross examination showed a well circumscribed, firm tumor measuring 3× 3 × 2,5 cm. Histologically, the tumor was composed of uniform, short spindle-shaped cells, proliferating in an edematous to fibrous stroma and numerous small to medium-sized thick-walled vessels. A panel of immunohistochemical stains was performed, and confirmed the diagnosis of Cellular angiofibroma.

**Conclusion:** In this report we aim to describe the clinical, pathological and immunohistochemical features of this rare entity through a literature review, and to discuss other vulvar mesenchymal lesions.

**Keywords:** Cellular angiofibroma, Vulva, Mesenchymal tumors, Histopathology, Immunohistochemistry

## Background

Cellular angiofibroma (CAF) is a rare benign mesenchymal lesion with a predilection for the genitourinary region. First described in 1997 [1], CAF is characterized by a spindle cell component and abundant small- to medium-sized thick-walled vessels [2]. Cases in males have been previously named "angiomyofibroblastoma-like tumor". Besides two small series, cellular angiofibroma has been described only in isolated case reports, we found only 68 patients with genital CAF (Table 1) [3, 4]. To date, this last condition still remains a poorly known lesion that needs further investigations to closely define its clinical and pathological features.

We report a case of cellular angiofibroma, for which the clinical diagnosis was Bartholin's glandular cyst.

* Correspondence: mouna.khmou@yahoo.fr
Department of Pathology, Children's Hospital Faculty of Medicine and Pharmacy, Mohammed V University Ibn Sina University Hospital, Rabat, Morocco

## Case presentation

A healthy 37-year-old woman consulted for an asymptomatic vulvar nodule of 6 years duration. She was concerned because it had progressively enlarged over the last few months. There was no history of pain or bleeding. Local and colposcopic examinations revealed a 3,5 cm freely mobile non reducible nodule located in the left labia majora. Ultrasonography showed a superficial, well-demarcated, solid soft tissue tumor. A well circumscribed lesion measuring 3 cm in diameter was excised with a rim of normal tissue. Gross examination showed a well circumscribed, solid, whitish, glossy tumor measuring 3× 3 × 2,5 cm. Microscopically, the tumor was well circumscribed, surrounded by a fibrous pseudocapsule. On low-power examination, hypocellular and hypercellular areas, composed of uniform, short spindle-shaped cells, proliferating in an edematous to fibrous stroma (Fig. 1). Numerous small to medium-sized thick-walled vessels were also seen

**Table 1** Summary of the literature review of vulvar CAF reported

| Authors | Year | Age | Localisation | Treatment | Follow-up |
|---|---|---|---|---|---|
| Nucci et al. [1] | 1997 | 50 | Vulva | Complete excision | NA |
| | | 46 | Left labia majora | Complete excision | NR, 19 months |
| | | 39 | Right labia | Complete excision | NR, 12 months |
| | | 49 | Labia | Complete excision | NA |
| Colombat et al. [25] | 2001 | 37 | Left labia majora | Complete excision | NA |
| Lane et al. [10] | 2001 | 77 | Left labia | Complete excision | NR, 12 months |
| Curry et al. [18] | 2001 | 37 | Clitoral hood | NA | NR, 15 months |
| Dufau et al. [16] | 2002 | 53 | Labia majora | NA | NA |
| Dargent et al. [9] | 2003 | 46 | Right labial region | | NR, 19 months |
| | | 49 | Lateral part of the clitoris. | | NR, 7 months |
| McCluggage et al. [22] | 2002 | 49 | Left labia majora | Complete excision | Reccurence 6 months later |
| Iwasa et al. [3] | 2004 | 49 | Labia majora | Complete excision | NA |
| | | 39 | Vulva | NA | NA |
| | | 46 | Labia majora | Complete excision | NR, 16 months |
| | | 50 | Vulva | Complete excision | Lost |
| | | 42 | Vulva | Complete excision | NR, 75 months |
| | | 42 | Perineum | NA | NA |
| | | 75 | Vulva | Complete excision | Died of breast cancer |
| | | 41 | Vulva | Complete excision | NR 54 months |
| | | 68 | Vulva | Complete excision | NR, 17 months |
| | | 59 | Labia majora | Complete excision | NR, 41 month |
| | | 49 | Vulva | NA | NA |
| | | 37 | Hymen Local | Excision + positive margins | NR, 24 months |
| | | 38 | Vagina | NA | NA |
| | | 46 | Vulva | Complete excision | NR, 35 months |
| | | 47 | Labium majus | Complete excision | NR, 44 months |
| | | 47 | Vulva | NA | NA |
| | | 48 | Labium majus | Complete excision | NR, 8 months |
| | | 24 | Vagina | NA | NR, 6 months |
| | | 58 | Vagina | Complete excision | NA |
| | | 50 | Vulva | Complete excision | NR, 6 months |
| | | 58 | Vulva | Complete excision | NR, 9 months |
| | | 50 | Vulva | NA | NA |
| W G McCluggage et al. [21] | 2004 | 20 | Not specified | Complete excision | NR, 20 month, |
| | | 25 | Posterior vaginal introitus | Complete excision | NR, 3 months |
| | | 65 | Left labia minora | Complete excision | NR, 12 months |
| | | 41 | Left labia majora | Complete excision | NR, 4 months |
| | | 59 | Right side of vulva | Complete excision | NR, 18 months |
| | | 32 | Right labia | Complete excision | NA |
| Micheletti et al. [8] | 2005 | 51 | vulva | Complete excision | NR, 4 months |
| Kerkuta et al. [7] | 2005 | 31 | small left labial | Complete excision | NR, 10 month |
| Chen et al. [11] | 2010 | 58 | Vulva | Complete excision | NR, 75 months |
| | | 52 | Vulva Local | Complete excision | Dead of carcinoma |
| | | 34 | Vulva | Complete excision | NA |

**Table 1** Summary of the literature review of vulvar CAF reported *(Continued)*

| | | 32 | Vulva | Complete excision | NA |
|---|---|---|---|---|---|
| | | 25 | Vulva | Complete excision | NR, 42 months |
| | | 43 | Vulva | Complete excision | NR, 2 months |
| | | 59 | Vulva | Complete excision | NR, 14 months |
| | | 46 | Vulva | Complete excision | NR, 4 months |
| | | 71 | Vulva | Complete excision | NA |
| | | 39 | Vulva | Complete excision | NR, 7 months |
| | | 46 | Vulva | Complete excision | NA |
| Flucke et al. [4] | 2011 | 41 | Perineal | Complete excision | NA |
| | | 39 | Vaginal introitus | Excision + positive margins | NR, 75 months |
| | | 50 | Vulva | Excision + positive margins | NR, 55 months |
| | | 51 | Labium majus | Marginal excision | NR, 66 months |
| | | 44 | Labium majus | Complete excision | NA |
| | | 50 | Vulva | Excision + positive margins | NA |
| | | 48 | Vulva | Complete excision | NA |
| | | 42 | Vulva | Complete excision | NA |
| | | 63 | Clitoris | Excision + positive margins | NR, 38 months |
| | | 27 | Labium majus | Marginal excision | NA |
| | | 42 | Vulva | Complete excision | NR, 30 month |
| | | 46 | Labium majus | Marginal excision | NA |
| | | 55 | Vulva | Complete excision | NR, 12 months |
| | | 57 | Vulva | NA | NR, 6 months |
| | | 47 | Vulva | Excision + positive margins | NA |
| | | 39 | Vaginal fornix | Marginal excision | NA |
| Present case | 2015 | 37 | Left labia majora | Complete excision | NR, 20 month |

*NR* No Recurrence
*NA* information not available

(Fig. 2). Mature adipocytes were noted in the periphery in small clusters. There was no necrosis and few or no mitotic figures (Fig. 3). Immunohistochemical staining was positive for vimentin, CD34 (Fig. 4), focally for actin, and negative for protein S-100, and desmin. These findings are consistent with the diagnosis of cellular angiofibroma. At 14 months postoperatively, the patient is doing well with no signs of recurrence.

## Discussion

Tumors primarily arising from the vulvo-vaginal area are relatively rare and they include soft tissue specific and non-specific tumors, as well as a spectrum of fibro-epithelial tumors [5, 6]. Cellular angiofibroma is an uncommon benign mesenchymal neoplasm, originally described in the genital region, and occurs equally in both genders [4]. A marked predilection for the vulva is observed [2], our review of the literature yielded 68 cases reported, involving the female genital tract (Table 1). Women are affected most often in the fifth decade, whereas males are mainly in the seventh decade [3]. Clinically, cellular angiofibroma is often mistaken for a Bartholin gland, labial, or submucosal cyst [7].

Etiopathologically, some authors suggested that these lesions are stem cell–derived, with a capacity for adipose and myofibroblastic differentiation in accordance with

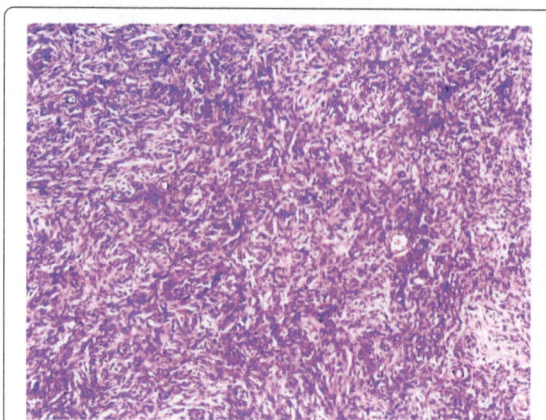

**Fig. 1** low-power view showing uniform, short spindle-shaped cells

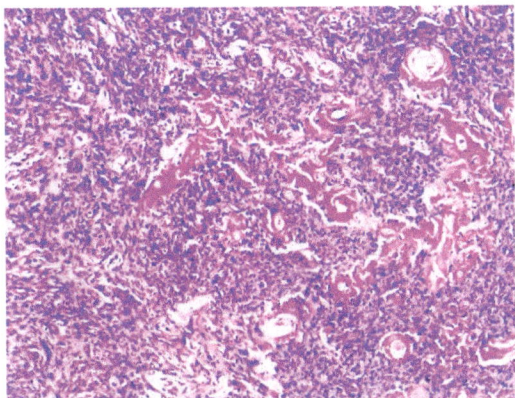

**Fig. 2** Numerous small to medium-sized with thick and hyalinized walls

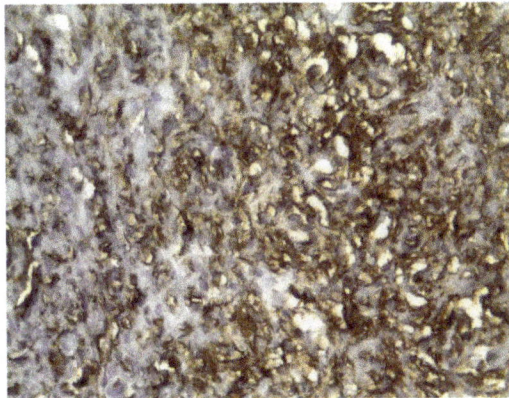

**Fig. 4** tumour cells exhibiting diffuse positivity with CD34

the influence of hormones, microenvironments, cytokines and growth factors [8].

Histologically, CAF is typically well circumscribed, composed of two principal components: bland spindle cells and prominent small to medium-sized vessels with mural hyalinization [3]. The spindle cells are arranged in short intersecting fascicles lying between short bundles of wispy collagen [9]. Hypocellular areas can be seen, often associated with stromal edema or hyalinization. Typically, significant pleomorphism and abnormal mitoses were absent [3]. The accompanying blood vessels tend to be thick-walled and even hyalinized [10]. Mature individual or small clusters of adipocytes can be present, most often located in the periphery of the lesion [2, 3]. Fletcher et al. recently have reported a study of 13 cases of cellular angiofibroma with atypia and sarcomatous transformation [11]. The sarcomatous component can show variable features (atypical lipomatous tumor, pleomorphic liposarcoma, and pleomorphic

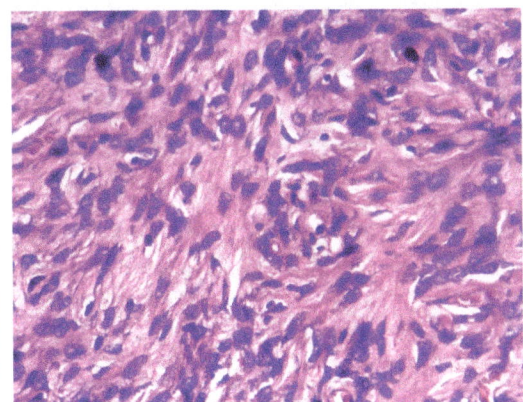

**Fig. 3** Bland spindle cells with uniform nuclei and pale indistinct cytoplasm

sarcoma). This phenomenon seems not to predispose to recurrence based on limited clinical follow-up available [2, 11].

Immunohistochemically, the tumor cells consistently are vimentin positive [9]. The expression of CD34 is seen in 60 % [3]. Characteristically, they do not express S-100 protein, actin, desmin, or EMA, although a discrete staining for the last three markers has been reported [3, 9]. Lastly, the tumor cells have been found to be estrogen (ER) and progesterone receptor (PR) positive. However, the significance of the positive estrogen and progesterone receptors in CAF is unknown [7]. In fact, a subset of mesenchymal cells of the distal female genital tract normally expresses estrogen and progesterone receptor and, the neoplastic cells arising from the vulva, may also show immunoreactivity for ER and/or PR [12]. Thus, ER or PR immunoreactivity cannot be used to distinguish CAF and its histological mimics [13]

No specific chromosomal abnormality is found in CAF, although cytogenetic analysis revealed, in a few reported cases, the loss of RB1 and FOXO1A1 genes due to the deletion of the 13q14 region [14]. This typical loss of genetic material is also shared by myofibroblastoma [15].

CAF, myofibroblastoma and angiomyofibroblastoma are usually considered as specific soft tissue tumors of the vulvo-vaginal area [16]. These tumors may show overlapping morphological, immunohistochemical and cytogenetic features, and thus differential diagnosis is mandatory [17, 15].

Clinically, the age of onset of CAF occurs approximately 10 years later in life than aggressive angiomyxoma, myofibroblastoma and angiomyofibroblastoma [18]. Histologically, aggressive angiomyxoma is poorly circumscribed, typically infiltrates adjacent soft tissue, and characterized by being composed of relatively uniform spindle cells, embedded in a myxoid matrix [10].

AMF is a benign tumor which belongs to the category of the "stromal tumors of the lower female genital tract", together with cellular angiofibroma and myofibroblastoma [19]. It is characterized by the presence of multinucleate cells and epithelioid or plasmacytoid cells which tend to aggregate around blood vessels which are thin-walled [21]. However recent cytogenetic analyses have shown that only CAF and myofibroblastoma are genetically related lesions because angiomyofibroblastoma lacks 13q14 deletion [20].

Myofibroblastoma is composed of ovoid- to spindle- or stellate-shaped cells, arranged in a variety of architectural patterns and set in a finely collagenous stroma. Hyalinized blood vessels are a diagnostic clue helpful in distinguishing cellular angiofibroma from myofibroblastoma [15].

Based on morphological, immunohistochemical and cytogenetic analyses, it has been postulated that CAF and myofibroblastoma of the lower female genital tract are closely related lesions that form a continuous spectrum of a single entity with different morphologic presentations, likely arising from a common precursor mesenchymal cell [19].

Desmin seems to be a discriminating marker, as aggressive angiomyxoma, myofibroblastoma and angiomyofibroblastoma are positive for this antibody [3, 15].

Other neoplasms that are not specific to the vulva, such as solitary fibrous tumour, spindle cell lipoma, smooth muscle tumours, nerve sheath tumours, and perineurioma, also enter into the differential diagnosis [22].

Spindle cell lipoma is composed of brightly, eosinophilic ropy and refractile stromal collagen bands with fewer capillary-sized thin-walled vessels, compared with palely eosinophilic and wispy collagen fibers associated with numerous thick-walled vessels in CAF [3, 18]. Solitary fibrous tumor (SFT) can be differentiated by the presence of thin-walled branching vascular pattern that may be described as hemangiopericytoma-like vessels, and dense collagen bundles [12, 23]. SFT shows positivity for CD34, CD99, bcl-2, and ER and/or PR, and negativity for SMA and desmin [24].

Other mesenchymal lesions (schwannoma, perineurioma and leiomyoma) can be ruled out in accordance with the histology and immunohistochemistry [8].

CAF behaves in a benign fashion and local excision with clear margins is the treatment of choice. This lesion shows no tendency for metastasis based on the limited clinical follow-up available [2, 3, 7]. However, there is one case of recurrent CAF, reported by McCluggage et al., in which a 49-year-old woman had recurrent swelling develop at the site of the previous excision 6 months later [22]. Our patient is well without evidence of local recurrence 20 months after excision.

## Conclusions

CAF represents a rare distinct clinico-pathological condition, that pathologists should be aware of morphological variation (Atypia and Sarcomatous transformation) to prevent diagnostic errors and therefore an aggressive therapy. As far as we are aware, no case of metastatic CAF has been described.

### Abbreviations
AMF, Angiomyofibroblastoma; CAF, Cellular angiofibroma; EMA, Epithelial membrane antigen; ER, estrogen receptor; PR, progesterone receptor.

### Acknowledgements
None.

### Funding
This article has no funding source.

### Authors' contributions
MK analyzed and interpreted the patient data, drafted the manuscript and made the figures. NL and ZA performed the histological examination, proposed the study, supervised MK and revised the manuscript. AM and LR have made substantial contributions to analysis and interpretation of patient data. All authors read and approved the final manuscript.

### Competing interest
The authors declare that they have no competing interests.

### Consent for publication
Written informed consent was obtained from the patient for publication of this Case Report and any accompanying images. A copy of the written consent is available for review by the Editor-in-Chief of this journal.

### Ethics approval and consent to participate
Not applicable.

### References
1. Nucci MR, Granter SR, Fletcher CD. Cellular angiofibroma: a benign neoplasm distinct from angiomyofibroblastoma and spindle cell lipoma. Am J Surg Pathol. 1997;21(6):636–44.
2. Val-Bernal JF, Azueta A, Parra A, Mediavilla E, Zubillaga S. Paratesticular cellular angiofibroma with atypical (bizarre) cells: case report and literature review. Pathol Res Pract. 2013;209(6):388–92.
3. Iwasa Y, Fletcher CD. Cellular angiofibroma: clinicopathologic and immunohistochemical analysis of 51 cases. Am J Surg Pathol. 2004;28(11): 1426–35.
4. Flucke U, van Krieken JH, Mentzel T. Cellular angiofibroma: analysis of 25 cases emphasizing its relationship to spindle cell lipoma and mammary-type myofibroblastoma. Mod Pathol. 2011;24(1):82–9.
5. McCluggage WG. Recent developments in vulvovaginal pathology. Histopathology. 2009;54(2):156–73.
6. Kazakov DV, Spagnolo DV, Stewart CJ, Thompson J, Agaimy A, Magro G, Bisceglia M, Vazmitel M, Kacerovska D, Kutzner H, Mukensnabl P, Michal M. Fibroadenoma and phyllodes tumors of anogenital mammary-like glands: a series of 13 neoplasms in 12 cases, including mammary-type juvenile fibroadenoma, fibroadenoma with lactation changes, and neurofibromatosis-associated pseudoangiomatous stromal hyperplasia with multinucleated giant cells. Am J Surg Pathol. 2010;34:95–103.
7. Kerkuta R, Kennedy CM, Benda JA, Galask RP. Vulvar cellular angiofibroma: a case report. Am J Obstet Gynecol. 2005;193(5):1750–2.
8. Micheletti AM, Silva AC, Nascimento AG, Da Silva CS, Murta EF, Adad SJ. Cellular angiofibroma of the vulva: case report with clinicopathological and immunohistochemistry study. Sao Paulo Med J. 2005;123(5):250–2.

9.  Dargent JL, de Saint AN, Galdón MG, Valaeys V, Cornut P, Noël JC. Cellular angiofibroma of the vulva: a clinicopathological study of two cases with documentation of some unusual features and review of the literature. J Cutan Pathol. 2003;30(6):405–11.

10.  Lane JE, Walker AN, Mullis Jr EN, Etheridge JG. Cellular angiofibroma of the vulva. Gynecol Oncol. 2001;81(2):326–9.

11.  Chen E, Fletcher CD. Cellular angiofibroma with atypia or sarcomatous transformation: clinicopathologic analysis of 13 cases. Am J Surg Pathol. 2010;34(5):707–14.

12.  Mandato VD, Santagni S, Cavazza A, Aguzzoli L, Abrate M, La Sala GB. Cellular angiofibroma in women: a review of the literature. Diagn Pathol. 2015;(19)10:114.

13.  Lourenço C, Oliveira N, Ramos F, Ferreira I, Oliveira M. Aggressive angiomyxoma of the vagina: a case report. Rev Bras Ginecol Obstet. 2013; 35(12):575–82.

14.  Ptaszyński K, Szumera-Ciećkiewicz A, Bartczak A. Cellular angiofibroma with atypia or sarcomatous transformation - case description with literature review. Pol J Pathol. 2012;63(3):207–11.

15.  Magro G, et al. Vulvovaginal myofibroblastoma: expanding the morphological and immunohistochemical spectrum. A clinicopathologic study of 10 cases. Hum Pathol. 2012;43(2):243-53.

16.  McCluggage WG. A review and update of morphologically bland vulvovaginal mesenchymal lesions. Int J Gynecol Pathol. 2005;24(1):26-38.

17.  Dufau JP, Soulard R, Gros P. Cellular angiofibroma, angiomyofibroblastoma and aggressive angiomyxoma: members of a spectrum of genital stromal tumours?. Ann Pathol. 2002;22(3):241-3.

18.  Curry JL, Olejnik JL, Wojcik EM. Cellular angiofibroma of the vulva with DNA ploidy analysis. Int J Gynecol Pathol. 2001;20(2):200-3.

19.  Magro G, et al. Mammary and vaginal myofibroblastomas are genetically related lesions: fluorescence in situ hybridization analysis shows deletion of 13q14 region. Hum Pathol. 2012;43(11):1887-93.

20.  Magro G et al. Vulvovaginal angiomyofibroblastomas morphologic, immunohistochemical, and fluorescence in situ hybridization analysis for deletion of 13q14 region. Hum Pathol. 2014;45(8):1647-55).

21.  McCluggage WG, Ganesan R, Hirschowitz L, Rollason TP. Cellular angiofibroma and related fibromatous lesions of the vulva: report of a series of cases with a morphological spectrum wider than previously described. Histopathology. 2004;45(4):360-8.

22.  McCluggage WG, Perenyei M, Irwin ST. Recurrent cellular angiofibroma of the vulva. J Clin Pathol. 2002;55(6):477-9.

23.  Fletcher CDM, Bridge JA, Hogendoorn PCW et al Classification of Tumours of Soft Tissue and Bone 4th edn. IARC Press: Lyon, France, 2013, p :80-82.

24.  Mosquera JM, Fletcher CD. Expanding the spectrum of malignant progression in solitary fibrous tumors: a study of 8 cases with a discrete anaplastic component–is this dedifferentiated SFT?. Am J Surg Pathol. 2009; 33(9):1314-21.

25.  Colombat M, Liard-Meillon ME, de Saint-Maur P, Sevestre H, Gontier MF. L'angiofibrome cellulaire, une tumeur vulvaire rare: à propos d'un cas. Ann Pathol 2001;21:145.

# 21

# Prognostic and predictive significance of podocalyxin-like protein expression in pancreatic and periampullary adenocarcinoma

Margareta Heby, Jakob Elebro, Björn Nodin, Karin Jirström and Jakob Eberhard[*]

## Abstract

**Background:** Adenocarcinoma of the periampullary region is associated with poor prognosis and new prognostic and treatment predictive biomarkers are needed for improved treatment. Membranous expression of podocalyxin-like 1(PODXL), which is a cell-adhesion glycoprotein and stem cell marker, has been found to correlate with an aggressive tumour phenotype and adverse outcome in several cancer types. The aim of the present study was to examine the clinicopathological correlates, prognostic and predictive significance of tumour-specific PODXL expression in a retrospective cohort of pancreatic and periampullary carcinoma, morphologically divided into intestinal type (I-type) and pancreatobiliary type (PB-type) tumours.

**Methods:** Immunohistochemical expression of PODXL was analysed in tissue microarrays with primary tumours and a subset of paired lymph node metastases from 175 patients operated with pancreaticoduodenectomy for periampullary adenocarcinoma. Chi square test was applied to analyse the relationship between PODXL expression and clinicopathological parameters. Kaplan Meier analysis and Cox regression models were applied to estimate differences in 5-year overall survival (OS) and recurrence-free survival (RFS) in strata according to membranous and non-membranous PODXL expression.

**Results:** Membranous PODXL expression was significantly higher in primary PB-type (49.5 %) as compared with I-type (17.5 %) tumours. In PB-type tumours, PODXL expression was significantly associated with female sex ($p = 0.005$), location to the pancreas ($p = 0.005$), and poor differentiation grade ($p = 0.044$). Membranous PODXL expression was significantly associated with a reduced RFS (HR = 2.44, 95 % CI 1.10–5.44) and OS (HR = 2.32, 95 % CI 1.05–5.12) in I-type tumours and with a reduced RFS (HR = 1.63, 95 % CI 1.07–2.49) but not OS in PB-type tumours. PODXL remained a significant independent prognostic factor only in I-type tumours (HR = 5.12, 95 % CI 1.43–18.31 for RFS and HR = 7.31, 95 % CI 2.12–25.16 for OS). Patients with I-type tumours displaying membranous PODXL expression had a significant beneficial effect of adjuvant chemotherapy regarding 5-year OS.

**Conclusion:** Membranous expression of PODXL is significantly higher in PB-type than in I-type periampullary adenocarcinomas and an independent factor of poor prognosis in the latter. The results further indicate a beneficial effect of adjuvant chemotherapy on I-type tumours with membranous PODXL expression, suggesting the potential utility of PODXL as a biomarker for improved treatment stratification of these patients.

**Keywords:** Periampullary adenocarcinoma, Pancreatic cancer, Podocalyxin-like 1, Immunohistochemistry, Biomarkers, Prognosis, Response prediction

* Correspondence: jakob.eberhard@med.lu.se
Department of Clinical Sciences Lund, Division of Oncology and Pathology,
Lund University, Skåne University Hospital, 221 85 Lund, Sweden

# Background

Adenocarcinoma of the periampullary region, including tumours originating in the distal bile duct, pancreas, ampulla of Vater and the periampullary duodenum, are a heterogeneous group of neoplasms and despite advances in surgery, radiotherapy, chemotherapy and targeted agents, patients still suffer from a poor prognosis. The incidence of these tumours has markedly increased over the past decades and in 2012 pancreatic cancers of all types were the seventh most common cause of cancer deaths, resulting in 330.000 deaths globally [1]. The overall 5-year survival is 5 %, all stages of the disease combined, and the median survival has been reported to be 5–8 months [2–4]. There are no early detection tests and most patients with localized disease have no recognizable symptoms or signs, resulting in late diagnosis in the majority of cases. Only15-20 % of the tumours are resectable at presentation [5], resectability often being limited by early local invasion of the surrounding anatomical structures, such as mesenteric arteries, or distant metastasis. There are two major morphological types of periampullary adenocarcinomas, i.e. pancreatobiliary (PB-type) adenocarcinomas (including pancreatic cancer, distal bile duct cancer, and some of the ampullary carcinomas) and intestinal type (I-type) periampullary adenocarcinomas (including duodenal carcinoma and some of the ampullary carcinomas). Morphological type seems to provide more important prognostic information in resected periampullary carcinoma than the tumour origin, with PB-type tumours being associated with significantly shorter survival rates than I-type tumours [6, 7]. The present diagnostic and prognostic information provided by histopathological parameters is far from sufficient, strongly implicating the need for additional molecular-based biomarkers to better define clinically relevant subgroups of these tumours for improved treatment stratification.

Podocalyxin-like protein (PODXL) is a member of the CD34 family of transmembrane sialomucins. PODXL is expressed on the apical surface of glomerular epithelial cells and podocytes [8], where it plays an integral role in maintaining adequate filtration [9], and it is also expressed on vascular endothelia [10] and hematopoietic stem cells [11, 12]. PODXL is upregulated in several types of cancer, and strong expression, in particular in the cell membrane, has been demonstrated to signify more aggressive tumours and poor prognosis in e.g. breast cancer [13], colorectal cancer [14-17] ovarian cancer [18], urinary bladder cancer [19], and glioblastoma [20].

PODXL has been found to be more frequently expressed (44 %) in pancreatic ductal adenocarcinoma as compared with other types of adenocarcinomas of the gastrointestinal and biliary tracts [21]. In another study, sialofucosylated PODXL was demonstrated to be a functional E- and L-selectin ligand expressed by metastatic pancreatic cancer

cells *in vitro*, and was also found to be overexpressed, with membranous localization, in 69 % of 105 pancreatic ductal adenocarcinomas [22]. To our knowledge, the prognostic or predictive impact of PODXL expression in pancreatic or periampullary adenocarcinoma has not yet been described. The aim of the present study was therefore to examine the clinicopathological correlates, prognostic and predictive significance of tumour-specific PODXL expression in a retrospective cohort of pancreatic and periampullary adenocarcinoma, with particular reference to morphological subtypes thereof.

# Methods
## Patients

The study consists of a retrospective consecutive cohort of 175 patients with primary periampullary adenocarcinomas, surgically treated with pancreaticoduodenectomy at the University hospitals of Lund and Malmö, Sweden, from January 1 2001 until December 31 2011 [23–25]. Out of 175 cases in the entire cohort, there were 110 pancreatobiliary-type and 65 intestinal-type adenocarcinomas. Survival data were collected from the Swedish National Civil Register. Follow-up started at the date of surgery and ended at death, at 5 years after surgery or at December 31, 2013, whichever came first. Information on neoadjuvant and adjuvant treatment and recurrence was obtained from patient records.

All haematoxylin & eosin stained slides from all cases were re-evaluated by one pathologist (JEL), blinded to the original report and outcome. The decision on tumour origin and morphological type was based on several criteria, as previously described [23].

The study has been approved by the Ethics Committee of Lund University (ref nr 445/07).

## Tissue microarray construction

Tissue microarrays (TMAs) were constructed using a semi-automated arraying device (TMArrayer, Pathology Devices, Westminister, MD, USA). A standard set of three tissue cores (1 mm) were obtained from each of the 175 primary tumours and from lymph node metastases from 105 of the cases, whereby one to three lymph node metastases were sampled in each case. Paired samples with non-malignant pancreatic tissue from the resection specimens were also obtained from 50 of the cases, using a standard set of two 1 mm tissue cores.

## Immunohistochemistry and staining evaluation

For immunohistochemical analysis of PODXL expression, 4 μm TMA-sections were automatically pre-treated using the PT Link system and then stained in an Autostainer Plus (DAKO; Glostrup, Copenhagen, Denmark) with the affinity-purified polyclonal, monospecific PODXL antibody (HPA002110; Atlas Antibodies AB, Stockholm,

Sweden) diluted 1: 250. This antibody, originally generated within the Human Protein Atlas (HPA) project, has also been used in and validated in several previous biomarker studies on e.g. colorectal, bladder, pancreatic and testicular cancer [14, 19, 22, 26]. The expression of PODXL was recorded as negative (0), weak cytoplasmic positivity in any proportion of cells (1), moderate cytoplasmic positivity in any proportion of cells (2), distinct membranous positivity in < = 50 % of cells (3) and distinct membranous positivity in >50 % of cells (4) as previously described [14-16, 19]. Staining of PODXL was evaluated by two independent observers (MH and KJ) who were blinded to clinical and outcome data. Scoring differences were discussed in order to reach consensus.

### Statistical analysis

Chi square test was applied to analyse the relationship between PODXL expression and clinicopathological parameters. Two patients with PB-type adenocarcinomas who had received neoadjuvant chemotherapy were excluded from the correlation and survival analyses. Three additional patients were excluded from the survival analyses; two with I-type adenocarcinomas who died within one month from surgery due to complications and one with PB-type adenocarcinoma who emigrated 5 months after surgery.

Kaplan Meier analysis and log rank test were applied to estimate differences in 5-year overall survival (OS) and recurrence-free survival (RFS) in strata according to membranous and non-membranous PODXL expression. Hazard ratios (HR) for death and recurrence within 5 years were calculated by Cox regression proportional hazard´s modelling in unadjusted analysis and in a multivariable model adjusted for age, sex, T-stage, N-stage, differentiation grade, lymphatic invasion, vascular invasion, perineural invasion, infiltration in peripancreatic fat, resection margins, tumour origin, and adjuvant chemotherapy. A backward conditional method was used for variable selection in the adjusted model. To estimate the interaction effect between adjuvant treatment and PODXL expression in order to measure any possible difference in treatment effect based on PODXL expression, the following interaction variable was constructed; any adjuvant treatment (+/−) × PODXL (+/−).

All tests were two sided. *P-values* <0.05 were considered significant. All statistical analyses were performed using IBM SPSS Statistics version 20.0 (SPSS Inc., Chicago, IL, USA).

### Results

#### PODXL expression in non-malignant pancreas, primary tumours and lymph node metastases

Sample immunohistochemical images of PODXL expression are shown in Fig. 1. PODXL expression could be assessed in in 63/65 (96.9 %) primary I-type carcinomas and 24/30 (80.0 %) lymph node metastases, and in 107/108 (99.1 %) primary PB-type carcinomas and 63/75 (84.0 %) corresponding lymph node metastases. PODXL expression could be assessed in 49/50 (98 %) paired non-malignant samples, all displaying negative or very weak PODXL expression in acini and ducts. The distribution of PODXL expression in primary tumours and metastases, which did not differ significantly, by histological subtype, is shown in Fig. 2. Membranous PODXL expression was denoted in 11/63 (17.5 %) primary and 2/24 (8.3 %) metastatic I-type carcinomas, and in 53/107 (49.5 %) primary and 23/63 (36.5 %) metastatic PB-type carcinomas. In I-type tumours, membranous PODXL in the metastasis was seen in 1/21 (4.8 %) cases denoted as having non-membranous expression in the primary tumour, and non-membranous PODXL expression in the metastasis was denoted in 2/3 (66.7 %) cases with primary tumours displaying membranous PODXL expression. In PB-type tumours, the number of cases with non-membranous to membranous conversion was 2/32 (6.2 %) and with membranous to non-membranous conversion 10/31 (32.3 %). In all further statistical analyses, a dichotomized variable of non-membranous (score 0, 1, 2) versus membranous (score 3, 4) PODXL expression in the primary and/or metastatic component is applied. According to this combined variable, 12/63 (19.0 %) I-type cases and 55/107 (51.4 %) PB-type cases displayed membranous PODXL expression in any component.

#### Associations of PODXL expression with clinicopathological factors

The associations between PODXL expression and clinicopathological factors in I-type and PB-type tumours, respectively, are shown in Table 1. In I-type tumours, there were no significant associations between PODXL expression and clinicopathological factors. In PB-type tumours, membranous PODXL expression was significantly associated with female sex ($p = 0.005$), with location to the pancreas ($p = 0.005$), and with poor differentiation grade ($p = 0.044$). There was no statistically significant association between PODXL expression and other clinicopathological factors including age at diagnosis, tumour size, T-stage, N-stage, resection margins, presence of vascular- lymphatic and neural invasion and growth in peripancreatic fat.

#### Prognostic and potential predictive value of PODXL expression

As demonstrated in Fig. 3, Kaplan-Meier analysis revealed significant associations of membranous PODXL expression with a reduced RFS (logrank $p = 0.024$) and OS (logrank $p = 0.032$) in I-type tumours and with a reduced RFS (logrank $p = 0.022$) but not OS in PB-type tumours. These associations were confirmed in univariable Cox regression

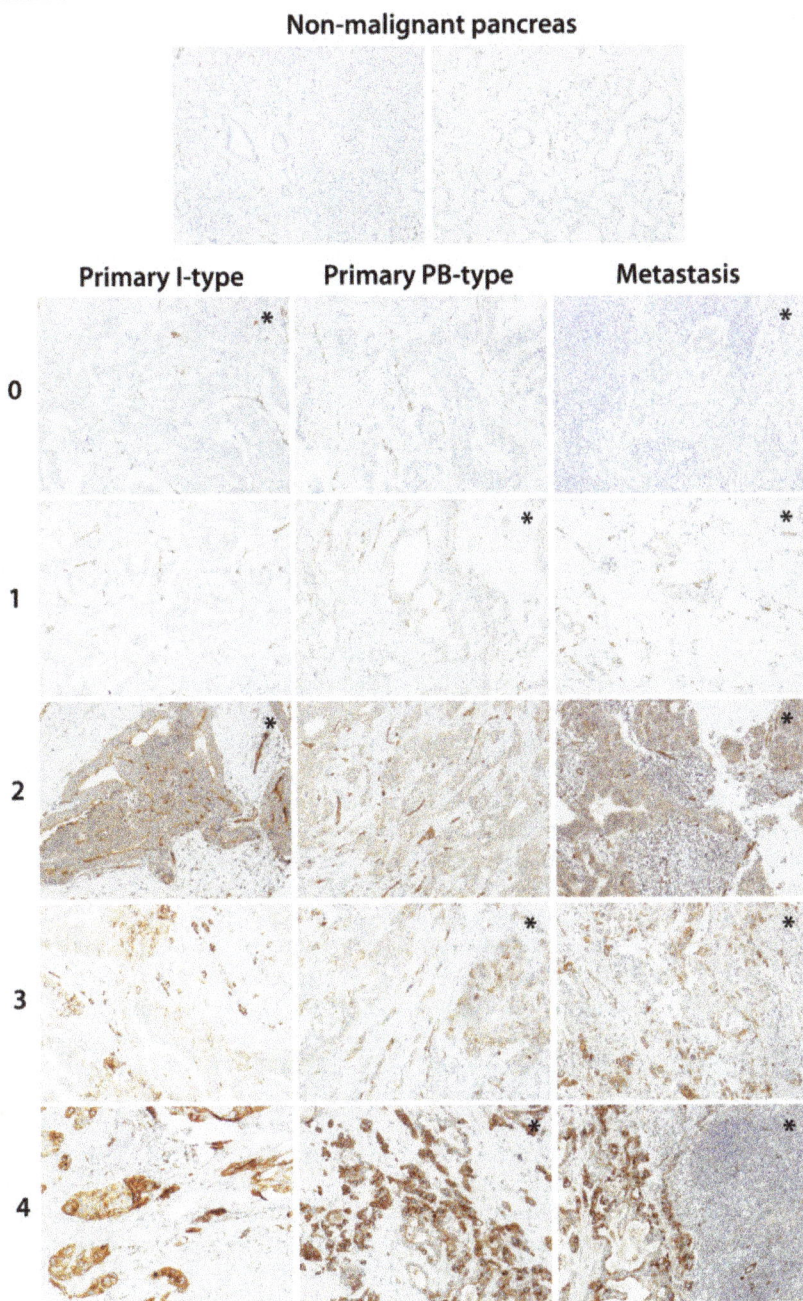

**Fig. 1** Sample immunohistochemical images. Immunohistochemical images of PODXL- negative non-malignant pancreatic tissue from two cases (*top row*), primary intestinal-type (*I-type*) tumours (*left column*), primary pancreatobiliary-type (*PB-type*) tumours (*mid-column*) and metastases (*right column*) with different PODXL staining scores (*0–4*). Asterisks indicate paired samples; i.e. from the same case/resection specimen. Score 0 = negative staining, score 1 = weak cytoplasmic positivity in any proportion of cells, score 2: moderate-strong cytoplasmic positivity in any proportion of cells, score 3: distinct membranous positivity in < = 50 % of cells and score 4 = distinct membranous positivity in >50 % of cells. All images with 10X original magnification

analysis for both RFS (Table 2) and OS (Table 3) in I-type tumours (HR = 2.44, 95 % CI 1.10–5.44, and HR = 2.32, 95 % CI 1.05–5.12, respectively) and for RFS (Table 2), but not OS (Table 3) in PB-type tumours (HR = 1.63, 95 % CI 1.07–2.49, logrank $p = 0.022$). In multivariable analysis, PODXL remained a significant prognostic factor only in

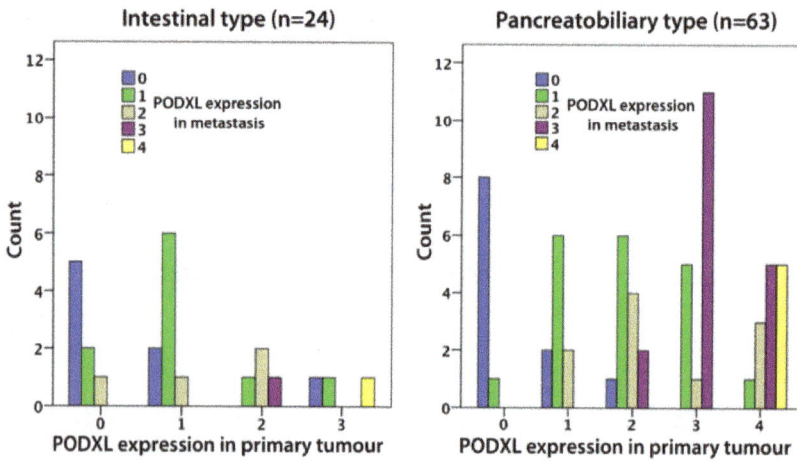

**Fig. 2** PODXL expression in primary tumours and metastases

I-type tumours (HR = 5.12, 95 % CI 1.43–18.31 for RFS, Table 2, and HR = 7.31, 95 % CI 2.12–25.16 for OS, Table 3).

Next, we examined the potential predictive impact of PODXL expression on survival in strata according to adjuvant treatment. As demonstrated in Fig. 4, patients with I-type tumours displaying membranous PODXL expression had a significant beneficial effect of adjuvant chemotherapy regarding 5-year OS. When ampullary PB-type tumours, expressing membranous PODXL in a similar proportion to I-type tumours, were included in the analysis, the beneficial value of adjuvant chemotherapy was even more pronounced (Fig. 4). Hazard ratios for 5-year OS according to adjuvant treatment and PODXL expression are shown in Additional file 1. The results demonstrate that survival did not differ significantly by membranous PODXL-expression in patients with I-type tumours or the extended group of I-type + ampullary PB-type tumours having received adjuvant chemotherapy. In contrast, the adverse prognostic impact of membranous PODXL expression was even more evident in patients not receiving adjuvant chemotherapy compared to the entire group (unadjusted HR = 4.38, 95 % CI 1.57–12.18 in I-type tumours, and unadjusted HR = 7.13; 95 % CI 2.64–19.26 in I-type + ampullary PB-type tumours). These associations remained significant in multivariable analysis, but there was no significant treatment interaction (Additional file 1). These associations were not significant in relation to RFS (data not shown) or in PB-type tumours (data not shown). The prognostic and predictive impact of membranous PODXL expression was similar when only its expression in the primary tumour was considered (data not shown). The prognostic value of the full range of PODXL scores (0–4) in relation to RFS and OS, in the entire cohort and by morphological subtype, is shown in Additional file 2. All survival analyses were also performed using a dichotomized

variable of score 0–1 vs 2–4, with allover less significant results (data not shown).

## Discussion

Pancreatic cancer is an extremely lethal type of cancer. On average, patients die from the disease within 6 months from diagnosis. Therefore it is of uttermost importance to find both predictive and prognostic factors so as to improve treatment. The results from this study provide a first demonstration of the prognostic and potential predictive value of PODXL in pancreatic, distal bile duct, ampullary and duodenal adenocarcinoma. PODXL-expression was found to be significantly higher in PB-type as compared with I-type tumours, with the exception for ampullary PB-type tumours. These findings are in line with the expected and provide further evidence of PODXL being associated with a more aggressive tumour phenotype and a biomarker of poor prognosis in human cancer.

The study cohort encompasses a retrospective cohort of 110 pancreatobiliary-type and 65 intestinal-type adenocarcinomas, including paired normal tissue and lymph node metastases from a subset of cases, thus providing a thorough characterization of PODXL expression in a wide range of periampullary adenocarcinomas. In the present study, membranous PODXL expression was denoted in 49.5 % of primary PB-type carcinomas, which is somewhat lower than in the previous study by Dallas et al., including tumours from 105 cases assembled in TMAs, wherein membranous PODXL expression was found in 69 % of the cases [22]. In primary I-type carcinomas, membranous PODXL expression was denoted in 17.5 %, which is well in line with previous TMA-based studies on colorectal cancer wherein membranous expression was found in 13.4 % and 9.6 % respectively [14, 15]. This observation further supports the theory that I-type carcinomas of the

**Table 1** Associations between membranous and non-membranous PODXL expression with clinciopathological parameters in intestinal type and pancreatobiliary type tumours, respectively

| | Intestinal type | | | Pancreatobiliary type | | |
|---|---|---|---|---|---|---|
| | PODXL NM | PODXL M | P | PODXL NM | PODXL M | P |
| | (n = 51) | (n = 12) | | (n = 52) | (n = 55) | |
| Age | | | | | | |
| (median, range) | 66.0 (38.0–83.0) | 67.5 (44.0–74.0) | 0.972 | 66.0 (44.0–81.0) | 68.0 (44.0–81.0) | 0.613 |
| Sex | | | | | | |
| Women | 28 (82.4) | 6 (17.6) | 0.761 | 17 (34.0) | 33 (66.0) | 0.005 |
| Men | 23 (79.3) | 6 (20.7) | | 35 (61.4) | 22 (38.6) | |
| Tumour origin | | | | | | |
| Duodenum | 12 (85.7) | 2 (14.3) | 0.610 | | | |
| Ampulla intestinal type | 39 (79.6) | 10 (20.4) | | | | |
| Ampulla pancreatobiliary type | | | | 14 (73.7) | 5 (26.3) | 0.005 |
| Distal bile duct | | | | 23 (51.1) | 22 (48.9) | |
| Pancreas | | | | 15 (34.9) | 28 (65.1) | |
| Tumour size mm | | | | | | |
| (median, range) | 30.0 (5.0–90.0) | 26.5 (12.0–40.0) | 0.923 | 30.0 (5.0–70.0) | 30.0 (15.0–70.0) | 0.313 |
| Differentiation grade | | | | | | |
| Well-moderate | 26 (83.9) | 5 (16.1) | 0.565 | 24 (61.5) | 15 (38.5) | 0.044 |
| Poor | 25 (78.1) | 7 (21.9) | | 28 (41.2) | 40 (58.8) | |
| T-stage | | | | | | |
| T1 | 4 (100.0) | 0 (0.0) | 0.246 | 2 (100.0) | 0 (0.0) | 0.392 |
| T2 | 9 (81.8) | 2 (18.2) | | 4 (40.0) | 6 (60.0) | |
| T3 | 21 (84.0) | 4 (16.0) | | 34 (43.6) | 44 (56.4) | |
| T4 | 17 (73.9) | 6 (26.1) | | 12 (70.6) | 5 (29.4) | |
| N-stage | | | | | | |
| N0 | 28 (84.8) | 5 (5.2) | 0.936 | 17 (56.7) | 13 (43.3) | 0.315 |
| N1 | 13 (68.4) | 6 (31.6) | | 21 (46.7) | 24 (53.3) | |
| N2 | 10 (90.9) | 1 (9.1) | | 14 (43.8) | 18 (56.2) | |
| Margins | | | | | | |
| R0 | 15 (88.2) | 2 (11.8) | 0.375 | 3 (50.0) | 3 (50.0) | 0.944 |
| R1-Rx | 36 (78.3) | 10 (21.7) | | 49 (48.5) | 52 (51.5) | |
| Perineural growth | | | | | | |
| No | 38 (86.4) | 6 (13.6) | 0.099 | 14 (63.6) | 8 (36.4) | 0.115 |
| Yes | 13 (68.4) | 6 (31.6) | | 38 (44.7) | 47 (55.3) | |
| Invasion of lymphatic vessels | | | | | | |
| No | 26 (89.7) | 3 (10.3) | 0.107 | 16 (50.0) | 16 (50.0) | 0.850 |
| Yes | 25 (73.5) | 9 (26.5) | | 36 (48.0) | 39 (52.0) | |
| Invasion of blood vessels | | | | | | |
| No | 48 (82.8) | 10 (17.2) | 0.217 | 35 (50.0) | 35 (50.0) | 0.691 |
| Yes | 3 (60.0) | 2 (40.0) | | 17 (45.9) | 20 (54.1) | |
| Growth in peripancreatic fat | | | | | | |
| No | 35 (85.4) | 6 (14.6) | 0.227 | 13 (59.1) | 9 (40.9) | 0.271 |
| Yes | 16 (72.7) | 6 (27.3) | | 39 (45.9) | 46 (54.1) | |

**Table 1** Associations between membranous and non-membranous PODXL expression with clinciopathological parameters in intestinal type and pancreatobiliary type tumours, respectively (Continued)

| Adjuvant chemotherapy | | | | | | |
|---|---|---|---|---|---|---|
| None | 40 (88.9) | 5 (11.1) | 0.145 | 23 (46.0) | 27 (54.0) | 0.348 |
| 5-FU-analogue | 2 (40.0) | 3 (60.0) | | 5 (62.5) | 3 (37.5) | |
| Gemcitabine | 4 (57.1) | 3 (42.9) | | 20 (45.5) | 24 (54.5) | |
| Gemcitabine + capecitabine | 1 (100.0) | 0 (0.0) | | 1 (50.0) | 1 (50.0) | |
| Oxaliplatin + 5-FU analogue | 4 (100.0) | 0 (0.0) | | 1 (100.0) | 0 (0.0) | |
| Gemcitabine + oxaliplatin | 0 (0.0) | 1 (100.0) | | 2 (100.0) | 0 (0.0) | |

*M* membranous PODXL expression, *NM* non-membranous PODXL expression
*R0* radical resection, *R1* non-radical resection, *RX* uncertain resection margins

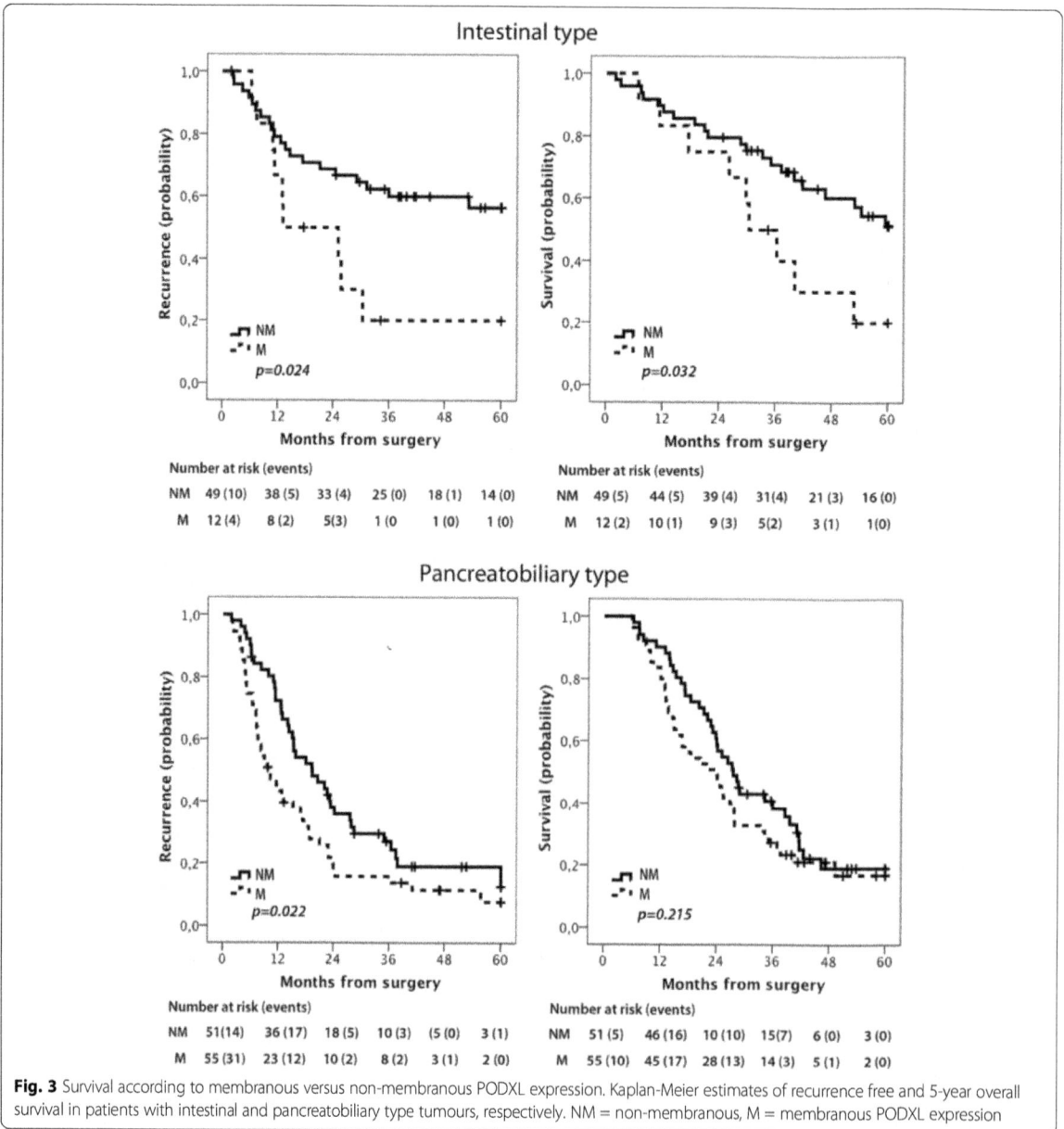

**Fig. 3** Survival according to membranous versus non-membranous PODXL expression. Kaplan-Meier estimates of recurrence free and 5-year overall survival in patients with intestinal and pancreatobiliary type tumours, respectively. NM = non-membranous, M = membranous PODXL expression

**Table 2** Unadjusted and adjusted hazard ratios for recurrence within five years in intestinal and pancreatobiliary type tumours

| | Intestinal type | | | Pancreatobiliary type | | |
|---|---|---|---|---|---|---|
| | n(events) | Unadjusted HR(95 % CI) | Adjusted HR(95 % CI) | n(events) | Unadjusted HR(95 % CI) | Adjusted HR(95 % CI) |
| Age | | | | | | |
| Continuous | 61 (29) | 1.00 (0.96–1.03) | 1.07 (1.02–1.13) | 106 (88) | 0.98 (0.96–1.01) | 1.00 (0.96–1.03) |
| Gender | | | | | | |
| Female | 34 (11) | 1.00 | 1.00 | 50 (42) | 1.00 | 1.00 |
| Male | 27 (18) | 2.31 (1.08–4.94) | 2.40 (0.94–6.14) | 56 (46) | 1.06 (0.70–1.61) | 0.88 (0.53–1.49) |
| Tumour origin | | | | | | |
| Duodenum | 13 (4) | 1.00 | 1.00 | – | – |
| Ampulla-Intestinal type | 48 (25) | 2.18 (0.76–6.27) | 6.82 (1.32–35.12) | – | – |
| Ampulla-Pancreatobiliary type | – | – | 19 (16) | 1.00 | 1.00 |
| Distal Bile duct | | – | – | 44 (38) | 1.10 (0.61–1.98) | 1.52 (0.78–2.94) |
| Pancreas | | – | – | 43 (34) | 1.06 (0.58–1.93) | 0.93 (0.49–1.77) |
| Tumour size | | | | | | |
| Continuous | 61 (30) | 1.00 (0.98–1.02) | 1.04 (1.00–1.09) | 106 (88) | 1.03 (1.02–1.05) | 1.02 (0.99–1.04) |
| T-stage | | | | | | |
| T1 | 4 (1) | 1.00 | 1.00 | 2 (1) | 1.00 | 1.00 |
| T2 | 10(3) | 1.28 (0.13–12.30) | 3.71 (0.34–40.64) | 10 (6) | 1.61 (0.19–13.36) | 0.66 (0.07–6.08) |
| T3 | 25 (9) | 1.86 (0.24–14.71) | 5.72 (0.50–65.06) | 77 (66) | 4.67 (0.64–33.96) | 1.21 (0.15–9.92) |
| T4 | 22 (16) | 5.44 (0.72–41.21) | 6.36 (0.21–195.20) | 17 (15) | 4.31 (0.56–33.10) | 1.83 (0.08–40.27) |
| N-stage | | | | | | |
| N0 | 33 (11) | 1.00 | 1.00 | 29 (21) | 1.00 | 1.00 |
| N1 (metastasis in 1–3 lgl) | 19 (11) | 2.07 (0.90–4.78) | 1.00 (0.37–2.70) | 45 (37) | 2.17 (1.25–3.78) | 2.04 (1.13–3.67) |
| N2 (metastasis in 4 or more lgl) | 9 (7) | 4.06 (1.55–10.59) | 6.88 (1.81–26.15) | 32 (30) | 3.11 (1.72–5.61) | 2.61 (1.42–4.83) |
| Differentiation grade | | | | | | |
| Well-moderate | 30 (11) | 1.00 | 1.00 | 39 (29) | 1.00 | 1.00 |
| Poor | 31 (18) | 2.16 (1.02–4.57) | 1.38 (0.40–4.79) | 67 (59) | 2.32 (1.45–3.71) | 2.02 (1.20–3.39) |
| Involved margins, status | | | | | | |
| R0 | 17 (3) | 1.00 | 1.00 | 6 (4) | 1.00 | 1.00 |
| R1 & Rx | 44 (26) | 4.51 (1.36–14.94) | 2.23 (0.62–8.03) | 100 (84) | 2.31 (0.84–6.36) | 2.39 (0.84–6.76) |
| Lymphatic growth | | | | | | |
| Absent | 28 (5) | 1.00 | 1.00 | 32 (23) | 1.00 | 1.00 |
| Present | 33 (24) | 6.16 (2.34–16.19) | 6.19 (1.76–21.82) | 74 (65) | 1.77 (1.09–2.88) | 1.05 (0.59–1.85) |
| Vascular growth | | | | | | |
| Absent | 56 (24) | 1.00 | 1.00 | 70 (55) | 1.00 | 1.00 |
| Present | 5 (5) | 8.16 (2.86–23.30) | 1.62 (0.39–6.65) | 36 (33) | 2.30 (1.47–3.61) | 2.08 (1.28–3.36) |
| Perineural growth | | | | | | |
| Absent | 42 (15) | 1.00 | 1.00 | 22 (14) | 1.00 | 1.00 |
| Present | 19 (14) | 2.72 (1.31–5.66) | 1.01 (0.27–3.81) | 84 (74) | 2.93 (1.57–5.46) | 2.04 (1.06–3.90) |
| Growth in peripancreatic fat | | | | | | |
| Absent | 40 (12) | 1.00 | 1.00 | 22 (13) | 1.00 | 1.00 |
| Present | 21 (17) | 4.74 (2.23–10.10) | 3.60 (1.43–9.07) | 84 (75) | 2.60 (1.42–4.75) | 1.45 (0.76–2.77) |

**Table 2** Unadjusted and adjusted hazard ratios for recurrence within five years in intestinal and pancreatobiliary type tumours (Continued)

| Adjuvant treatment | | | | | | |
|---|---|---|---|---|---|---|
| No | 43 (21) | 1.00 | 1.00 | 49 (40) | 1.00 | 1.00 |
| Yes | 18 (8) | 0.87 (0.38–1.96) | 0.12 (0.04–0.44) | 57 (48) | 1.08 (0.70–1.65) | 0.89 (0.54–1.49) |
| PODXL expression | | | | | | |
| Non-membranous | 49 (20) | 1.00 | 1.00 | 51 (40) | 1.00 | 1.00 |
| Membranous | 12 (9) | 2.44 (1.10–5.44) | 5.12 (1.43–18.31) | 55 (88) | 1.63 (1.07–2.49) | 1.53 (0.99–2.38) |

*R0* radical resection, *R1* non-radical resection, *RX* uncertain resection margins

pancreatic region resemble tumours with colorectal origin in a stronger way than PB-types. In line with the study by Ney et al., PODXL was negative or only weakly expressed in normal pancreatic parenchyma from the resection specimens [21].

In a previous study on colorectal cancer, wherein a PODXL expression was compared in full-face sections from 31 primary tumours and all available lymph node metastases ($n = 140$), there was an excellent concordance in that all primary tumours with non-membranous PODXL expression had metastases with non-membranous expression, whereas a few primary tumours with membranous PODXL expression had a varying proportion of metastatic lymph nodes with membranous and non-membranous PODXL expression [16]. These findings led to the conclusion that for prognostic or predictive purposes, analysis of the primary tumour would be sufficient [16]. In the present study, although negative conversion of membranous PODXL expression from primary tumour to lymph node metastasis was far more common than positive conversion, a few cases displayed the latter phenomenon. Of note, all analyses were based on TMA-samples, and therefore, future studies based on full-face sections are warranted to further examine the rate of positive conversion of membranous PODXL expression in pancreatic and periampullary cancers, so as to determine whether biomarker analysis of the primary tumour will be sufficient in the clinical setting.

In the present study membranous PODXL expression was an independent predictor of reduced 5-year overall and recurrence-free survival in I-type but not in PB-type tumours, although there was a significant association between membranous PODXL expression and a reduced RFS in the latter in unadjusted analysis. These findings are well in line with previous publications regarding the prognostic significance of PODXL expression in several other major types of cancer [13–15, 18–20]. In addition, and importantly, we found that patients with I-type tumours displaying membranous PODXL had a beneficial effect of adjuvant chemotherapy. When ampullary PB-type tumours, expressing membranous PODXL in a similar proportion to I-type tumours, were included in the analysis, the effect by adjuvant chemotherapy was even

more pronounced. This supports earlier data that patients with PODXL positive tumours benefit from adjuvant chemotherapy, irrespective of treatment regime, as seen in colorectal cancer [14, 15]. Moreover, these findings indicate that I-type tumours with high expression of PODXL are more likely to benefit from adjuvant therapy than PB-type tumours. Today, all patients with pancreatic and periampullary adenocarcinoma are recommended adjuvant treatment. Since adjuvant treatment often is associated with toxicity and adverse side effects, it is important to identify novel predictive and prognostic factors, such as PODXL, to support and improve clinical decisions. Therefore, the results from the present study indicate that PODXL could be used as a predictive marker for adjuvant treatment of periampullary cancer with intestinal morphology, and possibly also ampullary PB-type tumours. Of note, given the retrospective nature of the present study, the term "predictive" should be applied with caution. It must however be pointed out that the study cohort encompasses a consecutive series of clinically and histopathologically well-annotated pancreatoduodenectomy cases, of which only approximately half have been given adjuvant chemotherapy, which should allow for a fairly good assessment of both prognostic and predictive biomarkers even in the retrospective setting. Thus, the herein observed prognostic and potential predictive value of PODXL, in particular in I-type tumours, is of potential clinical relevance and merits further study in additional retrospective cohorts as well as in a controlled, prospective trial. Targeting PODXL with monoclonal antibodies may also be a future treatment option [27].

Membranous PODXL expression was considerably higher in PB-type as compared with I-type tumours, which is in line with the former being clinically more aggressive. In PB-type tumours, the prognostic value of PODXL was only significant for RFS, and not after adjustment for other clinicopathological factors, and there was no evident predictive value. The choice of prognostic cutoff, i.e. membranous vs non-membranous PODXL expression, can be considered appropriate for the herein used antibody, since the same antibody and cutoff has been used in the previous study on pancreatic cancer by Dallas et al. [22] and since this dichotomization yielded the strongest prognostic and predictive

**Table 3** Unadjusted and adjusted hazard ratios for death within five years in intestinal and pancreatobiliary type tumours

| | Intestinal type | | | Pancreatobiliary type | | |
| | n(events) | Unadjusted HR(95 % CI) | Adjusted HR(95 % CI) | n(events) | Unadjusted HR(95 % CI) | Adjusted HR(95 % CI) |
| --- | --- | --- | --- | --- | --- | --- |
| Age | | | | | | |
| Continuous | 61 (30) | 1.02 (0.98–1.06) | 1.07 (1.02–1.13) | 106 (82) | 0.99 (0.96–1.02) | 1.01 (0.98–1.05) |
| Gender | | | | | | |
| Female | 34 (13) | 1.00 | 1.00 | 50 (36) | 1.00 | 1.00 |
| Male | 27 (17) | 1.85 (0.89–3.84) | 2.12 (0.86–5.22) | 56 (46) | 1.20 (0.78–1.87) | 1.22 (0.76–1.95) |
| Tumour origin | | | | | | |
| Duodenum | 13 (5) | 1.00 | 1.00 | – | – | – |
| Ampulla-Intestinal type | 48 (25) | 1.49 (0.57–3.88) | 7.77 (1.86–32.39) | – | – | – |
| Ampulla-Pancreatobiliary type | | – | – | 19 (16) | 1.00 | 1.00 |
| Distal Bile duct | | – | – | 44 (32) | 0.74 (0.40–1.34) | 1.03 (0.50–2.15) |
| Pancreas | | – | – | 43 (34) | 0.91 (0.50–1.65) | 1.06 (0.52–2.19) |
| Tumour size | | | | | | |
| Continuous | 61 (30) | 1.00 (0.98–1.03) | 1.05 (1.01–1.10) | 106 (82) | 1.03 (1.01–1.05) | 1.01 (0.99–1.04) |
| T-stage | | | | | | |
| T1 | 4 (2) | 1.00 | 1.00 | 2 (1) | 1.00 | 1.00 |
| T2 | 10(3) | 0.65 (0.11–3.88) | 0.55 (0.07–4.50) | 10 (6) | 1.43 (0.17–11.85) | 0.77 (0.08–7.56) |
| T3 | 25 (9) | 0.94 (0.20–4.37) | 1.49 (0.19–11.34) | 77 (60) | 2.95 (0.41–21.34) | 0.84 (0.10–7.08) |
| T4 | 22 (16) | 2.55 (0.58–11.15) | 1.88 (0.19–18.25) | 17 (15) | 3.77 (0.50–28.71) | 2.12 (0.09–48.78) |
| N-stage | | | | | | |
| N0 | 33 (15) | 1.00 | 1.00 | 29 (18) | 1.00 | 1.00 |
| N1 (metastasis in 1–3 lgl) | 19 (9) | 1.17 (0.51–2.68) | 0.55 (0.20–1.50) | 45 (37) | 2.41 (1.35–4.29) | 2.85 (1.57–5.17) |
| N2 (metastasis in 4 or more lgl) | 9 (6) | 2.08 (0.80–5.37) | 8.96 (2.47–32.51) | 32 (27) | 2.59 (1.40–4.78) | 2.45 (1.30–4.63) |
| Differentiation grade | | | | | | |
| Well-moderate | 30 (12) | 1.00 | 1.00 | 39 (24) | 1.00 | 1.00 |
| Poor | 31 (18) | 1.98 (0.95–4.11) | 2.16 (0.77–6.03) | 67 (58) | 2.44 (1.50–3.95) | 2.13 (1.28–3.54) |
| Involved margins, status | | | | | | |
| R0 | 17 (4) | 1.00 | 1.00 | 6 (2) | 1.00 | 1.00 |
| R1 & Rx | 44 (26) | 2.56 (0.89–7.36) | 0.46 (0.12–1.69) | 100 (80) | 3.49 (0.86–14.25) | 2.57 (0.62–10.60) |
| Lymphatic growth | | | | | | |
| Absent | 28 (7) | 1.00 | 1.00 | 32 (22) | 1.00 | 1.00 |
| Present | 33 (23) | 3.61 (1.55–8.44) | 5.85 (1.93–17.77) | 74 (60) | 1.51 (0.92–2.48) | 0.96 (0.55–1.70) |
| Vascular growth | | | | | | |
| Absent | 56 (25) | 1.00 | 1.00 | 70 (47) | 1.00 | 1.00 |
| Present | 5 (5) | 7.78 (2.74–22.11) | 1.70 (0.40–7.31) | 36 (35) | 2.39 (1.54–3.72) | 2.45 (1.54–3.87) |
| Perineural growth | | | | | | |
| Absent | 42 (17) | 1.00 | 1.00 | 22 (14) | 1.00 | 1.00 |
| Present | 19 (13) | 2.15 (1.04–4.44) | 3.81 (1.55–9.37) | 84 (68) | 1.88 (1.05–3.38) | 0.92 (0.48–1.76) |
| Growth in peripancreatic fat | | | | | | |
| Absent | 40 (14) | 1.00 | 1.00 | 22 (14) | 1.00 | 1.00 |
| Present | 21 (16) | 3.49 (1.68–7.25) | 0.75 (0.06–9.94) | 84 (68) | 1.80 (1.00–3.25) | 1.25 (0.64–2.43) |
| Adjuvant treatment | | | | | | |
| No | 43 (24) | 1.00 | 1.00 | 49 (39) | 1.00 | 1.00 |

**Table 3** Unadjusted and adjusted hazard ratios for death within five years in intestinal and pancreatobiliary type tumours (Continued)

| Yes | 18 (6) | 0.60 (0.25–1.47) | 0.03 (0.01–0.16) | 57 (43) | 0.90 (0.58–1.39) | 0.67 (0.43–1.04) |
| --- | --- | --- | --- | --- | --- | --- |
| PODXL expression | | | | | | |
| Non-membranous | 49 (21) | 1.00 | 1.00 | 51 (38) | 1.00 | 1.00 |
| Membranous | 12 (9) | 2.32 (1.05–5.12) | 7.31 (2.12–25.16) | 55 (44) | 1.32 (0.85–2.03) | 1.10 (0.67–1.81) |

*R0* radical resection, *R1* non-radical resection, *RX* uncertain resection margins

value. It is however noteworthy that the category of tumours with moderate-strong cytoplasmic staining (score 2) is a somewhat ambiguous group with an intermediate prognosis, undoubtedly harbouring some cases with a prognosis equally poor to cases with membranous PODXL expression. While it is possible that in some of these cases, the presence of membranous expression may be masked by a strong cytoplasmic expression, this category of tumours may also constitute a different biological entity, possibly constituting an "intermediate" between tumours with negative/weak and membranous PODXL expression. In a comparative study on colorectal cancer, membranous expression of the herein used antibody and cytoplasmic expression of an in-house generated antibody were both found to be independent predictors of poor prognosis, and combined use of the antibodies was found to detect a group with an even worse prognosis [28].

Previous studies have demonstrated PODXL to be a functional ligand of E- and L- selectins in pancreatic cancer suggesting that its expression may promote haemotogenic spread of metastases by facilitating binding of circulating tumour cells to selectin-expressing host cells [22]. These findings further support the theory of PODXL overexpression being associated with more aggressive tumours [22]. Moreover, similar to the situation in colorectal [14, 15, 16] and urinary bladder [19] cancer, PODXL expression was observed predominantly on the invasive tumour front, also suggesting its importance in the metastatic spread of the disease. Of note, in the study on bladder cancer, the herein used polyclonal antibody was compared with two other monoclonal antibodies, all showing 100 % concordance regarding the detection of membranous PODXL expression, whereas the degree of cytoplasmic expression detected by the monoclonal antibodies was substantially weaker [19].

Our results are derived from TMA-based analyses on retrospectively collected tumour samples. Of note, the TMA-technique was also used in the study by Dallas et al. [22]. For characterization of key molecular alterations and expression of investigative biomarkers in tumours from large patient cohorts, whether retrospectively or prospectively defined, the TMA-technology is essential [29].

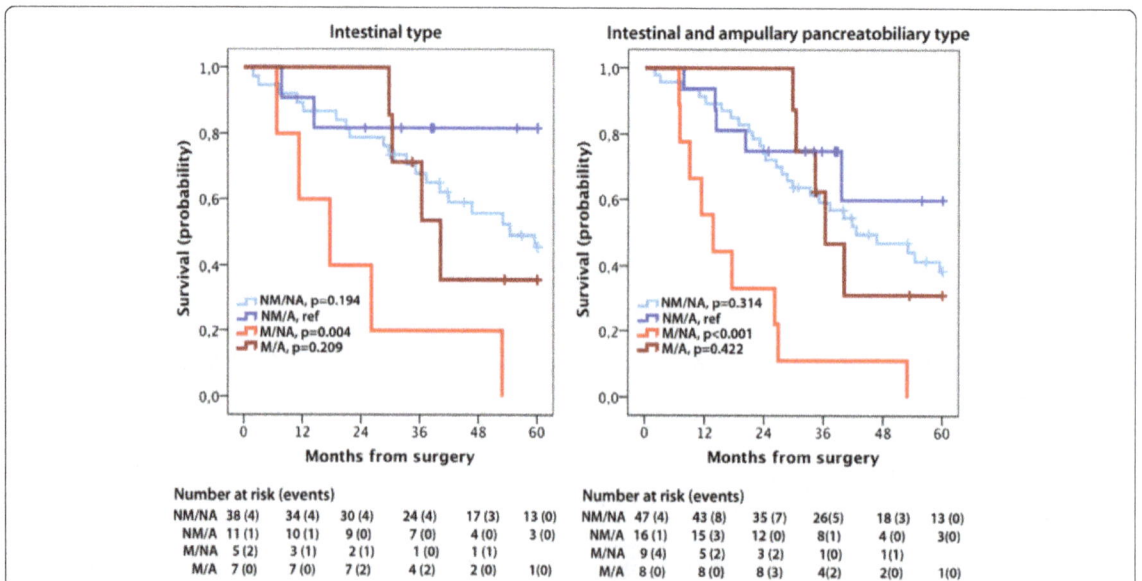

**Fig. 4** Survival according to PODXL expression and adjuvant chemotherapy. Kaplan-Meier estimates of 5-year overall survival in combined strata of membranous (*M*)/ non-membranous (*NM*) PODXL expression and adjuvant (*A*) /no adjuvant (*NA*) chemotherapy in patients with intestinal type tumours and intestinal type + ampullary pancreatobiliary type tumours, respectively. NM = non-membranous, M = membranous PODXL expression

However, some limitations related to the TMA-technique must be considered, most importantly its ability to accurately reflect the expression of heterogeneously expressed markers. To compensate for this one needs to ensure that tumour cores are sampled from different regions of the tumour. In the present study, the cores from the primary tumour were, whenever possible, obtained from different donor blocks, and different lymph nodes were sampled in cases with more than one metastatic node.

## Conclusions

Membranous expression of PODXL is significantly higher in pancreatobiliary type as compared with intestinal type periampullary adenocarcinomas and an independent factor of poor prognosis in the latter. The herein presented results also indicate a beneficial effect of adjuvant chemotherapy on intestinal type tumours with membranous PODXL expression, suggesting the potential utility of PODXL as a biomarker for improved treatment stratification of these patients.

## Additional files

**Additional file 1:** Cox proportional hazards analysis of the impact of PODXL expression on overall survival according to adjuvant treatment intestinal-type and intestinal-type + ampullary pancreatobiliary-type adenocarcinomas.

**Additional file 2:** Survival according to PODXL score. Kaplan-Meier estimates of recurrence free survival and 5-year overall survival, respectively, in (A,B) the entire cohort, (C, D) patients with intestinal type tumours and (E, F) patients with pancreatobiliary type tumours. Score 0 = negative staining, score 1 = weak cytoplasmic positivity in any proportion of cells, score 2: moderate-strong cytoplasmic positivity in any proportion of cells, score 3: distinct membranous positivity in < = 50 % of cells and score 4 = distinct membranous positivity in >50 % of cells.

### Abbreviations
PODXL: Podocalyxin-like protein 1; PB-type: Pancreatobiliary type adenocarcinoma; I-type: Intestinal type adenocarcinoma; TMA: Tissue microarray; OS: Overall survival; RFS: Recurrence free survival; HR: Hazard ratio; CI: Confidence interval.

### Competing interests
The authors declare that they have no competing interests.

### Authors' contributions
MH collected clinical data, annotated the immunohistochemical staining, performed the statistical analyses and drafted the manuscript. JEL collected clinicopathological data, assisted with TMA construction and helped draft the manuscript. BN constructed the tissue microarray and performed the IHC stainings. KJ conceived the study, evaluated the immunohistochemical staining and helped draft the manuscript. JEB collected clinical data, conceived the study and helped draft the manuscript. All authors read and approved the final manuscript.

### Acknowledgments
This study was supported by grants from the Knut and Alice Wallenberg Foundation, the Swedish Cancer Society, the Gunnar Nilsson Cancer Foundation, the Swedish Government Grant for Clinical Research, Lund University Faculty of Medicine and University Hospital Research Grants.

### References
1. C.P, SBWW. World Cancer Report 2014. In: Bernard W, editor. World Cancer Report 2014. Stewart CPW: IARC; 2014.
2. Heinemann V, Boeck S, Hinke A, Labianca R, Louvet C. Meta-analysis of randomized trials: evaluation of benefit from gemcitabine-based combination chemotherapy applied in advanced pancreatic cancer. BMC Cancer. 2008;8:82.
3. Jemal A, Siegel R, Ward E, Hao Y, Xu J, Thun MJ. Cancer statistics, 2009. CA Cancer J Clin. 2009;59(4):225–49.
4. Sultana A, Tudur Smith C, Cunningham D, Starling N, Neoptolemos JP, Ghaneh P. Meta-analyses of chemotherapy for locally advanced and metastatic pancreatic cancer: results of secondary end points analyses. Br J Cancer. 2008;99(1):6–13.
5. Herreros-Villanueva M, Hijona E, Cosme A, Bujanda L. Adjuvant and neoadjuvant treatment in pancreatic cancer. World J Gastroenterol. 2012;18(14):1565–72.
6. Westgaard A, Tafjord S, Farstad IN, Cvancarova M, Eide TJ, Mathisen O, et al. Pancreatobiliary versus intestinal histologic type of differentiation is an independent prognostic factor in resected periampullary adenocarcinoma. BMC Cancer. 2008;8:170.
7. Bronsert P, Kohler I, Werner M, Makowiec F, Kuesters S, Hoeppner J, et al. Intestinal-type of differentiation predicts favourable overall survival: confirmatory clinicopathological analysis of 198 periampullary adenocarcinomas of pancreatic, biliary, ampullary and duodenal origin. BMC Cancer. 2013;13:428.
8. Kerjaschki D, Sharkey DJ, Farquhar MG. Identification and characterization of podocalyxin–the major sialoprotein of the renal glomerular epithelial cell. J Cell Biol. 1984;98(4):1591–6.
9. Doyonnas R, Kershaw DB, Duhme C, Merkens H, Chelliah S, Graf T, et al. Anuria, omphalocele, and perinatal lethality in mice lacking the CD34-related protein podocalyxin. J Exp Med. 2001;194(1):13–27.
10. Horvat R, Hovorka A, Dekan G, Poczewski H, Kerjaschki D. Endothelial cell membranes contain podocalyxin–the major sialoprotein of visceral glomerular epithelial cells. J Cell Biol. 1986;102(2):484–91.
11. Doyonnas R, Nielsen JS, Chelliah S, Drew E, Hara T, Miyajima A, et al. Podocalyxin is a CD34-related marker of murine hematopoietic stem cells and embryonic erythroid cells. Blood. 2005;105(11):4170–8.
12. McNagny KM, Pettersson I, Rossi F, Flamme I, Shevchenko A, Mann M, et al. Thrombomucin, a novel cell surface protein that defines thrombocytes and multipotent hematopoietic progenitors. J Cell Biol. 1997;138(6):1395–407.
13. Somasiri A, Nielsen JS, Makretsov N, McCoy ML, Prentice L, Gilks CB, et al. Overexpression of the anti-adhesin podocalyxin is an independent predictor of breast cancer progression. Cancer Res. 2004;64(15):5068–73.
14. Larsson A, Johansson ME, Wangefjord S, Gaber A, Nodin B, Kucharzewska P, et al. Overexpression of podocalyxin-like protein is an independent factor of poor prognosis in colorectal cancer. Br J Cancer. 2011;105(5):666–72.
15. Larsson AH, Fridberg M, Gaber A, Nodin B, Leveen P, Jonsson GB, et al. Validation of podocalyxin-like protein as a biomarker of poor prognosis in colorectal cancer. BMC Cancer. 2012;12(1):282.
16. Larsson AH, Nodin B, Syk I, Palmquist I, Uhlen M, Eberhard J, et al. Podocalyxin-like protein expression in primary colorectal cancer and synchronous lymph node metastases. Diagn Pathol. 2013;8:109.
17. Kaprio T, Fermer C, Hagstrom J, Mustonen H, Bockelman C, Nilsson O, et al. Podocalyxin is a marker of poor prognosis in colorectal cancer. BMC Cancer. 2014;14:493.
18. Cipollone JA, Graves ML, Kobel M, Kalloger SE, Poon T, Gilks CB, et al. The anti-adhesive mucin podocalyxin may help initiate the transperitoneal metastasis of high grade serous ovarian carcinoma. Clin Exp Metastasis. 2012;29(3):239–52.
19. Boman K, Larsson AH, Segersten U, Kuteeva E, Johannesson H, Nodin B, et al. Membranous expression of podocalyxin-like protein is an independent factor of poor prognosis in urothelial bladder cancer. Br J Cancer. 2013;108(11):2321–8.
20. Binder ZA, Siu IM, Eberhart CG, Ap Rhys C, Bai RY, Staedtke V, et al. Podocalyxin-like protein is expressed in glioblastoma multiforme stem-like cells and is associated with poor outcome. PLoS One. 2013;8(10):e75945.
21. Ney JT, Zhou H, Sipos B, Buttner R, Chen X, Kloppel G, et al. Podocalyxin-like protein 1 expression is useful to differentiate pancreatic ductal adenocarcinomas from adenocarcinomas of the biliary and gastrointestinal tracts. Hum Pathol. 2007;38(2):359–64.
22. Dallas MR, Chen SH, Streppel MM, Sharma S, Maitra A, Konstantopoulos K. Sialofucosylated podocalyxin is a functional E- and L-selectin ligand expressed by metastatic pancreatic cancer cells. Am J Physiol Cell Physiol. 2012;303(6):C616–24.
23. Elebro J, Jirstrom K. Use of a standardized diagnostic approach improves the prognostic information of histopathologic factors in pancreatic and periampullary adenocarcinoma. Diagn Pathol. 2014;9(1):80.

24. Fristedt R, Elebro J, Gaber A, Jonsson L, Heby M, Yudina Y, et al. Reduced expression of the polymeric immunoglobulin receptor in pancreatic and periampullary adenocarcinoma signifies tumour progression and poor prognosis. PLoS One. 2014;9(11):e112728.

25. Elebro J, Heby M, Gaber A, Nodin B, Jonsson L, Fristedt R, et al. Prognostic and treatment predictive significance of SATB1 and SATB2 expression in pancreatic and periampullary adenocarcinoma. J Transl Med. 2014;12(1):289.

26. Cheung HH, Davis AJ, Lee TL, Pang AL, Nagrani S, Rennert OM, et al. Methylation of an intronic region regulates miR-199a in testicular tumor malignancy. Oncogene. 2011;30(31):3404–15.

27. Snyder KA, Hughes MR, Hedberg B, Brandon J, Hernaez DC, Bergqvist P, et al. Podocalyxin enhances breast tumor growth and metastasis and is a target for monoclonal antibody therapy. Breast Cancer Res. 2015;17(1):46.

28. Kaprio T, Hagstrom J, Fermer C, Mustonen H, Bockelman C, Nilsson O, et al. A comparative study of two PODXL antibodies in 840 colorectal cancer patients. BMC Cancer. 2014;14:494.

29. Torhorst J, Bucher C, Kononen J, Haas P, Zuber M, Kochli OR, et al. Tissue microarrays for rapid linking of molecular changes to clinical endpoints. Am J Pathol. 2001;159(6):2249–56.

# 22

# Expression of a-Tocopherol-Associated protein (TAP) is associated with clinical outcome in breast cancer patients

Xi Wang[1][*][†], Brian Z. Ring[2][†], Robert S. Seitz[3], Douglas T. Ross[4], Kirsten Woolf[1], Rodney A. Beck[5], David G. Hicks[1] and Shuyuan Yeh[1]

## Abstract

**Background:** The role of vitamin E in breast cancer prevention and treatment has been widely investigated, and the different tocopherols that comprise this nutrient have been shown to have divergent associations with cancer outcome. Our previous studies have shown that a-Tocopherol-associated protein (TAP), a vitamin E binding protein, may function as a tumor suppressor-like factor in breast carcinogenesis. The current study addresses the association of TAP expression with breast cancer clinical outcomes.

**Methods:** Immunohistochemical stain for TAP was applied to a tissue microarray from a breast cancer cohort consisting of 271 patients with a median follow-up time of 5.2 years. The expression of TAP in tumor cells was compared with patient's clinical outcome at 5 years after diagnosis. The potential role of TAP in predicting outcome was also assessed in clinically relevant subsets of the cohort. In addition, we compared TAP expression and Oncotype DX scores in an independent breast cancer cohort consisting of 71 cases.

**Results:** We demonstrate that the expression of TAP was differentially expressed within the breast cancer cohort, and that ER+/PR ± tumors were more likely to exhibit TAP expression. TAP expression was associated with an overall lower recurrence rate and a better 5-year survival rate. This association was primarily in patients with ER+ tumors; exploratory analysis showed that this association was strongest in patients with node-positive tumors and was independent of stage and treatment with chemotherapy. TAP expression in ER/PR negative or triple negative tumors had no association with clinical outcome. In addition, we did not observe an association between TAP expression and Oncotype DX recurrence score.

**Conclusions:** The significant positive association we found for a-Tocopherol-associated protein with outcome in breast cancer may help to better define and explain studies addressing a-tocopherol's association with cancer risk and outcome. Additionally, further studies to validate and extend these findings may allow TAP to serve as a breast-specific prognostic marker in breast cancer patients, especially in those patients with ER+ tumors.

**Keywords:** Breast cancer, a-Tocopherol-associated protein (TAP), Vitamin E

* Correspondence: xi_wang@urmc.rochester.edu
[†]Equal contributors
[1]Department of Pathology, University of Rochester Medical Center, Rochester, NY 14642, USA
Full list of author information is available at the end of the article

**Table 1** Cohort characteristics. *P* value for difference between proportion of clinical characteristic within TAP positive and negative patients determined with a two-proportion z-test, except for age and tumor size for which a *t*-test was employed

| | All cases | | TAP negative | | TAP positive | | |
| --- | --- | --- | --- | --- | --- | --- | --- |
| | No. of patients | % | No. of patients | % | No. of patients | % | *P* value |
| Total | 271 | | 183 | | 88 | | |
| Grade | | | | | | | |
| 1 | 34 | 12.5 | 20 | 10.9 | 14 | 15.9 | 0.33 |
| 2 | 105 | 38.7 | 59 | 32.2 | 46 | 52.3 | 0.02 |
| 3 | 92 | 33.9 | 78 | 42.6 | 14 | 15.9 | 0.03 |
| Unknown | 40 | 14.8 | 26 | 14.2 | 14 | 15.9 | nd |
| Stage | | | | | | | |
| I | 97 | 35.8 | 60 | 32.8 | 37 | 42 | 0.18 |
| II | 137 | 50.6 | 94 | 51.4 | 43 | 48.9 | 0.39 |
| III | 31 | 11.4 | 23 | 12.6 | 8 | 9.1 | 0.4 |
| Unknown | 6 | 2.2 | 6 | 3.3 | 0 | | nd |
| Age (avg, range) | | | | | | | |
| | 58.1 (26–89) | | 56.9 (26–87) | | 62.6 (35–89) | | <0.001 |
| T | | | | | | | |
| T1 | 138 | 50.9 | 82 | 44.8 | 56 | 63.6 | 0.01 |
| T2 | 101 | 37.3 | 74 | 40.4 | 27 | 30.7 | 0.19 |
| T3 | 14 | 5.2 | 12 | 6.6 | 2 | 2.3 | 0.41 |
| T4 | 8 | 3 | 6 | 3.3 | 2 | 2.3 | 0.47 |
| Unknown | 10 | 3.7 | 9 | 4.9 | 1 | 1.1 | nd |
| N | | | | | | | |
| N0 | 150 | 55.4 | 97 | 53 | 53 | 60.2 | 0.2 |
| N1 | 108 | 39.9 | 74 | 40.4 | 34 | 38.6 | 0.43 |
| N2 | 6 | 2.2 | 5 | 2.7 | 1 | 1.1 | 0.46 |
| Unknown | 7 | 2.6 | 7 | 3.8 | 0 | | nd |
| M | | | | | | | |
| M0 | 258 | 99.2 | 172 | 98.9 | 86 | 100 | 1 |
| M1 | 2 | 0.8 | 2 | 1.1 | 0 | | nd |
| Unknown | 11 | | 9 | | 2 | | nd |
| Tumor size (avg, cm) | | | | | | | |
| | 2.09 | | 2.39 | | 1.83 | | <0.001 |
| Received chemotherapy | | | | | | | |
| no | 133 | 49.1 | 75 | 41 | 58 | 65.9 | 1 |
| yes | 130 | 48 | 101 | 55.2 | 29 | 33 | 1 |
| Unknown | 8 | 3 | 7 | 3.8 | 1 | 1.1 | nd |
| ER | | | | | | | |
| ER- | 65 | 24 | 58 | 31.7 | 7 | 8 | 0.1 |
| ER+ | 197 | 72.7 | 120 | 65.6 | 77 | 87.5 | 0 |
| Unknown | 9 | 3.3 | 5 | 2.7 | 4 | 4.5 | nd |
| HER2 | | | | | | | |
| HER2- | 116 | 42.8 | 85 | 46.4 | 31 | 35.2 | 1 |
| HER2+ | 72 | 26.6 | 43 | 23.5 | 29 | 33 | 1 |
| Unknown | 83 | 30.6 | 55 | 30.1 | 28 | 31.8 | nd |

**Table 1** Cohort characteristics. *P* value for difference between proportion of clinical characteristic within TAP positive and negative patients determined with a two-proportion z-test, except for age and tumor size for which a *t*-test was employed *(Continued)*

| Hormone therapy | | | | | | | | |
|---|---|---|---|---|---|---|---|---|
| No | 77 | 26.7 | 57 | | 28.8 | 20 | 22.2 | 0.28 |
| yes | 187 | 64.9 | 120 | | 60.6 | 67 | 74.4 | 0.03 |
| Unknown | 24 | 8.3 | 21 | | 10.6 | 3 | 3.3 | nd |

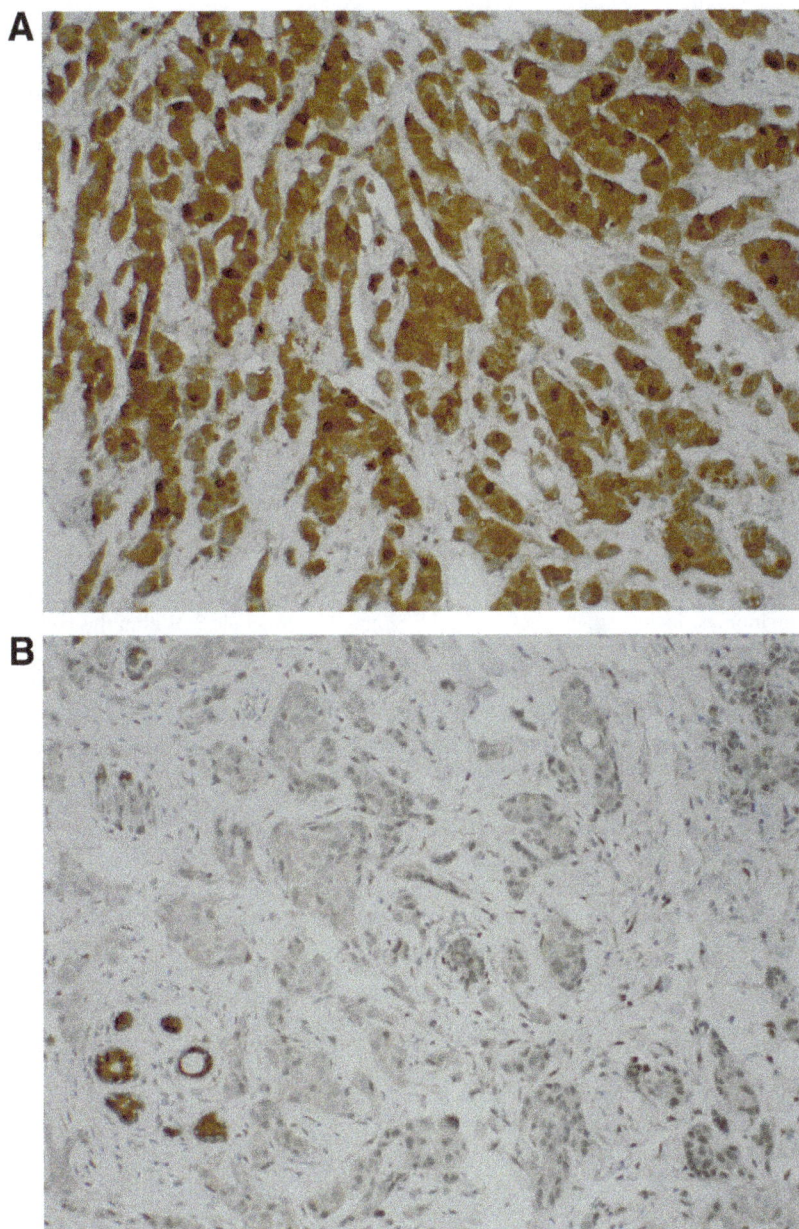

**Fig. 1** Invasive ductal carcinoma showing TAP staining positive (**a**), and negative with the positive internal control of normal/benign TDLU (**b**)

# Background

Breast cancer is the most common malignant tumor in women worldwide, comprising 16 % of all female cancers. Epidemiological studies have shown that vitamin E has a potential utility in the prevention and treatment of human malignancies, including breast cancer [1–3]. However clinical trials on the effectiveness of dietary supplementation with vitamin E or $\alpha$-tocopherol, the principle and most active vitamin E isoform in human plasma, as an aid in the prevention of cancer have not produced evidence of a consistent association with decreased cancer occurrence [4, 5]. The inconstancies between epidemiological studies and intervention trials may be due to differing roles for the tocopherols that comprise vitamin E or unexplained genetic diversity in the study populations affecting how they utilized vitamin E.

Our previous studies have shown that $\alpha$-Tocopherol-associated protein (TAP), a vitamin E binding protein [6], is selectively expressed in human breast, prostate, liver and brain tissue and its expression can be evaluated by immunohistochemical staining [7, 8]. We have shown that, while TAP can facilitate vitamin E retention in cancer cells and promote vitamin E-mediated anti-proliferation effects, it can also act as a tumor suppressor-like protein in a vitamin E-independent fashion. Overexpression of TAP in prostate cancer cells was shown to suppress cell growth; and a TAP siRNA knockdown in a prostate cell line led to increased cell growth [7]. In human breast, we identified that TAP is typically co-expressed with ER in sporadic normal/benign luminal cells in terminal ductal lobular units, and that TAP showed decreased expression in 57 % of invasive breast carcinomas, including 46 % of ER and PR positive carcinomas, and 80 % of high grade carcinomas [9]. Another study has shown that TAP mRNA level is negatively associated with tumor stage and lymph node status in breast cancer [10]. TAP expression therefore may be a candidate for a marker of less aggressive breast carcinoma.

Despite the advances in multidisciplinary treatment, breast cancer remains the second most common cause of death related to cancer in women. In addition to the routine pathologic characteristics of breast cancer, such as tumor size, grade, vascular invasion, lymph node metastasis, ER/PR/Her2 status etc., genes which may have an association with tumor biology and help in predicting recurrence, therapeutic response and survival have been studied widely. Currently there are at least nine gene expression signatures showing some correlation with certain clinical breast cancer outcomes [11–16]. The genes included in these panels are diverse but largely related to cell cycle regulation and proliferation, the ER pathway, and to a lesser degree, the immune system. Although these gene panels have similar outcomes performance, they exhibit a large degree of discordance in the

assignment of a particular breast tumor to a specific prognostic group [11]. More accurate prognostic predictive gene signatures will depend on better understanding of the genes specifically involved in breast cancer carcinogenesis.

To further investigate if TAP expression is associated with clinical outcome in breast carcinomas, we studied TAP expression in a breast cancer cohort of 271 patients diagnosed with invasive breast carcinomas with median follow up time of 5.2 years. In addition, in an independent cohort of 71 breast cancer cases, we compared TAP expression with the Oncotype DX recurrence score to determine if there was a correlation between TAP expression and this clinically available multigene prognostic/predictive assay.

# Methods

A tissue micro-array comprising 288 patient samples from a primary invasive breast cancer cohort from the Clearview Cancer Institute (CCI, AL, U.S.A.), consisting of all available patient samples collected from 1990 to 2001, was constructed. The patient average age was 58.9 (range 26–89), with an average tumor size 2.21 cm (range 0.2–8.0) and a median follow up time of 5.2 years. Ninety eight tumors were stage 1, 141 stage 2, and 33 stage 3. One hundred fifty four patients had negative lymph nodes, while 118 patients had positive lymph node(s). One hundred thirty two patients had received chemotherapy plus hormonal therapy, while 156 were untreated or treated with hormonal therapy only. No patients had been treated with Herceptin. Thirty six tumors were grade 1, 106 were grade 2 and 93 were grade 3. Within this cohort, 271 patients had complete follow-up and TAP expression data. The composition of this set of patients is as shown in Table 1.

An independent cohort of 71 invasive breast carcinomas for which Oncotype DX (Genomic Health, Inc.) recurrence scores had been determined were identified from the files of the Department of Pathology and Laboratory Medicine at Strong Memorial Hospital (Rochester, NY). All cases were hormone receptor positive, Her2 negative, and lymph node negative. A representative whole tissue section was cut from each tumor.

**Table 2** TAP and hormone receptor status, patient counts. $P$ value for difference between proportion of TAP positive and negative patients determined with a two-proportion z-test

|  | TAP- | TAP+ | P value |
|---|---|---|---|
| Hormone Receptor Negative (ER & PR-) | 48 | 6 | <0.001 |
| ER- | 58 | 7 | <0.001 |
| Hormone Receptor Positive (ER or PR+) | 127 | 78 | <0.001 |
| ER+ | 120 | 77 | 0.001 |
| HR positive/ HER2- | 56 | 29 | 0.003 |
| HR positive/ HER2+ | 31 | 28 | 0.35 |

This study was approved by the Huntsville Hospital Institutional Review Committee. Archived tumor samples were provided by the Clearview Cancer Institute of Huntsville Alabama and corresponding anonymized patient data was provided via an institutional review board–approved database. An IRB exemption for the use of the tissue samples was granted by the Huntsville Hospital Institutional Review Committee as all patient data were a) anonymized, b) consent was unnecessary, and c) only excess tissue was used.

Tissue arrays were processed as previously described [17]. TAP antibody was generated in house as previously published. Immunohistochemical staining for TAP was performed on tissue micro-array and whole tissue sections with the method we described previously [8]. TAP expression was classified as positive or negative, with positive expression defined as any cytoplasmic and/or nuclear staining (Fig. 1). Commercial antibodies for ER, PR, and HER2 were stained by a commercial service (US Labs Inc). ER and PR were considered positive if at least

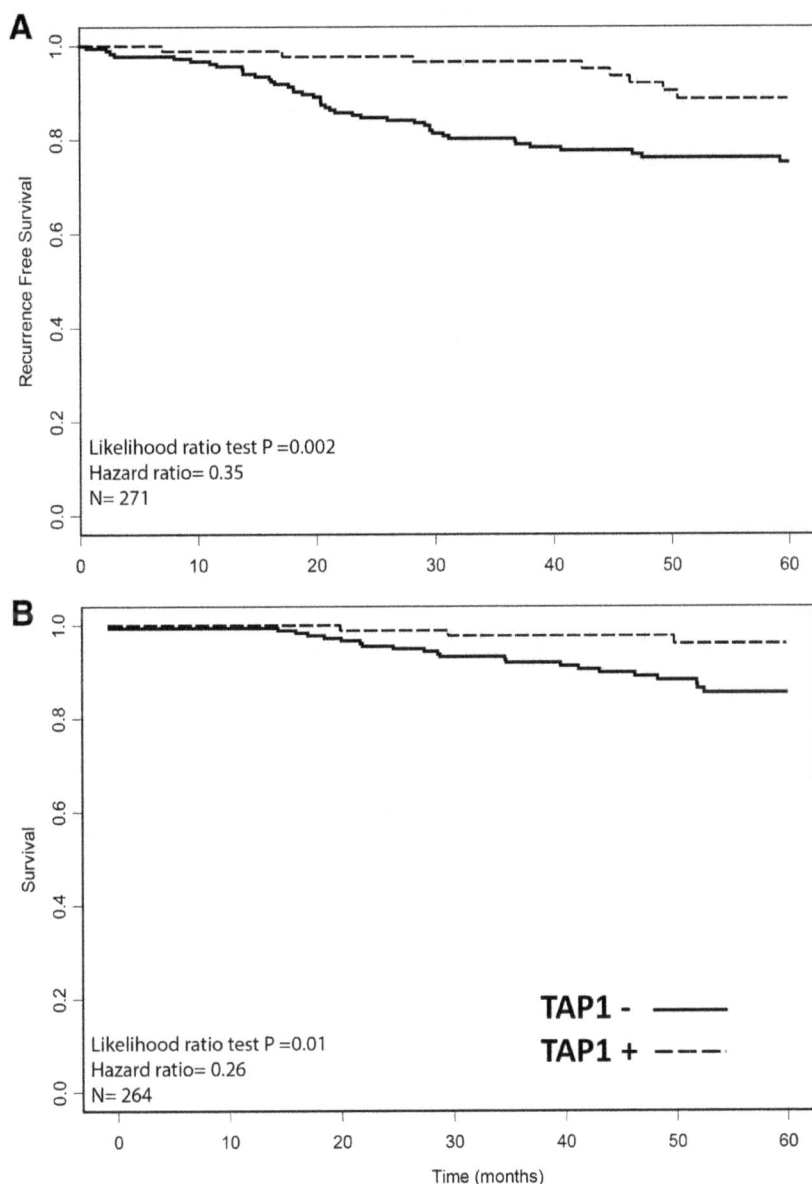

**Fig. 2** Patients with TAP-positive tumors had a lower 5-year recurrence rate (**a**) and better 5-year survival rate (**b**) than the patients with TAP-negative tumors. TAP-positive tumors are shown via a dotted line, TAP-negative tumors via a solid line

1 % of the cells examined exhibited any nuclear staining, and HER2 was scored positive when intense membrane staining in more than 10 % of invasive tumor cells was observed.

In assessing association with outcome, the likelihood ratio test was used in univariate analyses, and the Wald test for multivariate models. All $p$ values are presented as two sided, with a value of less than 0.05 being considered significant.

## Results

In the CCI breast cohort of 271 breast carcinoma samples, we observed positive TAP staining in 88 (32 %) and negative staining in 183 (68 %) tumors. Consistent with our previous findings, we found that ER+/PR ± tumors are more likely to exhibit TAP expression than hormone negative tumors (Table 2). Overall, patients with TAP-positive tumors had a lower 5-year recurrence rate ($N = 271$, $p = 0.002$) and better 5-year survival rate ($N = 264$, $p = 0.010$) (Fig. 2a, b). This positive association with outcome was conserved in all ER-positive tumors, regardless of PR status (5 year recurrence, HR = 0.35, $p = 0.02$, 5 year survival, HR = 0.141, $p = 0.014$) (Fig. 3a, b). This association was

also significant at 10 years post diagnosis (10 year survival HR = 0.21, $p = 0.0024$; 10 year recurrence HR = 0.55, $p = 0.023$). Looking further at the clinically relevant ER+/PR±/Her2- patients, significant associations were also observed (5 year recurrence, HR = 0.17, $p = 0.035$, 5 year survival, HR = <0.001, $p = 0.007$, $N = 81$). TAP was not prognostic of 5 year recurrence in ER+/HER2+ cases (HR = 0.38 $p = 0.22$, $N = 57$), ER-/HER2-(HR < 0.01, $p = 0.23$, $N = 32$), or ER-/HER2+ cases (HR = 4.1 $p = 0.28$, $N = 15$). Tumors negative for ER and PR had a non-significant association with 5-year recurrence and survival (Fig. 3c, d). In triple negative patients the association remained non-significant, though low patient numbers ($N = 25$) makes it difficult to draw conclusions from this subset analysis. Exploratory analysis showed that the association with outcome was even stronger in node-positive patients (5-year recurrence: $N = 118$, $p = 0.0001$; 5-year survival: $N = 114$, $p = 0.0036$), but it was not significant in node-negative patients (5-year recurrence: $N = 151$ and $p = 0.98$; 5-year survival: $N = 150$ and $p = 0.72$) (Fig. 4a-d). Within PR subsets (ER+/PR- and ER+/PR+), TAP did not have a significant association with recurrence ($p = 0.102$ and 0.098, respectively), though the hazard ratio remained low.

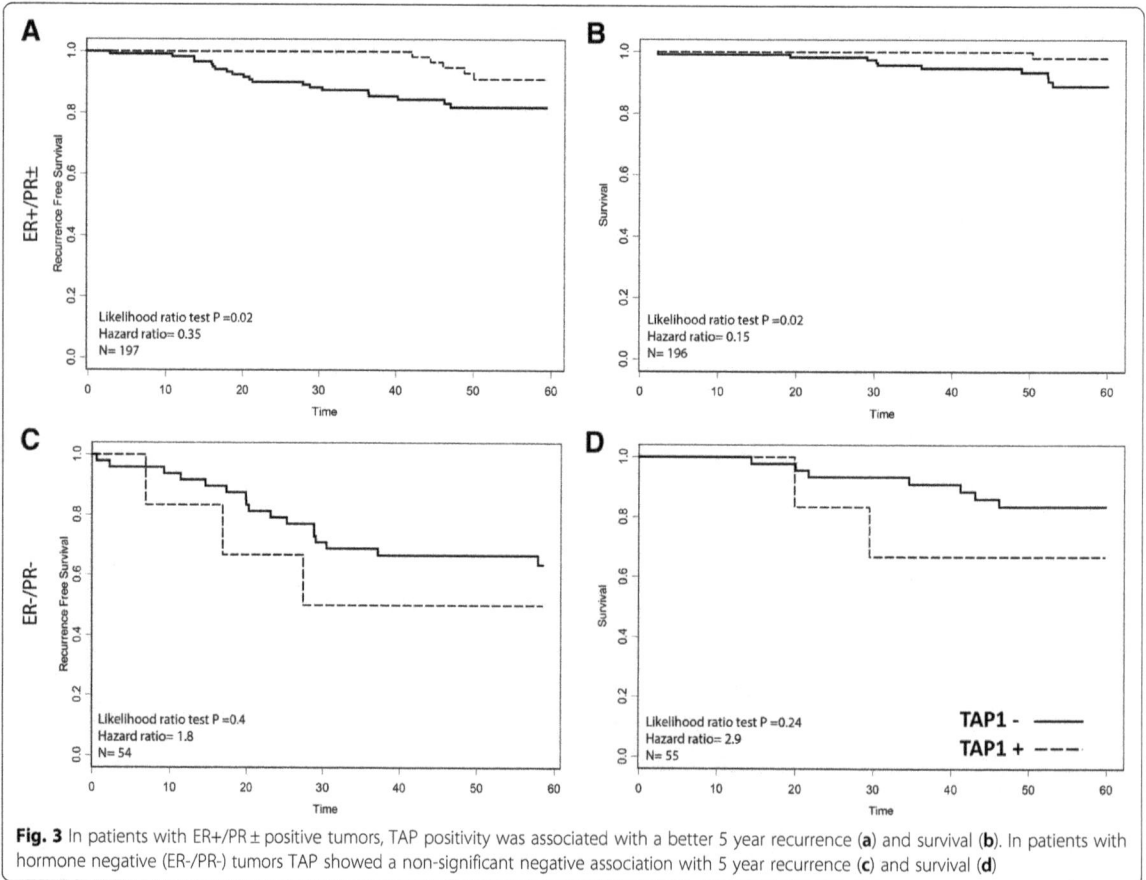

**Fig. 3** In patients with ER+/PR ± positive tumors, TAP positivity was associated with a better 5 year recurrence (**a**) and survival (**b**). In patients with hormone negative (ER-/PR-) tumors TAP showed a non-significant negative association with 5 year recurrence (**c**) and survival (**d**)

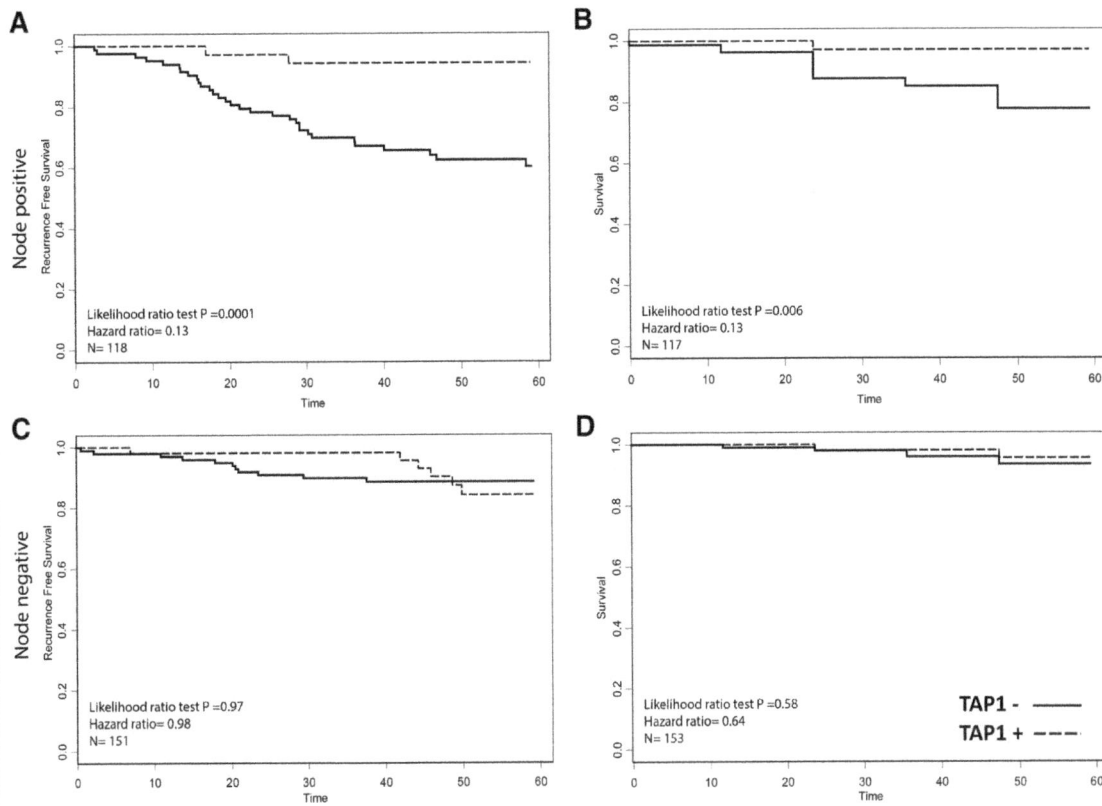

**Fig. 4** The association between TAP expression and better prognosis was even stronger in node-positive patients in 5 year recurrence (**a**) and survival (**b**), but was not significant in node-negative patients in 5 year recurrence (**c**) or survival (**d**)

Furthermore, TAP was independent of PR when assessed as a multivariable model (data not shown).

In an exploratory multivariate analysis of TAP status and common clinical variables, TAP was independent of age, stage, hormonal therapy and chemotherapy status with 5 year recurrence as the outcome measurement in all patients (Table 3). TAP was not independent of grade, which suggests that grade and TAP were measuring a shared aspect of cell biology. Indeed, there was a significant negative association between grade and TAP (p < 0.0001 via chi-square). TAP positive tumors were more likely to represent low grade tumors compared to TAP negative tumors. In patients with ER+/PR ± tumors, TAP expression was independent of stage and age in predicting 5 year recurrence; while in patients with ER+/PR±/Her2- tumors, TAP was not independent of stage (5 year recurrence HR = 0.18, $p = 0.110$). However, only 81 patients were included in this subset. When looking at 5 year survival, TAP expression was independent of age and stage, but not chemotherapy status or tumor grade.

In the study of tumors with a known Oncotype DX recurrence score, TAP was positive in 47 of the 71 tumors (66.2 %), with 29 of 43 (67.4 %) in a low risk group, 16 of 24 (66.7 %) in an intermediate risk group, and 2 of 4 (50 %) in a high risk group (Table 4). There was no association observed between TAP expression and Oncotype DX recurrence risk using a Fisher's exact test ($P = 0.60$).

The limitation of the study includes relatively small sample size in the CCI breast cohort and Oncotype DX cohort. Ki67 labeling index data and the status of vascular invasion were not available for analysis.

## Discussion

Genes involved in cell proliferation have been shown to comprise a major component of many of the available gene expression signatures used to predict clinical outcome in breast cancer patients [11–16]. TAP has also been implicated in the control of cellular proliferation and other aspects of tumor growth. Researchers demonstrated that vitamin E derivatives can inhibit cell proliferation and colony formation of breast cancer cell lines, and induce apoptosis of the tumor cells [18–21]. As a vitamin E binding protein, TAP can promote vitamin E retention and thus increase its concentration in cells. Our previous studies have demonstrated that TAP can promote vitamin E-induced inhibition of tumor cell

**Table 3** Association of TAP and other clinical variables with outcome using Cox proportional hazard regression. TAP, chemotherapy, grade, stage and age are shown as individual and multivariable models. Variables with a significant association with survival or recurrence are shown in bold

| | 5 year survival | | | 5 year recurrence | | | 5 year recurrence, ER+/PR± | | |
|---|---|---|---|---|---|---|---|---|---|
| | HR | p | N | HR | p | N | HR | p | N |
| **TAP** | 0.26 (0.08, 0.87) | 0.01 | 264 | 0.35 (0.16, 0.74) | 0.002 | 271 | 0.35 (0.13, 0.92) | 0.02 | 197 |
| Hormone therapy | 0.54 (0.25, 1.2) | 0.12 | 262 | 0.68 (0.38, 1.2) | 0.21 | 261 | 1.8 (0.55, 6.2) | 0.28 | 192 |
| **Chemotherapy** | 4.34 (1.63, 11.6) | 0.001 | 262 | 2.51 (1.37, 4.6) | 0.002 | 263 | 2.2 (1, 4.84) | 0.05 | 193 |
| **Grade** | 4.44 (1.74, 11.3) | <0.001 | 230 | 2.3 (1.34, 3.93) | 0.001 | 231 | 2.5 (1.24, 5.05) | 0.007 | 175 |
| **Stage** | 3.35 (1.82, 6.16) | <0.001 | 264 | 2.71 (1.76, 4.17) | <0.001 | 265 | 2.66 (1.47, 4.83) | 0.001 | 195 |
| Age | 0.98 (0.95, 1.01) | 0.193 | 264 | 0.98 (0.97, 1) | 0.054 | 265 | 0.97 (0.94, 1) | 0.058 | 195 |
| **TAP** | 0.28 (0.08, 0.95) | 0.04 | 264 | 0.38 (0.18, 0.81) | 0.012 | 265 | 0.37 (0.14, 0.98) | 0.045 | 195 |
| **Stage** | 3.25 (1.76, 6) | <0.001 | | 2.63 (1.71, 4.06) | <0.001 | | 2.57 (1.41, 4.69) | 0.002 | |
| TAP | 0.55 (0.16, 1.93) | 0.35 | 230 | 0.54 (0.23, 1.24) | 0.15 | 231 | 0.51 (0.19, 1.39) | 0.19 | 174 |
| **Grade** | 3.93 (1.52, 10.18) | 0.005 | | 2.05 (1.19, 3.52) | 0.01 | | 2.3 (1.15, 4.59) | 0.018 | |
| **TAP** | 0.28 (0.08, 0.94) | 0.039 | 264 | 0.38 (0.18, 0.82) | 0.014 | 265 | 0.37 (0.14, 0.98) | 0.045 | 195 |
| Age | 0.99 (0.96, 1.02) | 0.37 | | 0.98 (0.96, 1.01) | 0.16 | | 0.97 (0.94, 1.01) | 0.097 | |
| **TAP** | 0.27 (0.08, 0.90) | 0.032 | 262 | 0.37 (0.17, 0.78) | 0.0093 | 261 | 0.35 (0.13,0.93) | 0.036 | 192 |
| Hormone therapy | 0.58 (0.27, 1.3) | 0.17 | | 0.73 (0.41, 1.3) | 0.3 | | 1.77 (0.53, 5.9) | 0.35 | |
| **TAP** | 0.34 (0.1, 1.14) | 0.081 | 262 | 0.42 (0.2, 0.91) | 0.027 | 263 | 0.38 (0.14, 1.01) | 0.052 | 193 |
| **Chemotherapy** | 3.69 (1.37, 9.92) | 0.01 | | 2.16 (1.17, 4.01) | 0.014 | | 1.94 (0.87, 4.3) | 0.1 | |
| **TAP** | 0.33 (0.1, 1.13) | 0.078 | 262 | 0.41 (0.19, 0.89) | 0.023 | 263 | 0.38 (0.14, 1.03) | 0.057 | 193 |
| **Stage** | 2.77 (1.42, 5.4) | 0.003 | | 2.44 (1.53, 3.9) | 0 | | 2.42 (1.27, 4.61) | 0.007 | |
| Chemotherapy | 2.21 (0.79, 6.17) | 0.13 | | 1.35 (0.7, 2.59) | 0.37 | | 1.23 (0.53, 2.85) | 0.63 | |
| **TAP** | 0.32 (0.1, 1.1) | 0.07 | 262 | 0.41 (0.19, 0.89) | 0.024 | 263 | 0.39 (0.15, 1.06) | 0.065 | 193 |
| **Stage** | 2.8 (1.43, 5.47) | 0.003 | | 2.44 (1.53, 3.9) | 0 | | 2.53 (1.34, 4.76) | 0.004 | |
| Chemotherapy | 2.98 (0.89, 10) | 0.077 | | 1.34 (0.61, 2.94) | 0.47 | | 0.85 (0.31, 2.32) | 0.75 | |
| Age | 1.02 (0.98, 1.06) | 0.35 | | 1 (0.97, 1.03) | 0.98 | | 0.97 (0.94, 1.01) | 0.19 | |

proliferation and also regulate tumor cell growth in a vitamin E-independent fashion [7]. We also showed that TAP is selectively expressed in normal/benign breast luminal epithelium, but not in many other organ systems [8]. TAP expression is down-regulated at the mRNA and protein levels in several human breast cancer cell lines and in human breast carcinomas compared to a nonmalignant cell line and to normal/benign breast tissue. We extended these observations in current study, which showed that TAP expression is associated with an overall more favorable outcome, both in terms of tumor recurrence and survival rate in breast cancer patients. These findings, taken together, suggest that TAP is a regulator of cell proliferation that can affect breast carcinogenesis and tumor prognosis.

Breast cancer is a heterogeneous group of diseases. The biological features and clinical behavior of individual tumors are frequently different, even within the morphologically low grade, ER+/PR+/Her2- subtype, which is generally considered to be a group with a better prognosis. It is important to identify novel markers which

can predict clinical outcomes in this group. We have reported that TAP is co-expressed with ER in the normal/benign breast luminal epithelium of terminal ductal lobular units, where breast carcinogenesis is most likely to be initiated, and that TAP is down regulated in 46 % of ER and PR positive breast carcinomas, indicating that the loss of TAP expression may be associated with the process of hormonal carcinogenesis [9]. Here we have demonstrated that TAP expression in ER+/PR±/Her2- tumors is associated with a significantly better 5-year recurrence free and survival rate. This finding could be clinically significant in terms of further predicting tumor

**Table 4** Comparison of TAP positivity and OncoTypeDx Recurrence scores

| Recurrence Score | TAP + | TAP - | Total |
|---|---|---|---|
| 1 | 29 | 14 | 43 |
| 2 | 16 | 8 | 24 |
| 3 | 2 | 2 | 4 |
| Total | 47 | 24 | 71 |

behaviors of ER+/PR±/Her2- subtype breast carcinomas. Currently, there are few breast carcinogenesis-related oncogenes and tumor suppressor genes that are implicated in the clinical treatment and prognosis. Her2 and p53, the most widely evaluated cancer-related genes, are only altered in approximately 20-25 % of breast carcinomas, primarily in ER/PR negative tumors [22]. In contrast, TAP is altered in 57 % of breast carcinomas, including 46 % ER/PR+ tumors, thus may serve as a useful complement to existing biomarkers.

OncotypeDX has been used to guide clinical approaches for ER-positive, lymph node-negative breast cancer patients. Even though TAP expression is associated with better clinical outcome in ER-positive tumors, we did not identify any association between TAP expression and OncotypeDX recurrence scores in the additional cohort. This may suggest that TAP expression is associated with a different aspect(s) of tumor biology than is OncotypeDX and may be a useful complement in predicting patient outcome and tumor subclassification. Further study with a larger population of ER+ tumors is needed to help validate these findings.

Several studies have demonstrated a protective effect of vitamin E on the occurrence of several cancers (for review see [3]). However clinical trials have found little support for dietary supplementation [23]. The disparity of these results could be due to vitamin E not being cancer preventive at the supra-nutritional level, significant roles for other vitamin E isoforms, such as γ- and δ-tocopherols [24], or genetic diversity among dietary intervention trial participants contributing to unrecognized heterogeneity in how they utilized vitamin E. Our study found considerable heterogeneity among the tumors in expression of TAP, the vitamin E binding protein, and its significant association with cancer progression. This finding suggests a possible role for TAP in the interplay between vitamin E and cancer progression. Stratification of trial participation by TAP expression may be an interesting and important aspect for the elucidation of how dietary vitamin E supplementation may affect cancer risk and prognosis.

## Conclusions

In summary, we demonstrated that TAP, as a proliferation-related gene in breast carcinogenesis, is associated with a better 5-year clinical outcome, particularly in node-positive and ER+ breast cancer patients. TAP may serve as a prognostic marker, especially in those patients with ER+ low grade breast cancers, and may also serve to stratify studies assessing the role and utility of vitamin E or α-tocopherol supplementation for the prevention of cancer.

**Competing interests**
All authors declare no conflict of interests.

**Authors' contributions**
XW, RS, DTR, DGH and SY conceived of the study, and participated in its design and coordination. BZR performed the statistical analysis and figure preparation. KW and RAB performed the immunohistochemical assays. XW and BZR wrote the manuscript. All authors read and approved the final manuscript.

**Acknowledgements**
The authors wish to thank Yanling Wang for her technical assistance.

**Author details**
[1]Department of Pathology, University of Rochester Medical Center, Rochester, NY 14642, USA. [2]Institute for Genomic and Personalized Medicine, School of Life Science and Technology, Huazhong University of Science and Technology, Wuhan, China. [3]Insight Genetics Inc., Nashville, TN, USA. [4]CardioDx, Inc., Redwood City, CA, USA. [5]Conversant Biologics, Huntsville, AL, USA.

**References**
1. Wada S. Cancer preventive effects of vitamin E, vol. 13, 2011/04/07 edn.
2. Kline K, Yu W, Sanders BG. Vitamin E and breast cancer. J Nutr. 2004;134(12 Suppl):3458S–62S.
3. Ju J, Picinich SC, Yang Z, Zhao Y, Suh N, Kong AN, et al. Cancer-preventive activities of tocopherols and tocotrienols. Carcinogenesis. 2010;31(4):533–42.
4. Klein EA, Thompson Jr IM, Tangen CM, Crowley JJ, Lucia MS, Goodman PJ, et al. Vitamin E and the risk of prostate cancer: the Selenium and Vitamin E Cancer Prevention Trial (SELECT). JAMA. 2011;306(14):1549–56.
5. Lee IM, Cook NR, Gaziano JM, Gordon D, Ridker PM, Manson JE, et al. Vitamin E in the primary prevention of cardiovascular disease and cancer: the Women's Health Study: a randomized controlled trial. JAMA. 2005; 294(1):56–65.
6. Zimmer S, Stocker A, Sarbolouki MN, Spycher SE, Sassoon J, Azzi A. A novel human tocopherol-associated protein: cloning, in vitro expression, and characterization. J Biol Chem. 2000;275(33):25672–80.
7. Ni J, Wen X, Yao J, Chang HC, Yin Y, Zhang M, et al. Tocopherol-associated protein suppresses prostate cancer cell growth by inhibition of the phosphoinositide 3-kinase pathway. Cancer Res. 2005;65(21):9807–16.
8. Wang X, Ni J, Hsu CL, Johnykutty S, Tang P, Ho YS, et al. Reduced expression of tocopherol-associated protein (TAP/Sec14L2) in human breast cancer. Cancer Invest. 2009;27(10):971–7.
9. Johnykutty S, Tang P, Zhao H, Hicks DG, Yeh S, Wang X. Dual expression of alpha-tocopherol-associated protein and estrogen receptor in normal/ benign human breast luminal cells and the downregulation of alpha-tocopherol-associated protein in estrogen-receptor-positive breast carcinomas. Mod Pathol. 2009;22(6):770–5.
10. Tam KW, Ho CT, Lee WJ, Tu SH, Huang CS, Chen CS, et al. Alteration of alpha-tocopherol-associated protein (TAP) expression in human breast epithelial cells during breast cancer development. Food Chem. 2013;138(2–3):1015–21.
11. Reyal F, van Vliet MH, Armstrong NJ, Horlings HM, de Visser KE, Kok M, et al. A comprehensive analysis of prognostic signatures reveals the high predictive capacity of the proliferation, immune response and RNA splicing modules in breast cancer. Breast Cancer Res. 2008;10(6):R93.
12. Paik S, Shak S, Tang G, Kim C, Baker J, Cronin M, et al. A multigene assay to predict recurrence of tamoxifen-treated, node-negative breast cancer. N Engl J Med. 2004;351(27):2817–26.
13. Paik S, Tang G, Shak S, Kim C, Baker J, Kim W, et al. Gene expression and benefit of chemotherapy in women with node-negative, estrogen receptor-positive breast cancer. J Clin Oncol. 2006;24(23):3726–34.
14. Teschendorff AE, Naderi A, Barbosa-Morais NL, Pinder SE, Ellis IO, Aparicio S, et al. A consensus prognostic gene expression classifier for ER positive breast cancer. Genome Biol. 2006;7(10):R101.
15. van de Vijver MJ, He YD, van't Veer LJ, Dai H, Hart AA, Voskuil DW, et al. A gene-expression signature as a predictor of survival in breast cancer. N Engl J Med. 2002;347(25):1999–2009.
16. Wang Y, Klijn JG, Zhang Y, Sieuwerts AM, Look MP, Yang F, et al. Gene-expression profiles to predict distant metastasis of lymph-node-negative primary breast cancer. Lancet. 2005;365(9460):671–9.

17. Ring BZ, Seitz RS, Beck R, Shasteen WJ, Tarr SM, Cheang MC, et al. Novel prognostic immunohistochemical biomarker panel for estrogen receptor-positive breast cancer. J Clin Oncol. 2006;24(19):3039–47.

18. Anderson K, Simmons-Menchaca M, Lawson KA, Atkinson J, Sanders BG, Kline K. Differential response of human ovarian cancer cells to induction of apoptosis by vitamin E Succinate and vitamin E analogue, alpha-TEA. Cancer Res. 2004;64(12):4263–9.

19. Malafa MP, Neitzel LT. Vitamin E succinate promotes breast cancer tumor dormancy. J Surg Res. 2000;93(1):163–70.

20. Neuzil J, Weber T, Gellert N, Weber C. Selective cancer cell killing by alpha-tocopheryl succinate. Br J Cancer. 2001;84(1):87–9.

21. Yu W, Simmons-Menchaca M, Gapor A, Sanders BG, Kline K. Induction of apoptosis in human breast cancer cells by tocopherols and tocotrienols. Nutr Cancer. 1999;33(1):26–32.

22. Hamilton A, Piccart M. The contribution of molecular markers to the prediction of response in the treatment of breast cancer: a review of the literature on HER-2, p53 and BCL-2. Ann Oncol. 2000;11(6):647–63.

23. Stratton J, Godwin M. The effect of supplemental vitamins and minerals on the development of prostate cancer: a systematic review and meta-analysis. Fam Pract. 2011;28(3):243–52.

24. Lu G, Xiao H, Li GX, Picinich SC, Chen YK, Liu A, et al. A gamma-tocopherol-rich mixture of tocopherols inhibits chemically induced lung tumorigenesis in A/J mice and xenograft tumor growth. Carcinogenesis. 2010;31(4):687–94.

# 23

# Bone metastasis from malignant phyllodes breast tumor

Mohamed Reda El Ochi[1*], Mehdi Toreis[2], Mohamed Benchekroun[3], Zineb Benkerroum[4], Mohamed Allaoui[1], Mohamed Ichou[2], Basma El Khannoussi[5], Abderrahman Albouzidi[1] and Mohamed Oukabli[1]

## Abstract

**Background:** Phyllodes tumors are rare fibroepithelial tumors accounting for less than 1 % of all breast neoplasms. They are malignant in 20 % of cases. Only a few cases of malignant phyllodes tumors metastatic to bone have been reported.

**Case presentation:** Case 1: A 40 year-old white woman presented with three-week history of pain and functional impairment of the left lower limb. Her clinical past was remarkable for previous left mastectomy and radiotherapy for malignant phyllodes tumor performed one year ago. Computed tomography revealed a moth-eaten appearance of the left femoral head. The patient underwent computed guided femoral head biopsy. Pathological findings were consistent with metastatic malignant phyllodes tumor. The patient received ifosfamide and adriamycin chemotherapy. She is doing well without any evidence of progression on her imaging follow- up after 8 months.
Case 2: A 48 year-old white woman, with history of bilateral mastectomy and radiotherapy for malignant phyllodes tumor performed one and two year ago, presented with four-week left lower quadrant abdominal pain. Computed tomography and magnetic resonance imaging revealed a solid aggressive osteolytic mass of the left iliac bone with extensive soft tissue invasion. Biopsy of the tumor was performed and showed a sarcomatous proliferation consistent with metastatic malignant phyllodes tumor. The patient received the same chemotherapy regimen as in the first case but without any response on her imaging follow up after 6 months.

**Conclusion:** Malignant phyllodes tumor is a rare and aggressive fibroepithelial neoplasm. An accurate diagnosis of metastases should be based on clinicopathological correlation allowing exclusion of differential diagnoses. The goal of successful managing this tumor is early detection and complete resection prior to dissemination.

**Keywords:** Bone, Metastatic, Phyllodes, Tumor, Breast

## Background

Phyllodes tumors (PTs) are rare fibroepithelial tumors accounting for less than 1 % of all breast neoplasms [1, 2]. They are classified as benign, borderline and malignant [3].

Malignant PTs account for 20 % of all PTs [4] and may present with delayed metastases mainly in the lung [5].

Only a few cases of PT metastatic to bone have been reported [6]. To our knowledge, only 2 cases involving the iliac bone [6, 7] and 1 case involving the femur [8] are described in the literature. These papers have mainly focused on their radiological aspects. We report 2 cases of metastatic malignant PT of the breast involving the femoral head and the iliac bone and discuss the histopathological differential diagnoses.

## Case presentation

### Case 1: Clinical history

A 40 year-old white woman presented with a three-week history of pain and functional impairment of the left lower limb. Clinical examination showed limitation of the left lower limb movements. Her clinical past was remarkable for previous left mastectomy and for malignant PT performed one year ago. The mass measured 7x5x4 cm. Histological examination showed a biphasic proliferation characterized by a double layered epithelial component arranged in clefts surrounded by an hpercellular

* Correspondence: elochi20@yahoo.fr
[1]Department of Pathology, Mohamed V military Hospital, Hay Riad, Faculty of Medicine, Mohamed V University, BP10000 Rabat, Morocco
Full list of author information is available at the end of the article

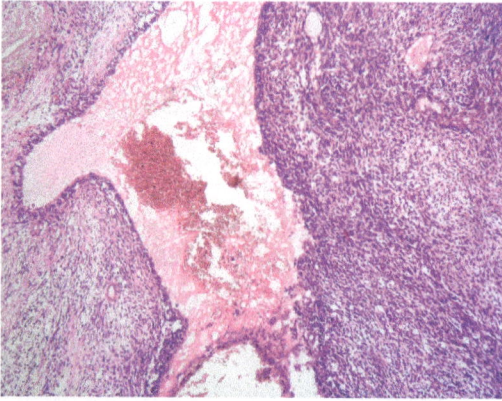

**Fig. 1** Malignant PT of the breast showing a leaf-like pattern with increased stromal cellularity and atypia (hematoxylin and eosin stain, original magnification × 100)

fibrosarcomatous component organized in leaf-like structures Fig. 1. There was stromal overgrowth, marked nuclear atypia and high mitotic activity (12 per 10 high-power fields). Surgical margins were complete and of at least 1 cm. Immunoreactivity with anti vimentin was found. Smooth muscle actin, desmin, CD34, S-100 protein, CD10, CKAE1/AE3, P63, estrogen and progesterone receptors were negative. Post operatively, the patient received radiation to the tumor bed at a dose of 50 Grays in 25 fractions without chemotherapy.

### Radiologic and histopathologic findings

Computed tomography and FDG-PET Scan revealed a moth-eaten appearance Fig. 2 and pathological FDG uptake of the left femoral head without other suspect lesions. The patient underwent computed guided femoral head biopsy. The post-operative course was uneventful. Microscopic examination showed a proliferation of fascicles of spindle cells with nuclear atypia and numerous mitotic figures Figs. 3 and 4. No areas of epithelial, osteoid or chondroid components were identified. Immunohistochemistry demonstrated only vimentin positivity. Pancytokeratin, smooth muscle actin, desmin, S100 protein, CD34, CD31, CD99, CD117, estrogen and progesterone receptors were all negative. Thus, a diagnosis of metastatic

malignant PT was made. The patient received ifosfamide and adriamycin chemotherapy. She is doing well without any evidence of progression on her imaging follow-up after 8 months.

### Case 2: Clinical history

A 48 year-old white woman presented with a four-week history of left lower quadrant abdominal pain. The patient's past medical history was significant for previous bilateral mastectomy for malignant PT one and two year ago Fig. 5. The tumors measured 10x8x5 cm in the right breast (first mastectomy) and 6×5×4,5 cm in the left breast. They showed stromal overgrowth, marked nuclear atypia and high mitotic activity (greater than 14 per 10 high-power fields). Surgical margins were complete and of at least 0,7 cm on the right breast and 1,2 cm on the left breast. Immunoreactivity was found only with vimentin and CD10. The patient received radiation only to the right tumor bed at a dose of 50 Grays in 25 fractions without chemotherapy.

### Radiologic and histopathologic findings

Computed tomography and magnetic resonance imaging revealed a solid aggressive osteolytic mass of the left iliac bone with extensive soft tissue invasion measuring 13 ×

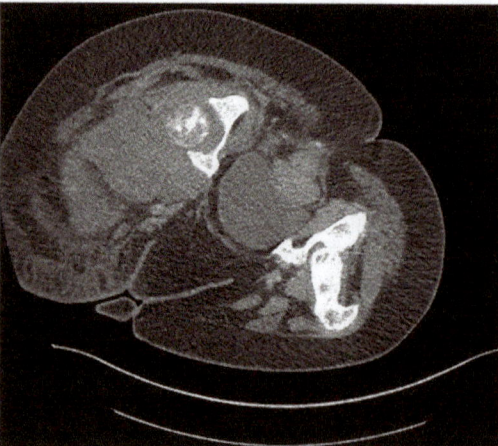

**Fig. 2** Axial computed tomography image showing a moth-eaten appearance of the femoral head

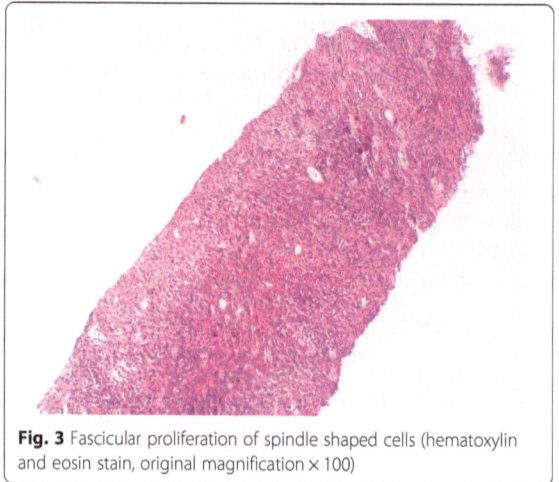

**Fig. 3** Fascicular proliferation of spindle shaped cells (hematoxylin and eosin stain, original magnification × 100)

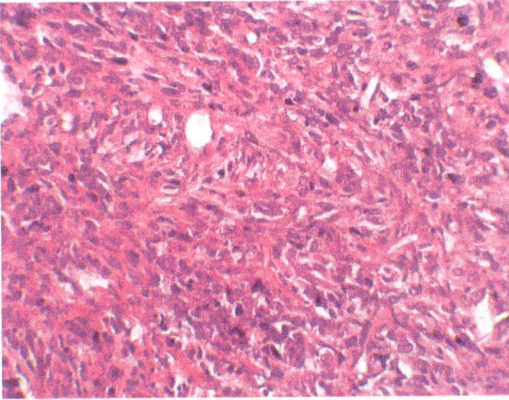

**Fig. 4** Tumor cells showing mild nuclear atypia (hematoxylin and eosin stain, original magnification × 400)

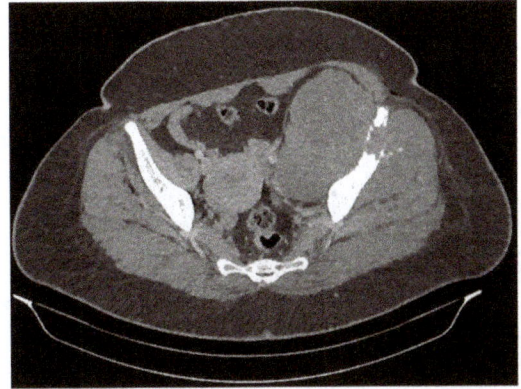

**Fig. 6** Axial computed tomography showing a solid aggressive osteolytic mass of the left iliac bone with extensive soft tissue invasion

11 cm Fig. 6. Biopsy of the tumor was performed and showed a sarcomatous proliferation similar to that described for the first case Figs. 7 and 8 with the same immunohistochemical profile. A diagnosis of metastatic malignant PT of the breast was made. The patient received the same chemotherapy regimen as in the first case but without any response after 7 months. The oncologist decided to use taxanes as second line chemotherapy with radiological stabilization on her imaging follow up.

## Discussion

PT is a rare fibroepithelial tumor accounting for less than 1 % of all breast neoplasms [1, 2]. They usually arise in women between ages 35 and 55 years and are classified as benign, borderline and malignant [2, 3].

Malignant types present approximately 20 % of all cases [4]. Actually, malignant PTs should be treated by conservative surgery with adequate negative surgical margins; the use of radiotherapy may be limited to patients with positive surgical margins [9, 10]. Distant metastases are seen in 10–20 % of cases [1]. They can occur even after technically adequate initial breast surgery [1]. The most reliable predictive factors for development of distant metastases are stromal overgrowth, nuclear pleomorphism and high mitotic activity [9, 11], whereas the role of tumor size and local recurrence is controversial [1, 11, 12]. Tan et al. found, by multivariate analysis, that stromal atypia, overgrowth, surgical margins and mitoses are independently predictive of clinical behaviour [13]. He developed a nomogram based on these criteria to predict recurrence-free survival, but the amalgamation of local

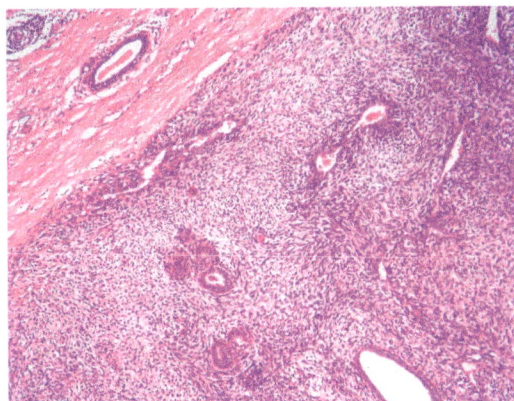

**Fig. 5** Malignant PT of the breast showing a periductal stromal growth with malignant features (hematoxylin and eosin stain, original magnification × 100)

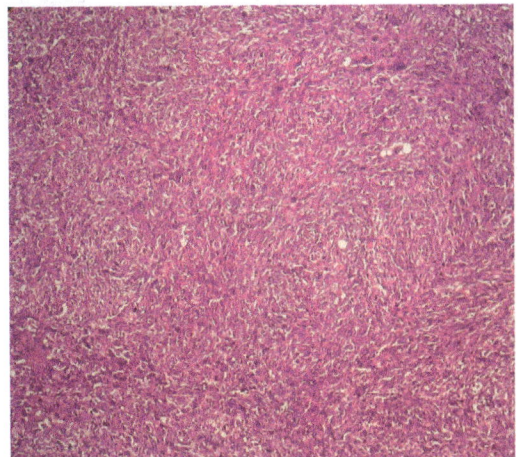

**Fig. 7** Proliferation of densely packed spindle cells (hematoxylin and eosin stain, original magnification × 100)

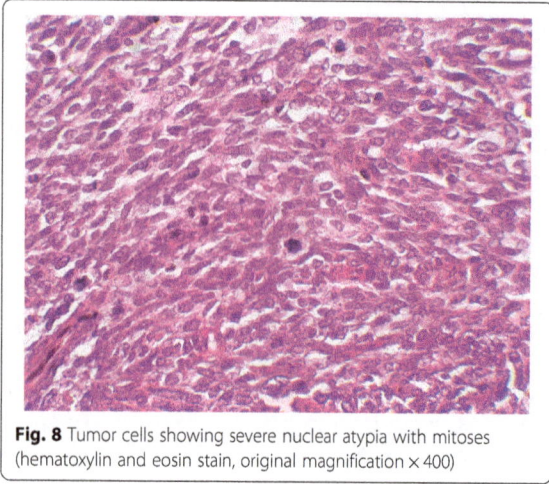

**Fig. 8** Tumor cells showing severe nuclear atypia with mitoses (hematoxylin and eosin stain, original magnification × 400)

with distant recurrences and the low rate of metastasis in this series could limit its ability in predicting dissemination. The recurrence free survival was 0,8 and 0,47 at 1 and 3 years for the first case, 0,76 and 0,4 at 1 and 3 years for the second case. Al-Masry et al. have shown that the expression of CD10 can be used to predict the occurrence of distant metastasis [14].

Metastatic PTs mainly develop from 3 to 10 years after the inital therapy, but they can be delayed or occur as soon as synchronous presentation [11]. The lung is the most common site of metastatic spread [2, 3, 15]. Only a few cases of PT metastatic to bone have been reported [6] with 2 cases involving the iliac bone [6, 7] and 1 case involving the femur [8].

Clinical features are not specific and vary among location of bone metastasis. Radiographs and computed tomography may show a solid mass adjacent to the involved bone and infiltrating the cortex and medulla in a permeative pattern [8]. The magnetic resonance imaging may better delineate the metastatic extent [8].

Pathological examination shows a malignant proliferation of fascicles of spindle cells with nuclear atypia and high mitotic index without epithelial component [15, 16].

Immunohistochemistry demonstrates only vimentin positivity. Pancytokeratin, smooth muscle actin, desmin, S100 protein, CD34, C31, CD99 and CD117 are generally negative [15, 16].

Positivity of estrogen and progesterone receptors had never been reported. These morphological and immunohistochemical findings play an important role in excluding sarcomas, myoepithelioma, metastatic sarcomatoid carcinoma, melanoma and gastrointestinal stromal tumor. Generally, it's difficult to make a specific diagnosis only by microscopic examination, but the final diagnosis should be based on clinicopathological correlation. There is no consensus regarding adjuvant therapy. Both

radiotherapy and chemotherapy are recommended in metastatic PTs [2, 6, 16]. Ifosfamide is the most active agent [16]; antiestrogen therapy is not indicated [3, 16]. Some studies revealed several potentially targetable pathway including epidermal growth factor receptor, angiogenesis (vascular endothelial growth factor A, angiopoietin-2, vascular cell adhesion molecule 1, platelet- derived growth factor receptor A, pituitary tumor-transforming1) and immunotherapy (programmed cell death protein 1, programmed death-ligand 1) for patients with locally advanced or metastatic tumors [4, 10]. Park et al. reported a major response to sunitinib and paclitaxel in a case of lung metastatic malignant PT of breast [17].

Little is known about the prognosis of bone metastasis from malignant PT. Nguyen [6] report one case involving the left iliac bone with good response after radiotherapy. The prognosis of malignant PT metastatic to the lung seems to be worse [2].

## Conclusion

In summary, malignant PT is a rare and aggressive fibroepithelial neoplasm. An accurate diagnosis of metastases should be based on clinicopathological correlation allowing exclusion of differential diagnoses. The goal of successful managing this tumor is early detection and complete resection prior to dissemination.

### Consent

Written informed consents were obtained from the patients for publication of these Cases Report and any accompanying images. Copies of the written consents are available for review by the Editor-in-Chief of this journal.

**Abbreviations**
PT: Phyllodes tumor.

**Competing interests**
The authors declare that they have no competing interests.

**Authors' contributions**
MRE, MT, BE and MA analyzed and interpreted the patient data, drafted the manuscript and made the figures. AA, BE and MO performed the histological examination, proposed the study, supervised MRE and revised the manuscript. ZB, MI and MB have made substantial contributions to analysis and interpretation of patient data. All authors read and approved the final manuscript.

**Author details**
[1]Department of Pathology, Mohamed V military Hospital, Hay Riad, Faculty of Medicine, Mohamed V University, BP10000 Rabat, Morocco. [2]Department of Medical Oncology, Mohamed V military Hospital, Hay Riad, Faculty of Medicine, Mohamed V University, Rabat, Morocco. [3]Department of of Orthopaedics and Traumatology, Mohamed V military Hospital, Hay Riad, Faculty of Medicine, Mohamed V University, Rabat, Morocco. [4]Department of of Gynecology and obstetrics, Mohamed V military Hospital, Hay Riad, Faculty of Medicine, Mohamed V University, Rabat, Morocco. [5]Department of Pathology, National Institute of Oncology, Hay Riad, Faculty of Medicine, Mohamed V University, Rabat, Morocco.

**References**

1. Parker S, Harries SA. Phyllodes tumours. Postgrad Med J. 2001;77:428–35.
2. Chen WH, Cheng SP, Tzen CY, Yang TL, Jeng KS, Liu CL, et al. Surgical treatment of phyllodes tumors of the breast: retrospective review of 172 cases. J Surg Oncol. 2005;91:185–94.
3. Lightner AL, Shurell E, Dawson N, Omidvar Y, Foster N. A single-center experience and review of the literature: 64 cases of phyllodes tumors to better understand risk factors and disease management. Am Surg. 2015;81:309–15.
4. Gatalica Z, Vranic S, Ghazalpour A, Xiu J, Ocal IT, McGill J. et al. Multiplatform molecular profiling identifies potentially targetable biomarkers in malignant phyllodes tumors of the breast. Oncotarget. 2015; doi:10.18632/oncotarget.6421.
5. Rowe JJ, Prayson RA. Metastatic malignant phyllodes tumor involving the cerebellum. J Clin Neurosci. 2015;22:226–7.
6. Nguyen BD. Imaging of pelvic bone metastasis from malignant phyllodes breast tumor. Radiology Case Report. 2006;1:15.
7. Goldschmidt RA, Resnik CS, Mills AS, Walsh JW. Case report 266. Diagnosis: metastasis to right ilium from cystosarcoma phylloides of breast. Skeletal Radiol. 1984;11:213–5.
8. Singer A, Tresley J, Velazquez-Vega J, Yepes M. Unusual aggressive breast cancer: metastatic malignant phyllodes tumor. Journal of Radiology Case report. 2013;7:24–37.
9. Carter BA, Page DL. Phyllodes tumor of the breast: local recurrence versus metastatic capacity. Hum Pathol. 2004;35:1051–2.
10. Spitaleri G, Toesca A, Botteri E, Bottiglieri L, Rotmensz N, Boselli S, et al. Breast phyllodes tumor: a review of literature and a single center retrospective series analysis. Crit Rev Oncol Hematol. 2013;88:427–36.
11. Kapiris I, Nasiri N, A'Hern R, Healy V, Gui GP. Outcome and predictive factors of local recurrence and distant metastases following primary surgical treatment of high-grade malignant phyllodes tumours of the breast. Eur J Surg Oncol. 2001;27:723–30.
12. Asoglu O, Ugurlu MM, Blanchard K, Grant CS, Reynolds C, Cha SS, et al. Risk factors for recurrence and death after primary surgical treatment of malignant phyllodes tumors. Ann Surg Oncol. 2004;11:1011–7.
13. Tan PH, Thike AA, Tan WJ, Thu MM, Busmanis I, Li H, et al. Predicting clinical behaviour of breast phyllodes tumours: a nomogram based on histological criteria and surgical margins. J Clin Pathol. 2012;65:69–76.
14. Al-Masri M, Darwazeh G, Sawalhi S, Mughrabi A, Sughayer M, Al-Shatti M. Phyllodes tumor of the breast: role of CD10 in predicting metastasis. Ann Surg Oncol. 2012;19:1181–4.
15. Al-Rabiy FN, Ali RH. Malignant phyllodes tumor with osteosarcomatous differentiation metastasizing to small bowel and causing intestinal obstruction. Diagn Histopathol. 2015;46:165–68.
16. Asoglu O, Karanlik H, Barbaros U, Yanar H, Kapran Y, Kecer M, et al. Malignant phyllodes tumor metastatic to the duodenum. World J Gastroenterol. 2006;12:1649–51.
17. Park IH, Kwon Y, Kim EA, Lee KS, Ro J. Major response to sunitinib (Sutene) in metastatic malignant phyllodes tumor of breast. Invest New Drugs. 2009;27:387–8.

# 24

# 5-type HPV mRNA versus 14-type HPV DNA test: test performance, over-diagnosis and overtreatment in triage of women with minor cervical lesions

Bjørn Westre[1], Anita Giske[1], Hilde Guttormsen[1], Sveinung Wergeland Sørbye[2]* and Finn Egil Skjeldestad[3]

**Abstract**

**Background:** Repeat cytology and HPV testing is used in triage of women with minor cytological lesions. The objective of this study was to evaluate 14-type HPV DNA and 5-type HPV mRNA testing in delayed triage of women with ASC-US/LSIL.

**Methods:** We compared a DNA test (Roche Cobas 4800) and an 5-type mRNA test (PreTect HPV-Proofer). In total 564 women were included in the study.

**Results:** The sensitivity among solved cases for CIN3+ were 100 % (15/15) for both tests. The sensitivity for CIN2+ of the HPV DNA test was 100 % (38/38) relative to 79 % (30/38) for the 5-type HPV mRNA test. The corresponding estimates of specificity for CIN2+ among solved cases were 84 % (393/466; 95 % CI: 81–88) and 91 % (451/498; 95 % CI: 88–93). The positive predictive values for CIN3+ were 13.5 % (15/111) for DNA+ and 19.5 % (15/77) for 5-type mRNA+. Significantly more women screened with 5-type mRNA than DNA returned to screening (81 % vs 71 %, $p < 0.01$). Subsequently, significantly fewer women were referred for colposcopy/biopsies/treatment (19 % (105/564) vs 29 % (165/564), $p < 0.01$).

**Conclusions:** 5-type HPV mRNA is more specific than 14-type HPV DNA in delayed triage of women with ASC-US/LSIL. The referral rate for colposcopy was 57 % higher for DNA+ relative to mRNA+ cases (165 vs 105), with the same detection rate of CIN3+, but the 5-type mRNA test had lower sensitivity for CIN2+. It is important to consider the trade-off between sensitivity and specificity of the diagnostic test when designing screening algorithms.

**Keywords:** HPV, DNA, mRNA, Screening, Triage, CIN, CIN2, CIN3, Cervical cancer

## Background

Cervical cancer is the third most common cancer in women worldwide [1]. Persistent infection of human papillomavirus (HPV) causes virtually all cases of cervical cancer [2]. In Europe most cervical cancer cases are caused by HPV types 16, 18, 31, 33, and 45 [1, 3]. Cervical cancer can be prevented by early detection and treatment of precancerous lesions [4]. Women with minor cytological cervical lesions have an increased risk of having, or developing, high-grade dysplasia compared to women with normal cytology. However, most minor cytological lesions regress spontaneously, and therefore careful triage is crucial in order to avoid unnecessary referrals and overtreatment [5]. In Norway, HPV test is used in delayed triage of women with atypical squamous cells of undetermined significance (ASC-US) or low-grade squamous intraepithelial lesions (LSIL) [6]. If the HPV test is positive, the woman is referred to colposcopy.

The HPV E6/E7 mRNA test PreTect HPV-Proofer which detects HPV E6/E7 mRNA from the five most prevalent types causing cervical cancer has been shown to have a higher clinical specificity and positive predictive value (PPV) than HPV DNA tests [7–14]. A high specificity and a low positivity rate of a triage test indicates a low

* Correspondence: sveinung.sorbye@unn.no
[2]Department of Clinical Pathology, University Hospital of North Norway, 9038 Tromsø, Norway
Full list of author information is available at the end of the article

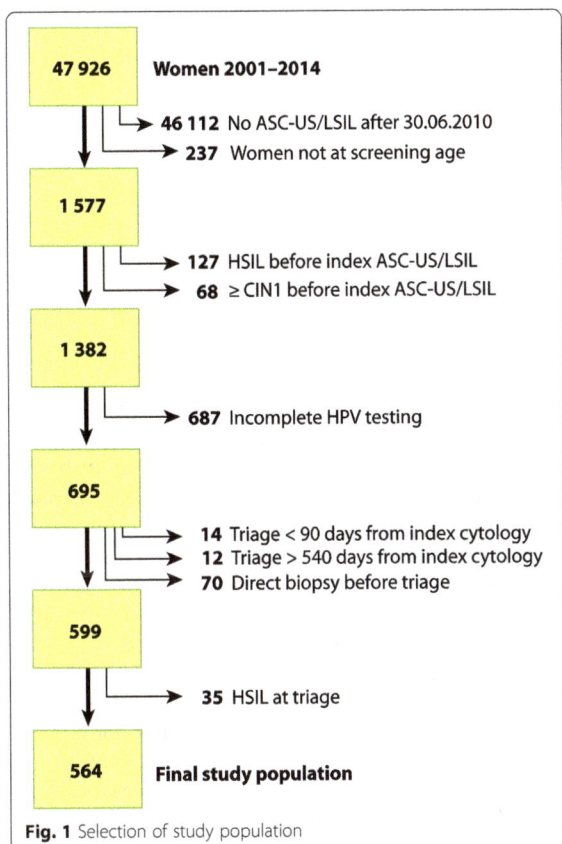

**Fig. 1** Selection of study population

referral rate for colposcopy [8]. In this study we performed a direct comparison of a 5-type HPV mRNA and a 14-type HPV DNA test in delayed triage of ASC-US/LSIL related to referral rates for colposcopy, biopsy rates, and histological outcomes.

**Methods**

Organized cervical cancer screening was introduced in Norway in 1995 with the recommendation that all women 25 to 69 years have a Pap smear collected every third year [15]. During the study period the Norwegian cervical cancer program recommended delayed triage with repeat cytology and HPV testing 6–12 months after the index diagnosis of ASC-US/LSIL. Women with high-grade squamous intraepithelial lesions (HSIL) or repeated ASC-US/LSIL with a positive HPV test were referred to colposcopy/biopsy immediately after triage. Women with a normal smear and a positive HPV test were recommended a repeat HPV test within 12 months, whereas women with an ASC-US/LSIL/normal smear with a negative HPV test were returned to the screening program at a three-year interval [9].

This study compared test performance of the HPV mRNA test PreTect HPV-Proofer (PreTect AS, Norway), which detects E6/E7 mRNA of 5 HPV types, and the HPV DNA test Cobas 4800 (Roche Molecular Diagnostics), which detects 14 HPV types. We followed the manufacturer's instructions in preparation of aliquots and detection of mRNA, while we analyzed HPV DNA in accordance with national guidelines [10]. The conventional cytology

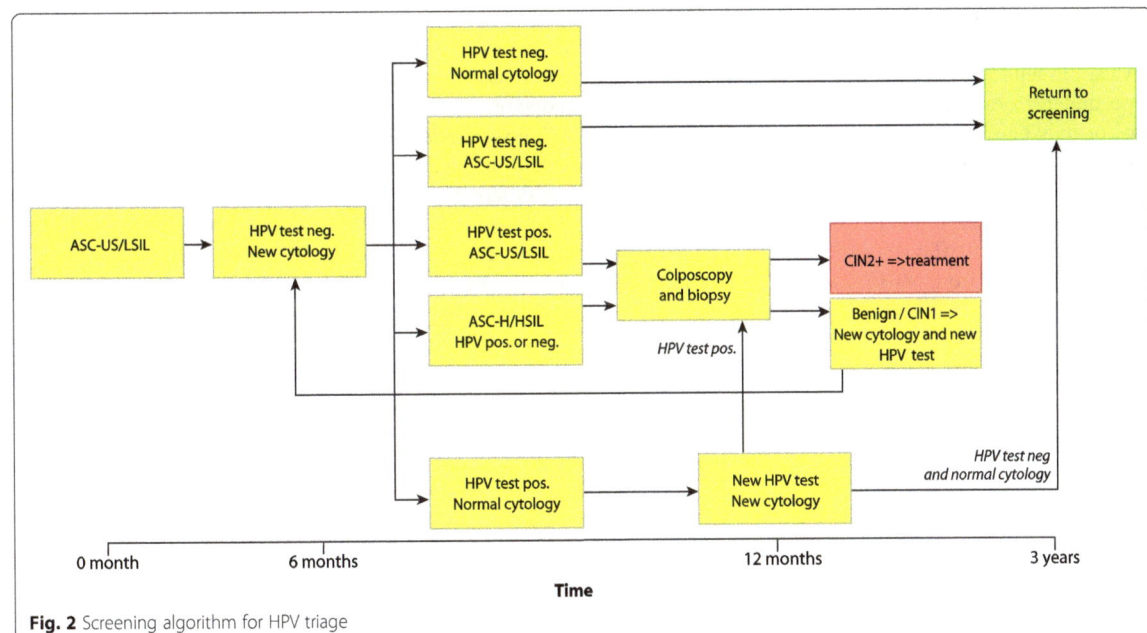

**Fig. 2** Screening algorithm for HPV triage

**Table 1** Outcome of triage by HPV test ($n = 564$)

| | DNA | | 5-type-mRNA | |
|---|---|---|---|---|
| | $N = 564$ | % (95 % CI) | $N = 564$ | % (95 % CI) |
| Back to screening | 399 | 70.7 (66.9–74.5) | 459 | 81.4 (78.2–84.6)* |
| Met for biopsy | 105 | 18.6 (15.4–21.8) | 77 | 13.7 (10.9–16.5) |
| Scheduled, not met for biopsy | 36 | 6.4 (4.4–8.4) | 15 | 2.7 (1.4–4.0)* |
| Incomplete follow-up | 24 | 4.3 (2.6–6.0) | 13 | 2.3 (1.1–3.5) |

*$p < 0.05$
*Triage* repeat cytology and HPV test 3–18 months after index ASC-US/LSIL cytology
*DNA* HPV DNA test (Cobas 4800)
*5-type-mRNA* HPV mRNA test (PreTect HPV-Proofer)

(Pap smear) consists of sampling cells from the cervical area. The sample is obtained using a brush, and the cells are placed directly onto a glass slide and spray fixed. Then the same brush is placed into a liquid medium (ThinPrep, Cytyc Corporation, Marlborough, USA) for HPV testing. In Norway, many hospitals have switched from conventional Pap smears to liquid-based cytology (LBC), but Ålesund Hospital still uses conventional Pap smears.

The Department of Pathology, Ålesund Hospital, located on the western coast of Norway, serves a background population of approximately 50 000 women at screening age 25–69 years and assesses 12 000 cervical smears annually. Since 1999 the department has used the clinical database SymPathy for administration of cytological and histological specimens. From January 1, 2001, through September 15, 2014, we identified 47 926 women with 160 466 valid smears, among which 1 577 women had a diagnosis of ASC-US/LSIL after June 30, 2010. Our study commenced on January 4, 2012, when the department introduced the HPV DNA test. After excluding women with a history of HSIL, or biopsy with cervical intraepitelial neoplasi grade 1 or worse (CIN1+), those under 25 or over 69 years of age, and cases with none or only one HPV test, 695 women were eligible for study participation (Fig. 1).

The Norwegian cervical cancer screening program recommended triage 6 to 12 months after the index ASC-US/LSIL [6, 9] (Fig. 2). We expanded the triage follow-up window from 90 to 540 days after the index

smear. Therefore women having triage <90 days ($n = 14$) or >540 days ($n = 12$) after index smear, and women having direct biopsy (reflex testing) before or at triage ($n = 70$), and women who had HSIL at triage ($n = 35$) were excluded, leaving 564 women for final analyses. Either a positive HPV DNA or a positive HPV mRNA test triggered colposcopy.

We defined solved cases as subjects who returned to the screening program from either a valid smear/negative HPV test, or having had a biopsy, which determined future follow-up/treatment. Corresponding dates were "outcome" dates for solved cases, while we censored cases not met for biopsy or incomplete follow-up at last day of study, September 15, 2014. Abnormal cervical cytology was classified using the Bethesda system. Cervical biopsies were reported using WHO histological classification of tumors of the uterine cervix (http://screening.iarc.fr/colpochap.php?-chap=2). All biopsies were reviewed by one experienced pathologist (BW). Biopsies with uncertain cellular changes were immunostained with p16 (INK4a) (Roche mtm laboratories AG). If there was a discrepancy between biopsy and treatment histology, the most severe histology was endpoint.

The sensitivity of the HPV tests is defined as the proportion of high-grade dysplasia (CIN2+) detected by the two different HPV tests. In the calculations of specificity, it is assumed that HPV negative samples without detected dysplasia during the follow-up period were disease-free.

All analyses were done in SPSS, version 22.0, with Chi-square test for categorical variables, $t$-test for continuous variables, and survival analyses for clinically solved cases. Significance level was set to $p < 0.05$.

**Table 2** Most severe histology from biopsy/cone specimen by HPV test

| Histology | HPV DNA | | 5-type-mRNA | |
|---|---|---|---|---|
| | $N = 105$ | % (95 % CI) | $N = 77$ | % (95 % CI) |
| Normal/CIN1 | 67 | 63.8 (54.6–73.0) | 47 | 61.0 (50.1–71.9) |
| CIN2 | 23 | 21.9 (14.0–29.8) | 15 | 19.5 (10.7–28.3) |
| CIN3+ | 15 | 14.3 (7.6–21.0) | 15 | 19.5 (10.7–28.3) |

*CIN* cervical intraepitelial neoplasi
*HPV DNA* HPV DNA test (Cobas 4800)
*5-type-mRNA* HPV mRNA test (PreTect HPV-Proofer)

### Results

At index cytology 84 % (473/564) were ASC-US and 16 % (91/564) LSIL. At the most recent screen prior to index cytology 79 % (444/564) of the women had a normal cytology within the screening interval, 4 % (24/564) had a normal cytology beyond the screening interval, whereas index cytology represented the first smear, ever,

**Table 3** Test performance of HPV DNA test (N = 504) and 5-type-mRNA test (N = 536) in solved cases

| Triage status | CIN2+ | CIN1- | Total |
|---|---|---|---|
| HPV DNA positive | 38 | 73 | 111[a] |
| HPV DNA negative | 0 | 393 | 393 |
| Total | 38 | 466 | 504 |
| | | | |
| Triage status | CIN2+ | CIN1- | Total |
| HPV mRNA positive | 30 | 47 | 77 |
| HPV mRNA negative | 8 | 451 | 459 |
| Total | 38 | 498 | 536 |

CIN2+ CIN2, CIN3, ACIS, and cervical cancer

CIN1- Normal and CIN1

[a]Of the 111 women with a positive HPV DNA test, six women had normal cytology and a negative HPV DNA test at second follow-up and returned to screening at 3-year interval

for 17 % (96/564) of the women. The mean age was 39 years (SD 10.5 years) and nearly 40 % (217/564) of the women were 25–34 years of age.

Mainly from triage, but also after follow-up of a normal cytology with a positive HPV test at triage, the 5-type mRNA test scheduled significantly more women back to screening, 81 % (459/564), than the DNA test, 71 % (399/564) (p < 0.01). There was no difference in incomplete follow-ups by screening test, HPV DNA test 4 % (24/564)/mRNA test 2 % (13/564) (p = 0.09). Accordingly, the DNA test targeted significantly more women for biopsy, 25 % (141/564) than the 5-type mRNA test, 16 % (92/564) (p < 0.01) (Table 1). In total 141 women were recommended colposcopy by the DNA test, and 105 (74 %) met for biopsy. Out of the 92 women scheduled for biopsy by the 5-type mRNA test, 77 (84 %) made a visit (p = 0.12).

There was no difference in histology outcome by screening test among women who had biopsy and/or treatment. Both tests identified 14 women with CIN3 and one woman with squamous cell carcinoma (Table 2). The positive predictive value (PPV) for CIN2+ was 34 % (38/111) for HPV DNA and 39 % (30/77) for the 5-type mRNA test. The PPVs for CIN3+ were 13.5 % (15/111) and 19.5 % (15/77) for the DNA and the 5-type mRNA test (Table 3). The increased referral rate to biopsy among DNA-tested women relative to mRNA-tested women resulted in 10 more cases of normal histology, 10 more cases of CIN1, and eight more cases of CIN2 (Table 4).

At triage, 65 % (386/564) were negative in both tests (DNA-/mRNA-), while 29 % (165/564) and 19 % (105/564) were positive with the DNA or 5-type mRNA test, respectively. In total, 98 women were double positive (DNA+/mRNA+). Among the 73 HPV DNA positive and 5-type mRNA negative women (DNA+/mRNA-), 69 were positive for HPV types other than 16 and 18, two for HPV16, and two for HPV18. Among women with a negative HPV DNA test, seven tests were positive with the 5-type mRNA test (DNA-/mRNA+), four HPV16 and three HPV other than 16 and 18. Among the 53 women testing positive for HPV16 (DNA+ and/or mRNA+), 44 tested positive in both tests (DNA+/mRNA+), 48 tested positive for HPV DNA, and 49 for 5-type mRNA. Similar results for HPV18, 11 women out of 14 were double positive (DNA+/mRNA+), 13 tested positive for HPV DNA, while 12 tested positive for 5-type mRNA. The largest difference was for HPV other types than HPV16 and HPV18. Only 39 out of 116 tested positive in both tests (DNA+/mRNA+), 110 tested positive for DNA, and 44 tested positive for 5-type mRNA.

**Table 4** HPV positivity, genotype, and HPV test by stage of triage and histology

| | HPV DNA | | | | | 5-type-mRNA | | | | |
|---|---|---|---|---|---|---|---|---|---|---|
| | | HPVNeg. | HPV 16 | HPV 18 | HPV other | | HPVNeg. | HPV 16 | HPV 18 | HPV other |
| Stages of triage | N | % | % | % | % | N | % | % | % | % |
| At triage[a] | 564 | 69.7 | 8.5 | 2.3 | 19.5 | 564 | 81.4 | 8.7 | 2.1 | 7.8 |
| Recommended biopsy[b] | 141 | | 28.4 | 8.5 | 63.1 | 92 | | 45.7 | 10.9 | 43.5 |
| Had biopsy[c] | 105 | | 36.2 | 7.6 | 56.2 | 77 | | 51.9 | 9.1 | 39.0 |
| By histology | N | | % | % | % | N | | % | % | % |
| Normal/CIN1 | 67 | | 26.9 | 7.5 | 65.7 | 47 | | 44.7 | 8.5 | 46.8 |
| CIN2 | 23 | | 39.1 | 13.0 | 47.8 | 15 | | 53.3 | 20.0 | 26.7 |
| CIN3 | 14 | | 71.4 | 0.0 | 28.6 | 14 | | 71.4 | 0.0 | 28.6 |
| Sq. cell carcinoma | 1 | | 0.0 | 0.0 | 100 | 1 | | 0.0 | 0.0 | 100 |

HPV DNA other HPV type 31, 33, 35, 39, 45, 51, 52, 56, 58, 59, 66, and 68

5-type-mRNA other HPV type 31, 33, and 45

CIN cervical intraepitelial neoplasi

[a]The Norwegian cervical cancer screening program recommended triage 6 to 12 months after the index ASC-US/LSIL

[b]Women with either a positive HPV DNA or a positive HPV mRNA test are recommended biopsy

[c]In total 141 women were recommended colposcopy by the DNA test, and 105 (74 %) met for biopsy. Out of the 92 women scheduled for biopsy by the 5-type mRNA test, 77 (84 %) made a visit (p = 0.12)

Table 4 summarizes HPV positivity, genotype, stage of triage and histology by HPV test. The DNA test detected 23 cases of CIN2, relative to 15 with the 5-type mRNA test. There was concordance between tests in eight cases of HPV16, three cases of HPV18, and three cases of HPV other than 16 and 18. One CIN2 case testing HPV16 in the DNA test tested HPV other than 16 and 18 in the 5-type mRNA test. The eight additional cases of CIN2 detected by the DNA test were all negative for HPV 16/18 and positive for other than 16 and 18: three in the age group 25–34 years and five in the 35–69 group. All cases with CIN3 ($n = 14$) were concordant for HPV type in both tests ($n = 10$ for HPV16, $n = 4$ for HPV other than 16 or 18).

In total 89 % (504/564) of the DNA cases were solved across the time frame of the study, relative to 95 % (536/564) of the 5-type mRNA-tested cases ($p < 0.01$). The cumulative proportions of cases solved within 12 and 36 months were significantly higher for 5-type mRNA-tested subjects, 92 % (95 % CI: 90–94) and 96 % (95 % CI: 94–98), than DNA-tested subjects, 85 % (95 % CI: 82–88) and 90 % (95 % CI: 87–93)).

The sensitivity among solved cases for CIN2+ of the HPV DNA test was 100 % (38/38) relative to 79 % (30/38, 95 % CI: 67–92) for the 5-type mRNA test. The corresponding estimates of specificity among solved cases were 84 % (393/466, 95 % CI: 81–88), and 91 % (451/498, 95 % CI: 88–93) (Table 3) ($p < 0.01$). In Tables 5, 6, 7 and 8 we provide data on triage cytology (ASC-US or LSIL) by HPV test for CIN2+ and CIN3 + .

## Discussion

Our study shows that the 5-type HPV mRNA test had significantly lower positivity rate (19 %) than the 14-type HPV DNA test (29 %), which led to a significantly higher referral rate to colposcopy for the HPV DNA test. Both tests diagnosed equal numbers of women with CIN3+, whereas the DNA test detected eight more cases of

**Table 6** Test performance of HPV DNA test and 5-type HPV mRNA test in repeated ASC-US in solved cases versus CIN3+

| Triage status | CIN3+ | CIN2- | Total |
|---|---|---|---|
| HPV DNA positive | 9 | 78 | 87 |
| HPV DNA negative | 0 | 28 | 28 |
| Total | 9 | 106 | 115 |

| Triage status | CIN3+ | CIN2- | Total |
|---|---|---|---|
| HPV mRNA positive | 9 | 54 | 63 |
| HPV mRNA negative | 0 | 50 | 50 |
| Total | 9 | 104 | 113 |

*CIN2+* CIN2, CIN3, ACIS, and cervical cancer
*CIN1-* Normal and CIN1

CIN2. All these CIN2 cases were of HPV types other than 16/18 in both tests, and they were negative for HPV mRNA 31, 33, and 45.

In agreement with other studies, the positivity rate of the HPV DNA test in triage of ASC-US/LSIL is nearly double compared to the 5-type HPV mRNA test (Table 9 [6, 7, 10–12, 16]). We found a 57 % higher referral rate using HPV DNA versus 5-type mRNA while others have reported a double referral rate ratio using HPV DNA compared to 5-type mRNA [6, 7, 10].

Most studies report a higher sensitivity for CIN2+ and CIN3+ using the HPV DNA test or 14-type HPV mRNA test (Hologic APTIMA) compared to the 5-type HPV mRNA test, whereas the specificity is significantly higher for 5-type HPV mRNA compared to HPV DNA (or 14-type HPV mRNA test) [6, 7, 16–18]. The higher specificity reflects the higher positive predictive value (PPV) for the HPV 5-type mRNA test relative to the HPV DNA test (or 14-type HPV mRNA test).

The major difference in test performance between the DNA and the 5-type mRNA test was HPV types other than 16/18, which were in most cases HPV mRNA-negative for 31/33/45. The choice of test is crucial to

**Table 5** Test performance of HPV DNA test and 5-type HPV mRNA test in repeated ASC-US in solved cases versus CIN2+

| Triage status | CIN2+ | CIN1- | Total |
|---|---|---|---|
| HPV DNA positive | 25 | 62 | 87 |
| HPV DNA negative | 0 | 28 | 28 |
| Total | 25 | 90 | 115 |

| Triage status | CIN2+ | CIN1- | Total |
|---|---|---|---|
| HPV mRNA positive | 18 | 45 | 63 |
| HPV mRNA negative | 5 | 45 | 50 |
| Total | 23 | 90 | 113 |

*CIN2+* CIN2, CIN3, ACIS, and cervical cancer
*CIN1-* Normal and CIN1

**Table 7** Test performance of HPV DNA test and 5-type HPV mRNA test in repeated LSIL in solved cases versus CIN2+

| Triage status | CIN2+ | CIN1- | Total |
|---|---|---|---|
| HPV DNA positive | 13 | 31 | 44 |
| HPV DNA negative | 0 | 5 | 5 |
| Total | 13 | 36 | 49 |

| Triage status | CIN2+ | CIN1- | Total |
|---|---|---|---|
| HPV mRNA positive | 12 | 17 | 29 |
| HPV mRNA negative | 1 | 19 | 20 |
| Total | 13 | 46 | 49 |

*CIN2+* CIN2, CIN3, ACIS, and cervical cancer
*CIN1-* Normal and CIN1

**Table 8** Test performance of HPV DNA test and 5-type HPV mRNA test in repeated LSIL in solved cases versus CIN3+

| Triage status | CIN3+ | CIN2- | Total |
|---|---|---|---|
| HPV DNA positive | 6 | 38 | 44 |
| HPV DNA negative | 0 | 5 | 5 |
| Total | 6 | 43 | 49 |
| | | | |
| Triage status | CIN3+ | CIN2- | Total |
| HPV mRNA positive | 6 | 23 | 29 |
| HPV mRNA negative | 0 | 20 | 20 |
| Total | 6 | 43 | 49 |

*CIN2+* CIN2, CIN3, ACIS, and cervical cancer
*CIN1-* Normal and CIN1

avoid over-diagnosis in triage of women with minor cytological lesions. Our data indicates that the difference in sensitivity/loss of CIN2 may be attributed to HPV types with a low oncogenic potential with slow progression into cancer. The next screening round will capture these women for follow-up/treatment if there is any progression. A triage HPV test with high specificity, targeting the HPV types with the highest potential for progression to cervical cancer, will reduce over-diagnosis and overtreatment, as observed in this study. Over-diagnosis is a cost-driver in unnecessary conizations and may lead to an increased risk of premature births and late abortions in subsequent pregnancies [19, 20] in this young population.

In our study the 5-type HPV mRNA test detected the same number of CIN3+, with a significant lower positivity rate and significant lower referral rate to colposcopy

than the HPV DNA test. The risk of cervical cancer in women with ASC-US/LSIL is low and even lower if the HPV mRNA test is negative [6, 16, 21]. In Europe, HPV16 predominates in both CIN3 and cervical cancer. Other HPV types have a slower progression into cancer [22]. In countries with an organized cervical cancer screening program the risk of development of cervical cancer is higher for HPV types 16, 18, 31, 33 and 45 than for other HPV types [23]. These observations support the use of a specific HPV mRNA test detecting the five main HPV types in triage of women with minor cytological lesions.

In a meta-analysis of the accuracy of 5-type HPV mRNA tests, the pooled sensitivity for CIN2+ of the 10 included studies was 75 % and 76 % for the triage of ASC-US and LSIL, respectively [14]. It is well known that many cervical lesions with moderate or severe dysplasia will regress spontaneously. Only 5 % of women with CIN2 will develop cervical cancer without treatment [24]. Only 31 % of colposcopically visible lesions with CIN3 will progress to invasive cancer within 30 years [25]. About 40 % of CIN2 will regress within two years, and the regression rate of CIN2 caused by other HPV types than HPV type 16 is even higher [26]. It is probable that the 5-type HPV mRNA test in triage of women with minor cervical lesions identifies the majority of the lesions that are destined to progress to cancer [27, 28]. When women with ASC-US/LSIL and a negative 5-type mRNA test are returned to screening in three years, we can reduce overtreatment of women with CIN1-2 caused by HPV types with a low risk of progression [22, 23, 26, 29].

**Table 9** Test-performance of the 5-type mRNA test and 13–14 types DNA tests in delayed triage and reflex testing of women with minor cytological lesions and CIN3+ as outcome

| Ref. | Data collection | Year publ. | Country | Study design | Timing HPV test | Length f-up (mo) | Diagnosis | HPV test | N | N HPV positive | N Met for biopsy | CIN3+ Sens. | Spes. | PPV | NPV |
|---|---|---|---|---|---|---|---|---|---|---|---|---|---|---|---|
| 6 | July 2005–Dec. 2009 | 2013 | Norway | Case-series | Delayed triage | ≤36 | Repeat ASCUS/LSIL | HC II 5 mRNA | 2150 1543 | 1504 510 | 1 184 435 | NR | | | |
| 7 | Jan. 2004–Dec. 2006 | 2011 | Italy | Head-to-head | Reflex testing | ≤2 | ASCUS/LSIL | HC II 5 mRNA | 795 755 | 614 204 | 377 132 | NR | | | |
| 10 | Jan. 2012–Sept. 2012 | 2014 | Norway[a] | Head-to-head | Delayed triage | ≤33 | Repeat ASCUS/LSIL | COBAS 5 mRNA | 281 281 | 92 37 | 65 26 | 100 75.0 | 77.8 91.6 | 6.2 11.5 | 100 99.6 |
| 11 | Aug. 2005–Jan. 2007 | 2008 | UK | Head-to-head | Reflex testing | Same day | ≤ mild dyskaryosis | HC II 5 mRNA | 567 558 | NR | NRe | 100 89.4 | 26.0 72.8 | 11.1 23.2 | 100 NR |
| 12 | Sept. 2007–Oct. 2009 | 2012 | UK | Head-to-head | Reflex Testing | Same day | ≤ mild dyskaryosis | HC II 5 mRNA | 670 641 | 526 272 | NRe | 100 80.9 | NR | 9.2 16.6 | 100 NR |
| 16 | NR | 2010 | Canada | Head-to-head | Reflex testing | ≤6 | ASCUS/LSIL | HC II 5 mRNA | 781 781 | 619 328 | NRe | NR | | | |
| A | Jan. 2012–Sep. 2013 | | Norway[a] | Head-to-head | Delayed testing | ≤33 | Repeat ASCUS/LSIL | COBAS 5 mRNA | 564 564 | 171 105 | 105 77 | 100 100 | 80.0 85.2 | 13.9 16.3 | 100 100 |

*A* Present study
*Sens* Sensitivity; *Spes.* Specificity; *PPV* positive predictive value; *NPV* negative predictive value; *NR* Not reported; *NRe* Not relevant. All women had colposcopy regardless of HPV result
[a]Only solved cases are included in test-performance analysis

The experience in the Department of Pathology, Ålesund Hospital, is that the 5-type HPV mRNA test has a high specificity and a high positive predictive value. This makes it useful for triage of women with minor cervical lesions.

## Conclusions

5-type HPV mRNA is more specific than HPV DNA in triage of women with repeated ASC-US/LSIL. The referral rate for colposcopy after repeated ASC-US/LSIL was 57 % higher for DNA+ relative to mRNA+ cases, with the same detection rate of CIN3+. It is important to consider the trade-off between sensitivity and specificity of the diagnostic test when designing screening algorithms.

## Abbreviations

ASC-H, atypical squamous cells – cannot exclude HSIL; ASC-US, atypical squamous cells of undetermined significance; CIN, cervical intraepithelial neoplasia, also known as cervical dysplasia; CIN1, CIN2, CIN3, cervical intraepithelial neoplasia grade 1, 2 or 3, also known as low grade, moderate or severe cervical dysplasia; CIN2+, CIN2, CIN3, adenocarcinoma in situ (ACIS) or cervical cancer DNA: Deoxyribonucleic acid; HPV, human papillomavirus; HPV DNA test, cobas 4800 detects DNA from 14 high-risk HPV types (16, 18, 31, 33, 35, 39, 45, 51, 52, 56, 58, 59, 66 and 68) at clinically relevant infection levels; HPV mRNA test, PreTect HPV-Proofer detects E6/E7 mRNA of 5 HPV types (16, 18, 31, 33 and 45); HSIL, High grade squamous intraepithelial lesion; LBC, liquid-based cytology; LSIL, low grade squamous intraepithelial lesion; mRNA, messenger RNA; NPV, negative predictive value; Pap smear, the Papanicolaou test, also known as Pap test, cervical smear or cervical cytology; PPV, positive predictive value; RNA, ribonucleic acid; WHO, the World Health Organization

## Acknowledgements

Not applicable.

## Funding

This research was supported by a grant from the Helse Møre og Romsdal Trust. The funders had no role in study design, data collection and analysis, decision to publish, or preparation of the manuscript.

## Authors' contributions

BW, SWS and FES participated in the design of the study. AG and HG screened all the PAP-smears and performed HPV mRNA testing. BW reviewed all the histological diagnosis. SWS and FES performed the statistical analysis. All authors read and approved the final manuscript.

## Authors' information

Not applicable.

## Competing interests

The authors declare that they have no competing interests.

## Consent for publication

Not applicable.

## Ethics approval and consent to participate

The Regional Committee for Medical and Health Research Ethics, North Norway, has approved the protocol as a quality assurance study in laboratory work fulfilling the requirements for data protection procedures within the department (2012/276/REK Nord). Norwegian regulations exempt quality assurance studies from written informed consent from the patients (https://lovdata.no/dokument/SF/forskrift/2000-12-15-1265).

## Author details

[1]Department of Pathology, Ålesund Hospital, Møre and Romsdal Health Trust, Ålesund, Norway. [2]Department of Clinical Pathology, University Hospital of North Norway, 9038 Tromsø, Norway. [3]Research Group Epidemiology of Chronic Diseases, Department of Community Medicine, UiT The Arctic University of Norway, Tromsø, Norway.

## References

1. Arbyn M, Castellsague X, de Sanjose S, Bruni L, Saraiya M, Bray F, et al. Worldwide burden of cervical cancer in 2008. Ann Oncol. 2011;12:2675–86.
2. Ramakrishnan S, Partricia S, Mathan G. Overview of high-risk HPV's 16 and 18 infected cervical cancer: pathogenesis to prevention. Biomed Pharmacother. 2015;70:103–10.
3. de Sanjose S, Quint WG, Alemany L, Geraets DT, Klaustermeier JE, Lloveras B, et al. Human papillomavirus genotype attribution in invasive cervical cancer: a retrospective cross-sectional worldwide study. Lancet Oncol. 2010;11:1048–56.
4. Saslow D, Solomon D, Lawson HW, Killackey M, Kulasingam SL, Cain J, et al. American Cancer Society, American Society for Colposcopy and Cervical Pathology, and American Society for Clinical Pathology screening guidelines for the prevention and early detection of cervical cancer. Am J Clin Pathol. 2012;137:516–42.
5. Arbyn M, Martin-Hirsch P, Buntinx F, Van Ranst M, Paraskevaidis E, Dillner J. Triage of women with equivocal or low-grade cervical cytology results: a meta-analysis of the HPV test positivity rate. J Cell Mol Med. 2009;13:648–59.
6. Nygard M, Roysland K, Campbell S, Dillner J. Comparative effectiveness study on human papillomavirus detection methods used in the cervical cancer screening programme. BMJ Open. 2014;4:e003460.
7. Benevolo M, Vocaturo A, Caraceni D, French D, Rosini S, Zappacosta R, Terrenato I, Ciccocioppo L, Frega A, Giorgi Rossi P. Sensitivity, specificity, and clinical value of human papillomavirus (HPV) E6/E7 mRNA assay as a triage test for cervical cytology and HPV DNA test. J Clin Microbiol. 2011;49(7):2643–50. doi:10.1128/JCM.02570-10.
8. Koliopoulos G, Chrelias C, Pappas A, Makridima S, Kountouris E, Alepaki M, Spathis A, Stathopoulou V, Panayiotides I, Panagopoulos P, Karakitsos P, Kassanos D. The diagnostic accuracy of two methods for E6&7 mRNA detection in women with minor cytological abnormalities. Acta Obstet Gynecol Scand. 2012;91(7):794–801. doi:10.1111/j.1600-0412.2012.01414.x.
9. Sorbye SW, Fismen S, Gutteberg T, Mortensen ES. Triage of women with minor cervical lesions: data suggesting a "test and treat" approach for HPV E6/E7 mRNA testing. PLoS One. 2010;5:e12724.
10. Sorbye SW, Fismen S, Gutteberg TJ, Mortensen ES, Skjeldestad FE. HPV mRNA is more specific than HPV DNA in triage of women with minor cervical lesions. PLoS One. 2014;9:e112934.
11. Szarewski A, Ambroisine L, Cadman L, Austin J, Ho L, Terry G, et al. Comparison of predictors for high-grade cervical intraepithelial neoplasia in women with abnormal smears. Cancer Epidemiol Biomarkers Prev. 2008;17:3033–42.
12. Szarewski A, Mesher D, Cadman L, Austin J, Ashdown-Barr L, Ho L, et al. Comparison of seven tests for high-grade cervical intraepithelial neoplasia in women with abnormal smears: the Predictors 2 study. J Clin Microbiol. 2012;50:1867–73.
13. Trope A, Sjoborg K, Eskild A, Cuschieri K, Eriksen T, Thoresen S, et al. Performance of human papillomavirus DNA and mRNA testing strategies for women with and without cervical neoplasia. J Clin Microbiol. 2009;47:2458–64.
14. Verdoodt F, Szarewski A, Halfon P, Cuschieri K, Arbyn M. Triage of women with minor abnormal cervical cytology: meta-analysis of the accuracy of an assay targeting messenger ribonucleic acid of 5 high-risk human papillomavirus types. Cancer Cytopathol. 2013;121:675–87.
15. Nygård JF, Skare GB, Thoresen SO. The cervical cancer screening programme in Norway, 1992–2000: changes in Pap smear coverage and incidence of cervical cancer. J Med Screen. 2002;9:86–91.
16. Ratnam S, Coutlee F, Fontaine D, Bentley J, Escott N, Ghatage P, et al. Clinical performance of the PreTect HPV-Proofer E6/E7 mRNA assay in comparison with that of the Hybrid Capture 2 test for identification of women at risk of cervical cancer. J Clin Microbiol. 2010;48:2779–85.
17. Arbyn M, Ronco G, Anttila A, Meijer CJ, Poljak M, Ogilvie G, et al. Evidence regarding human papillomavirus testing in secondary prevention of cervical cancer. Vaccine. 2012;30 Suppl 5:F88–99.

18. Arbyn M, Roelens J, Cuschieri K, Cuzick J, Szarewski A, Ratnam S, et al. The APTIMA HPV assay versus the Hybrid Capture 2 test in triage of women with ASC-US or LSIL cervical cytology: a meta-analysis of the diagnostic accuracy. Int J Cancer. 2013;132:101–8.

19. Arbyn M, Kyrgiou M, Simoens C, Raifu AO, Koliopoulos G, Martin-Hirsch P, et al. Perinatal mortality and other severe adverse pregnancy outcomes associated with treatment of cervical intraepithelial neoplasia: meta-analysis. BMJ. 2008;337:a1284. doi:10.1136/bmj.a1284.:a1284.

20. Bruinsma FJ, Quinn MA. The risk of preterm birth following treatment for precancerous changes in the cervix: a systematic review and meta-analysis. BJOG. 2011;118:1031–41.

21. Sorbye SW, Fismen S, Gutteberg TJ, Mortensen ES. HPV mRNA test in women with minor cervical lesions: experience of the University Hospital of North Norway. J Virol Methods. 2010;169:219–22.

22. Tjalma WA, Fiander A, Reich O, Powell N, Nowakowski AM, Kirschner B, et al. Differences in human papillomavirus type distribution in high-grade cervical intraepithelial neoplasia and invasive cervical cancer in Europe. Int J Cancer. 2013;132:854–67.

23. Powell NG, Hibbitts SJ, Boyde AM, Newcombe RG, Tristram AJ, Fiander AN. The risk of cervical cancer associated with specific types of human papillomavirus: a case–control study in a UK population. Int J Cancer. 2011;128:1676–82.

24. Ostor AG. Natural history of cervical intraepithelial neoplasia: a critical review. Int J Gynecol Pathol. 1993;12:186–92.

25. McCredie MR, Sharples KJ, Paul C, Baranyai J, Medley G, Jones RW, et al. Natural history of cervical neoplasia and risk of invasive cancer in women with cervical intraepithelial neoplasia 3: a retrospective cohort study. Lancet Oncol. 2008;9:425–34.

26. Castle PE, Schiffman M, Wheeler CM, Solomon D. Evidence for frequent regression of cervical intraepithelial neoplasia-grade 2. Obstet Gynecol. 2009;113:18–25.

27. Basu P, Roychowdhury S, Bafna UD, Chaudhury S, Kothari S, Sekhon R, et al. Human papillomavirus genotype distribution in cervical cancer in India: results from a multi-center study. Asian Pac J Cancer Prev. 2009;10:27–34.

28. Kraus I, Molden T, Holm R, Lie AK, Karlsen F, Kristensen GB, et al. Presence of E6 and E7 mRNA from human papillomavirus types 16, 18, 31, 33, and 45 in the majority of cervical carcinomas. J Clin Microbiol. 2006;44:1310–7.

29. Zappacosta R, Gatta DM, Marinucci P, Capanna S, Lattanzio G, Caraceni D, et al. Role of E6/E7 mRNA test in the diagnostic algorithm of HPV-positive patients showing ASCUS and LSIL: clinical and economic implications in a publicly financed healthcare system. Expert Rev Mol Diagn. 2015;15:1–14.

# 25

# Enrichment of the embryonic stem cell reprogramming factors Oct4, Nanog, Myc, and Sox2 in benign and malignant vascular tumors

Clarissa N. Amaya and Brad A. Bryan[*]

### Abstract

**Background:** The "stem cell theory of cancer" states that a subpopulation of cells with stem cell-like properties plays a central role in the formation, sustainment, spread, and drug resistant characteristics of malignant tumors. Recent studies have isolated distinct cell populations from infantile hemangiomas that display properties equivalent to aberrant progenitor cells, suggesting that, in addition to malignant tumors, benign tumors may also contain a stem cell-like component.

**Methods:** In this study, the expression levels of the embryonic stem cell reprogramming factors Oct4, Nanog, Myc, Sox2, and Klf4 were examined via immunohistochemistry in a panel of 71 benign, borderline, and malignant vascular tumors including capillary hemangioma, cavernous hemangioma, granulomatous hemangioma, venous hemangioma, hemangioendothelioma, hemangiopericytoma, and angiosarcoma. Antigenicity for each protein was quantified based on staining intensity and percentage of tissue positive for each antigen, and subsequently compared to data obtained from two control tissue sets: 10 vascular tissues and a panel of 58 various malignant sarcomas.

**Results and discussion:** With the exception of Myc (which was only present in a subset of benign, borderline, and malignant tumors), Oct4, Nanog, Sox2, and Klf4 were detectable at variable levels across both normal and diseased tissues. Semi-quantitative evaluation of our immunohistochemical staining revealed that protein expression of Oct4, Nanog, Myc, and Sox2, but not Klf4, was significantly increased in benign, borderline, and malignant vascular tumors relative to non-diseased vascular tissue controls. Interestingly, the enhanced levels of Oct4, Nanog, Myc, and Sox2 protein were approximately equivalent between benign, borderline, and malignant vascular tumors.

**Conclusions:** These findings provide supporting evidence that enrichment for proteins involved in pluripotency is not restricted solely to malignant tumors as is suggested by the "stem cell theory of cancer", but additionally extends to common benign vascular tumors such as hemangiomas.

## Background

The origin of cancer remains unclear, however the "cancer stem cell theory" postulates that a subpopulation of cancer cells with stem cell-like properties is responsible for sustaining long term tumor growth [1]. In addition, cancer stem cells give rise to metastases and can act as a reservoir that potentially leads to relapse after treatment has eliminated all observable signs of the cancer. These cancer stem cells are believed to be genotypically and/or phenotypically related to normal stem cells and share many of the features of normal stem cells such as self-renewal, drug resistance, and a proliferative potential to generate a multi-potent cellular lineage [2, 3]. The core transcription factors that control "stemness" in embryonic stem cells include Oct4, Sox2, Nanog, Myc, and Klf4, and the combination of these factors has been shown to successfully reprogram differentiated somatic cells into pluripotent stem cells [4]. There is substantial evidence that cancer stem cells express these specific markers and their activity contributes to the oncogenic properties inherent in this disease [5].

---

* Correspondence: brad.bryan@ttuhsc.edu
Department of Biomedical Sciences, Paul L. Foster School of Medicine, Texas Tech University Health Sciences Center, El Paso, TX, USA

In addition to malignant tumors, benign prostate, breast, and angiomyolipoma tumors express various stem cell markers, suggesting the expression of these markers is not limited exclusively to malignant tumors [6–9]. It was recently reported that benign infantile hemangiomas, which are the most common tumors of infancy, express higher levels of neural crest and stem cell markers at the mRNA level than dermal microvascular endothelial cells [10], and within this tumor type resides multiple cellular subpopulations expressing Oct4 and Nanog proteins [11]. Moreover, it was recently revealed that a clonogenic subpopulation of cells isolated from cutaneous infantile hemangiomas was capable of differentiating into endothelial cells, smooth muscle, or adipocytes [12], suggesting that a stem cell-like component may drive the etiology of this benign vascular tumor. These fascinating findings suggest that the "stem-cell theory of cancer" may serve as a more generalized theory than is currently accepted, and extend to benign vascular tumors.

Thus, in this study we used immunohistochemical analysis to examine the expression of the stem cell reprogramming factors Oct4, Sox2, Nanog, Myc, and Klf4 in 71 diverse benign and malignant vascular tumors. Our findings surprisingly revealed that, relative to normal endothelial tissues, staining of benign and malignant vascular tumors demonstrated significantly higher expression of these stem cell reprogramming factors.

## Methods

### Immunohistochemistry (IHC)

Blood vessel disease spectrum tissue arrays containing various vascular tumors and non-diseased controls were purchased from US Biomax, Inc. (#SO8010). The sarcoma tissue arrays were purchased from Novus Biologicals (#NBP2 = 30332). For detection of protein expression, tissue arrays were labeled with anti-Myc (Cat# ab32072; Abcam), anti-Oct4 (Cat# ab18976; Abcam), anti-Sox2 (Cat# ab97959; Abcam), anti-Klf4 (Cat# ab118961; Abcam), and anti-Nanog (Cat# ab80892; Abcam) antibodies. Antigenicity was detected using Alkaline Phosphatase reactivity (CellMarque). Positive (primary antibody included) and negative (primary antibody excluded) controls from human intestine (Klf4), human testicle (Oct4 and Nanog), rat brain (Sox2), or human colon cancer (Myc) which have been reported by the Human Protein Atlas (HPA) (www.proteinatlas.org) were subjected to immunohistochemistry to validate the specificity of each antibody tested (Additional file 1: Figure S1). In addition, immunohistochemistry for each antigen was performed on adipose tissue as a negative control, given the HPA revealed no to very low expression of each protein in this tissue type (Additional file 1: Figure S1). Immunopositivity was quantified by two metrics: the percentage of tissue with positive staining (<25 %, 25–50 %, 50–75 %, or >75 %) and the

staining intensity (0 = no staining, + = weak staining, ++ = moderate staining, +++ = high staining). IHC scores were determined by multiplying the staining intensity (0 = 0, + = 1, ++ = 2, +++ = 3) by the percent of tissue stained (<25 % = 1, 25–50 % = 2, 50–75 % = 3, >75 % = 4) based on previously described methods [13]. For statistical analysis, the Mann-Whitney rank sum test was used. Statistical significance was determined if the two-sided P value of the test was < 0.05. Use of human tissues for research was approved by TTUHSC board review #11027.

## Results

Included in this study were 71 diseased vascular tissue samples originally collected from human patients, representing malignant (seven angiosarcomas, two hemangiopericytomas), borderline (six hemangioendothelioma), and benign (five infantile hemangioma, one capillary hemangioma, 45 cavernous hemangiomas, three granulomatous hemangiomas, one venous hemangioma) vascular tumors and one thrombophlebitis. Known characteristics of patients grouped according to biopsy classification are reported in Table 1. As controls, we included two tissue sets in this analysis: 1) ten non-diseased blood vessel tissues and 2) a diverse panel of 58 human sarcoma tumors. The non-diseased blood vessel tissues were chosen to evaluate the expression of stem cell reprogramming factors in normal vasculature, while the various sarcomas were selected to compare the levels of stem cell reprogramming factors in borderline and malignant vascular sarcomas to that of other malignant mesenchymal tumors.

IHC staining for the stem cell reprogramming factors Oct4, Nanog, Myc, Klf4, and Sox2 was performed in the vascular tumor samples as well as the two control tissue sets. Representative images of each staining are depicted in Figs. 1, 2, 3, 4 and 5. With the exception of Myc, each of these proteins was detectable at variable levels across non-diseased vascular tissues, ranging from 50 % of normal tissues displaying Nanog and Klf4 immunoreactivity to 90 % of normal tissues displaying Oct4 immunoreactivity (Table 2). Expression of these "stem cell regulators" in non-diseased adult tissue is not surprising given that the HPA reports detection of Oct4, Nanog, Klf4, and Sox2 in approximately 70, 11, 29, and 51 % of normal human tissues, respectively. Though HPA reports Myc expression in

**Table 1** Vascular tumor and control patient characteristics

| Variable | Overall | Malignant | Borderline | Benign | Normal |
|---|---|---|---|---|---|
| # patient samples | 81 | 9 | 6 | 56 | 10 |
| Age [mean years (s.d.)] | 41 ± 17 | 53 ± 19 | 36 ± 15 | 40 ± 17 | 34 ± 14 |
| Age [median years (range)] | 42 (80) | 53 (64) | 35 (44) | 42 (71) | 32 (44) |
| Sex | 42 F, 39 M | 4 F, 5 M | 6 F, 0 M | 27 F, 29 M | 5 F, 5 M |

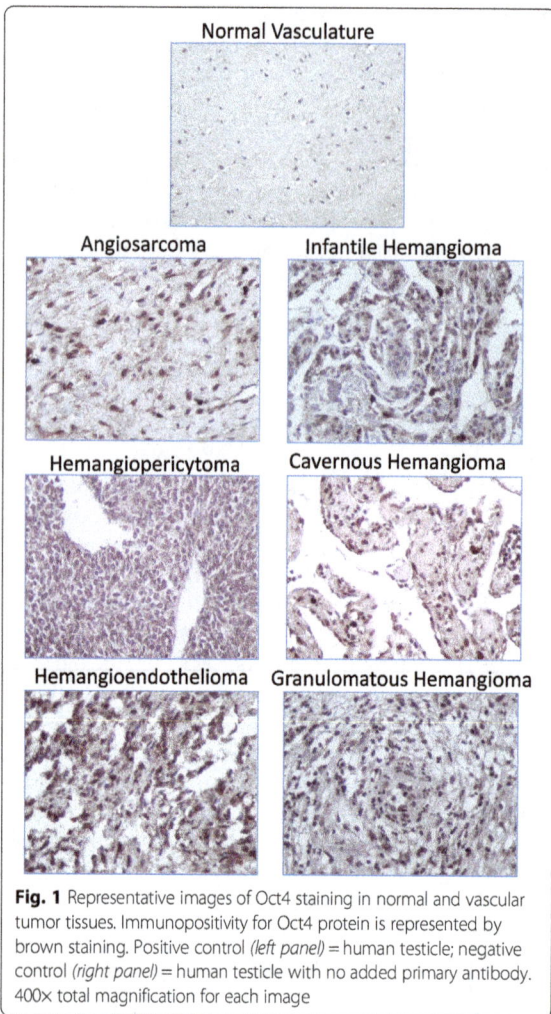

**Fig. 1** Representative images of Oct4 staining in normal and vascular tumor tissues. Immunopositivity for Oct4 protein is represented by brown staining. Positive control *(left panel)* = human testicle; negative control *(right panel)* = human testicle with no added primary antibody. 400× total magnification for each image

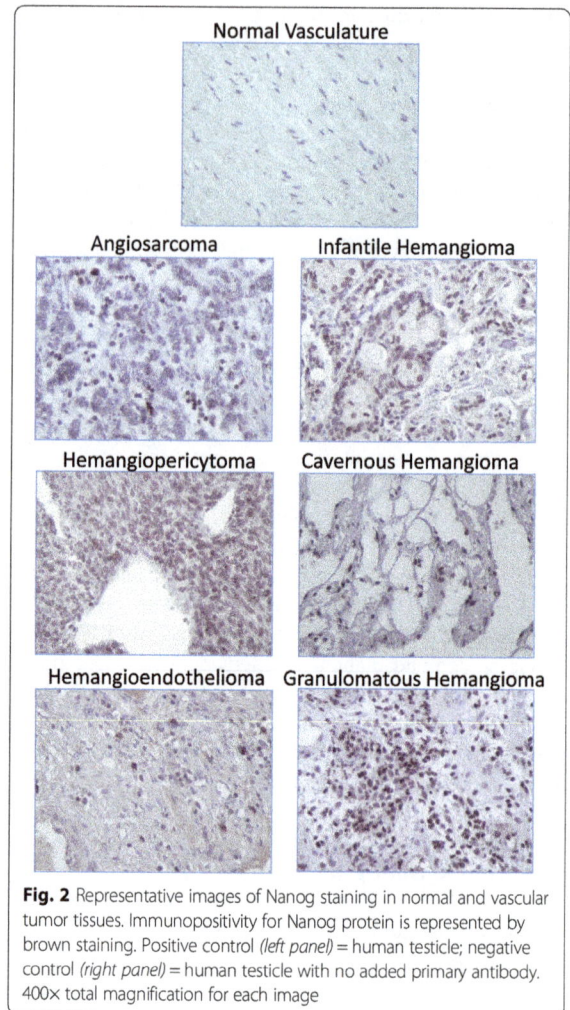

**Fig. 2** Representative images of Nanog staining in normal and vascular tumor tissues. Immunopositivity for Nanog protein is represented by brown staining. Positive control *(left panel)* = human testicle; negative control *(right panel)* = human testicle with no added primary antibody. 400× total magnification for each image

56 % of normal human tissues, we did not detect this protein in any non-diseased vascular tissues tested in this analysis. While immunostaining for these stem cell regulators was observed in non-diseased vasculature, the IHC score for these tissues was relatively low given that staining intensity for each stem cell marker was weak to moderate and often occurred in a very small fraction (<25 %) of the cells comprising the tissue (Fig. 6, Additional file 2: Table S1).

In contrast to the non-diseased vascular rich tissue controls, benign vascular tumors and the single thrombophlebitis sample exhibited significantly increased staining (in both intensity and percentage of positive tissue) for Oct4, Nanog, Myc, and Sox2, with no statistically significant increase in antigenicity for Klf4 (Fig. 6, Additional file 2: Table S1). It is worth noting that unlike the absence of Myc expression in normal vasculature, 46 % of the benign tumors tested were positive for Myc protein. The data obtained from malignant and borderline vascular tumors

were remarkably similar to that demonstrated from the benign vascular tumors. Malignant and borderline vascular sarcomas displayed 100 % immunoreactivity for Oct4, Nanog, and Sox2, while Myc protein was present in 50 % of malignant and borderline vascular tumors (Table 2). The IHC scores for all proteins tested except Klf4 were significantly increased in the malignant and borderline vascular tumors relative to the non-diseased controls, and were surprisingly very similar to the levels observed in benign vascular tumors. The elevated IHC scores observed for malignant and borderline vascular tumors correlated to the results obtained in a diverse panel of malignant sarcoma cells, revealing immunoreactivity for Oct4, Nanog, and Sox2 in 100 % of various sarcoma tissues and 72 % for Myc and Kfl4 (Additional file 2: Table S2). While Klf4 protein expression was not significantly different between any of the vascular tumors or vascular tissue controls, this protein did show a significantly increased mean IHC score

Enrichment of the embryonic stem cell reprogramming factors Oct4, Nanog, Myc, and Sox2...

209

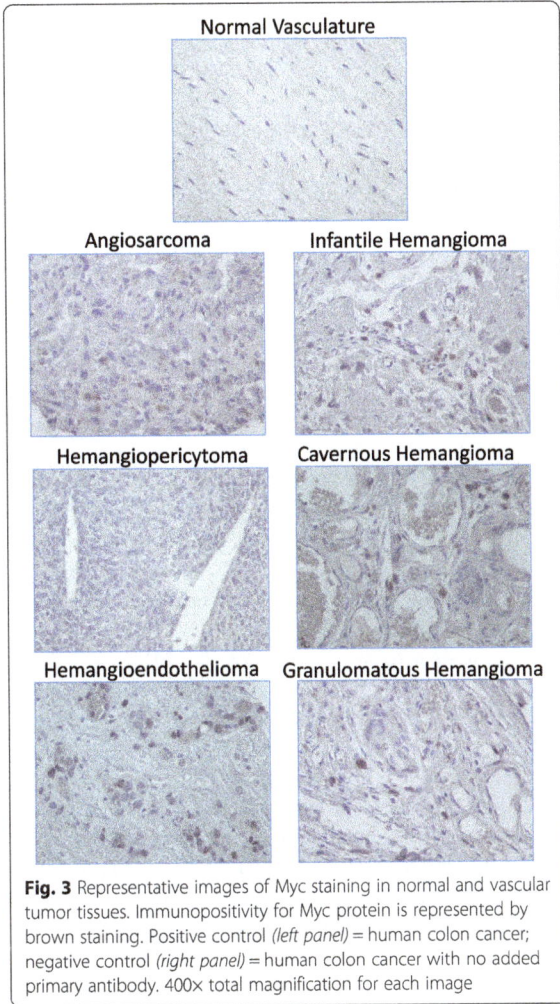

**Fig. 3** Representative images of Myc staining in normal and vascular tumor tissues. Immunopositivity for Myc protein is represented by brown staining. Positive control *(left panel)* = human colon cancer; negative control *(right panel)* = human colon cancer with no added primary antibody. 400× total magnification for each image

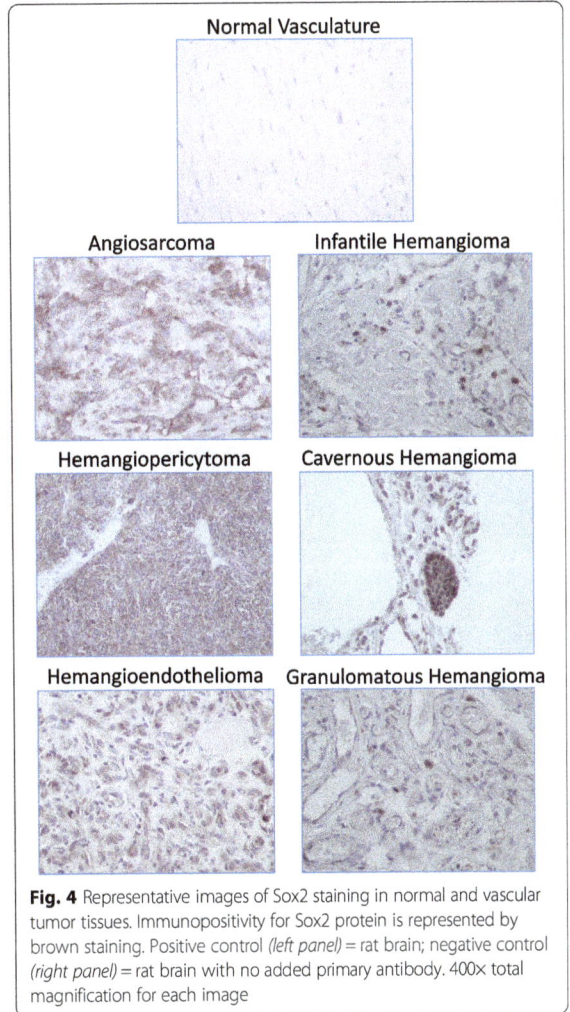

**Fig. 4** Representative images of Sox2 staining in normal and vascular tumor tissues. Immunopositivity for Sox2 protein is represented by brown staining. Positive control *(left panel)* = rat brain; negative control *(right panel)* = rat brain with no added primary antibody. 400× total magnification for each image

in the sarcoma tissue control set (Fig. 6, Additional file 2: Table S2). The expression of Oct4, Nanog, Myc, Sox2, and Klf4 in the current study correlated well with data reported in the HPA which reveals expression of Oct4 in 88 % of cancers, Sox2 in 88 % of cancers, Myc in 78 % of cancers, Klf4 in 28 % of cancers, and Nanog in 7 % of cancers.

## Discussion

This study directly stems from the results of a handful of recent publications which suggest that the benign vascular tumor, infantile hemangioma, harbors a subpopulation of stem cell-like progenitor cells. mRNA and protein expression of neural crest and stem cell markers was previously confirmed in a panel of hemangioma samples, revealing variable expression levels for Oct4, Myc, Sox2, and Nanog [10, 11]. These publications suggest that infantile hemangiomas may contain cells that are capable of differentiating into all three embryonic germ layers and

additionally point to a possible mechanism of clonality in these tumors. Indeed, implantation of isolated CD133+ stem cell populations from infantile hemangiomas produce hemangioma-like tumors in xenograft animal models [14], however Oct4 and Nanog positive subpopulations from infantile hemangiomas failed to form teratomas in SCID/NOD mice [11], a hallmark of embryonic stem cell-derived tumors [15], suggesting they do not function like true embryonic stem cells. Substantial lines of evidence controversially suggest that congenital and infantile hemangiomas originate from metastatic spread of placental chorangiomas [16–20], creating a possibility in which the etiology of some childhood hemangiomas (at least in their earliest stages) may be more similar to metastatic tumors than benign tumors. Thus, our observations that both infantile hemangiomas and malignant vascular tumors such as angiosarcomas and hemangiopericytomas expressed stem cell reprogramming factors at significantly increased

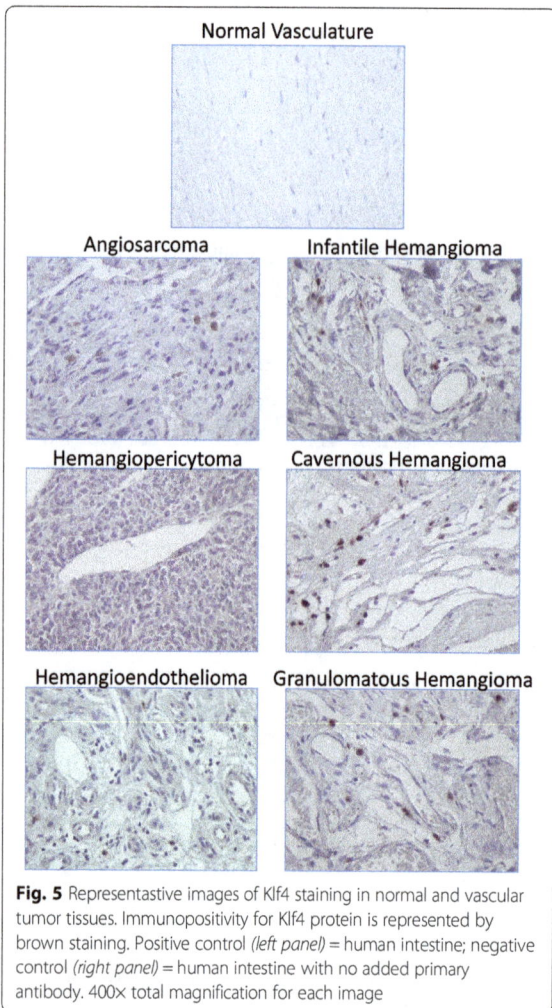

**Fig. 5** Representastive images of Klf4 staining in normal and vascular tumor tissues. Immunopositivity for Klf4 protein is represented by brown staining. Positive control *(left panel)* = human intestine; negative control *(right panel)* = human intestine with no added primary antibody. 400× total magnification for each image

quite surprising. These benign tumors often occur in the third to fourth decade of life, thus their origin cannot be attributed easily to distal neoplasms as arguably may occur in infantile hemangiomas. These expression patterns in diverse benign vascular tumors are intriguing given that the presence of "stemness" proteins in malignant tumors is well established in the literature and forms the basis for the "stem cell theory of cancer"; however our data provide strong evidence that these proteins could potentially contribute to the formation and/or properties associated with a diverse array of benign vascular tumors. Though more studies must be performed for definitive arguments either way, it is possible that the "stem cell theory of cancer" is too narrowly defined in its current state and may need to be broadened to include benign neoplasms. This subject should be treaded lightly and with careful future evaluation as, while Oct4 has been shown to maintain pluripotency during early embryogenesis, its role as a pure stem cell marker has been questioned given that it is also expressed in differentiated cells [21, 22]. Nanog expression has been reported in E18 stage rat myocardial tissues, and is detectable in post-natal stages up to 30 days after birth and after acute myocardial infarction [23, 24].

Compared to the abundance of research performed in carcinomas and hematopoietic cancers, relatively minimal work has been reported evaluating the presence of stem cells as driving components in malignant mesenchymal tumors, and much of these efforts have focused exclusively on pediatric bone and musculoskeletal sarcomas [25–27]. For instance, osteosarcomas and Ewing's sarcomas express Oct4 and Nanog [25, 28, 29] and rhabdomyosarcomas express Oct4, Nanog, and Sox2 [30]. Moreover, the EWS-FLI1 fusion gene, present in nearly 85 % of Ewing's sarcomas, induces the expression of Oct4, Nanog, and Sox2 in human pediatric mesenchymal stem cells but not their adult counterparts [31]. Though drug resistant progenitor-like cell populations have been reported for angiosarcomas [32, 33], only expression of Myc as an embryonic stem cell marker has been thoroughly examined in malignant vascular tumors [34]. It has been reported that Myc gene amplification and overexpression occurs in post-irradiation induced angiosarcomas, but not in primary cutaneous angiosarcomas or in other radiation-associated vascular proliferations [35, 36]; however several other studies provide evidence that Myc amplification and overexpression is not a definitive marker of radiation-induced tumorigenesis in angiosarcomas [37–39]. Our data additionally demonstrates that Oct4, Nanog, Sox2, Klf4, and Myc are widely expressed at high levels across a wide variety of sarcomas and benign vascular tumors at elevated levels. While the data reported in this study in no way indicate that the cells expressing these markers are cancer stem cells (which generally make up single digit or less percentages of the total cancer cell population in a tumor), the

and relatively similar levels compared to non-diseased vascular tissue, is not entirely surprising.

In contrast, our highly novel observations that other benign vascular tumors such as adult capillary, cavernous, granulomatous, and venous hemangiomas as well as the single thrombophlebitis sample displayed expression of Oct4, Nanog, Myc, and Sox2 in similarly elevated rates and intensities as seen in malignant sarcomas was

**Table 2** Percentage of tumors with positive antigenicity for embryonic stem cell reprogramming factors

| Protein | Normal | Benign | Borderline | Malignant | Various Sarcomas |
|---------|--------|--------|------------|-----------|------------------|
| Oct4 | 90 % | 100 % | 100 % | 100 % | 100 % |
| Nanog | 50 % | 98 % | 100 % | 100 % | 100 % |
| Myc | 0 % | 46 % | 50 % | 50 % | 72 % |
| Sox2 | 60 % | 98 % | 100 % | 100 % | 100 % |
| Klf4 | 50 % | 59 % | 67 % | 63 % | 72 % |

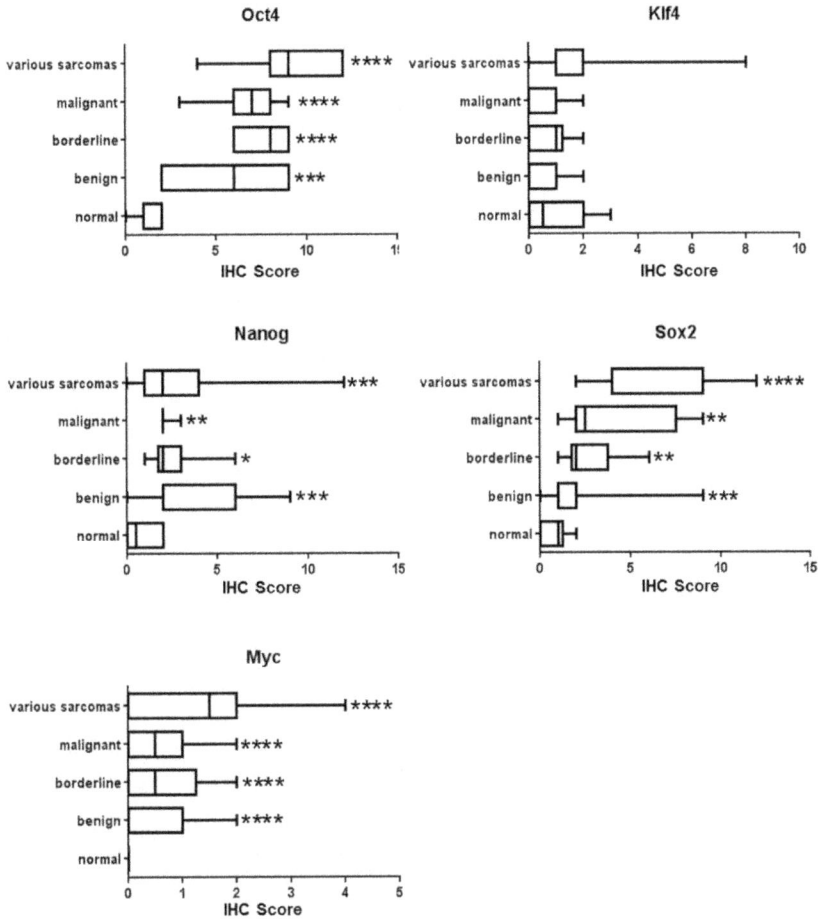

**Fig. 6** Antigenicity for embryonic stem cell reprogramming factors in normal tissue and vascular tumors. Box and whisker plots depicting the IHC scores for Oct4, Nanog, Myc, Sox2, and Klf4 in normal vasculature, benign, borderline or malignant vascular tumors, or across a panel of various sarcomas. The Mann-Whitney rank sum test was used to determine statistical significance. Significance was determined if the two-sided P value of the test was < 0.05. Asterisks indicate level of significance relative to normal vasculature (* $p < 0.05$, ** $p < 0.05$, *** $p < 0.005$, **** $p < 0.0005$)

statistically significant increases in Oct4, Nanog, Sox2, and Myc expression in benign and malignant tumors relative to normal tissues provides correlative support that overexpression of these proteins could contribute to their overall tumorigenic properties.

## Conclusion

In conclusion, the data presented in this study demonstrate that the protein expression of embryonic stem cell reprogramming factors is enriched in benign, borderline, and malignant vascular tumors. This finding could translate to future therapeutic targeting of tumor cell populations that express embryonic stem cell reprogramming factors to disrupt tumor cell clonality, long term growth, and drug resistance.

## Additional files

**Additional file 1: Figure S1.** Positive and negative staining controls. For each indicated antigen detected by immunohistochemistry, three controls were performed. The Negative Control column represents images acquired following immunohistochemistry against the indicated antigen on adipocyte tissue, which has been shown by the HPA to express no to low levels of each protein. The No Primary Antibody column represents images acquired following immunohistochemistry using no primary antibody on tissues as indicated in the Materials and Methods section to demonstrate that the detection system was no causing background staining on the samples. The Positive Control column represents images acquired from immunohistochemistry using the indicated antibody on tissues as indicated in the Materials and Methods section that are known to strongly express each antigen. (DOC 488 kb)

**Additional file 2: Table S1.** Immunopositivity for stem cell reprogramming factors in malignant and benign vascular tumors. **Table S2.** Immunopositivity for stem cell reprogramming factors in a panel of diverse sarcomas. (DOC 214 kb)

## Abbreviations
CD133: Cluster of differentiation 133 protein; EWS-FLI1: Ewings sarcoma oncogene-friend leukemia virus integration 1; HPA: Human protein atlas; IHC: Immunohistochemistry; Klf4: Kruppel-like factor 4; Myc: Myelocytomatosis viral oncogene homolog; Nanog: Homeobox protein Nanog; Oct4: Octamer-binding transcription factor 3/4; SCID/NOD: Severe combined immunodeficiency disease/non-obese diabetic; SOX2: Sex determining region Y box 2 protein; TTUHSC: Texas Tech University Health Sciences Center.

## Competing interests
The authors declare that they have no competing interests.

## Authors' contributions
AM carried out all IHC analysis and statistical analysis. BB designed the study, drafted the manuscript. Both authors read and approved the final manuscript.

## Authors' information
Not applicable.

## Acknowledgements
We would like to thank Dolores Diaz of the TTUHSC Histology Core for assistance with IHC methodology.

## Funding
This analysis was funded through a Liddy Shriver Sarcoma Initiative Grant and TTUHSC seed funding to BB.

## References

1. Bjerkvig R, Tysnes BB, Aboody KS, Najbauer J, Terzis AJ. Opinion: the origin of the cancer stem cell: current controversies and new insights. Nat Rev Cancer. 2005;5(11):899–904.
2. Dean M, Fojo T, Bates S. Tumour stem cells and drug resistance. Nat Rev Cancer. 2005;5(4):275–84.
3. Kreso A, Dick JE. Evolution of the cancer stem cell model. Cell Stem Cell. 2014;14(3):275–91.
4. Patel M, Yang S. Advances in reprogramming somatic cells to induced pluripotent stem cells. Stem Cell Rev. 2010;6(3):367–80.
5. Ben-Porath I, Thomson MW, Carey VJ, Ge R, Bell GW, Regev A, et al. An embryonic stem cell-like gene expression signature in poorly differentiated aggressive human tumors. Nat Genet. 2008;40(5):499–507.
6. da Arnaud Cruz P, Marques O, Rosa AM, de Fatima Faria M, Rema A, Lopes C. Co-expression of stem cell markers ALDH1 and CD44 in non-malignant and neoplastic lesions of the breast. Anticancer Res. 2014;34(3):1427–34.
7. Lim SD, Stallcup W, Lefkove B, Govindarajan B, Au KS, Northrup H, et al. Expression of the neural stem cell markers NG2 and L1 in human angiomyolipoma: are angiomyolipomas neoplasms of stem cells? Mol Med. 2007;13(3–4):160–5.
8. Prajapati A, Gupta S, Mistry B, Gupta S. Prostate stem cells in the development of benign prostate hyperplasia and prostate cancer: emerging role and concepts. BioMed Res Intl. 2013;2013:107954.
9. Ugolkov AV, Eisengart LJ, Luan C, Yang XJ. Expression analysis of putative stem cell markers in human benign and malignant prostate. Prostate. 2011;71(1):18–25.
10. Spock CL, Tom LK, Canadas K, Sue GR, Sawh-Martinez R, Maier CL, et al. Infantile hemangiomas exhibit neural crest and pericyte markers. Ann Plast Surg. 2015;74(2):230–6.
11. Itinteang T, Tan ST, Brasch HD, Steel R, Best HA, Vishvanath A, et al. Infantile haemangioma expresses embryonic stem cell markers. J Clin Pathol. 2012;65(5):394–8.
12. Huang L, Nakayama H, Klagsbrun M, Mulliken JB, Bischoff J. Glucose transporter 1-positive endothelial cells in infantile hemangioma exhibit features of facultative stem cells. Stem Cells. 2015;33(1):133–45.
13. Krajewska M, Smith LH, Rong J, Huang X, Hyer ML, Zeps N, et al. Image analysis algorithms for immunohistochemical assessment of cell death events and fibrosis in tissue sections. J Histochem Cytochem : Off J Histochemistry Soc. 2009;57(7):649–63.
14. Khan ZA, Boscolo E, Picard A, Psutka S, Melero-Martin JM, Bartch TC, et al. Multipotential stem cells recapitulate human infantile hemangioma in immunodeficient mice. J Clin Investig. 2008;118(7):2592–9.
15. Xu C, Inokuma MS, Denham J, Golds K, Kundu P, Gold JD, et al. Feeder-free growth of undifferentiated human embryonic stem cells. Nat Biotechnol. 2001;19(10):971–4.
16. Bakaris S, Karabiber H, Yuksel M, Parmaksiz G, Kiran H. Case of large placental chorioangioma associated with diffuse neonatal hemangiomatosis. Pediatr Dev Pathol: Off J Soc Pediatr Pathol Paediatr Pathol Soc. 2004;7(3):258–61.
17. Baruteau J, Joomye R, Muller JB, Vinceslas C, Baraton L, Joubert M, et al. Chorioangiomatosis: a rare etiology of nonimmune hydrops fetalis. Obstetric and pediatric implications for patient care. Arch Pediatr: Organe Off de la Soc Francaise de Pediatrie. 2009;16(10):1341–5.
18. Maymon R, Hermann G, Reish O, Herman A, Strauss S, Sherman D, et al. Chorioangioma and its severe infantile sequelae: case report. Prenat Diagn. 2003;23(12):976–80.
19. Miliaras D, Conroy J, Pervana S, Meditskou S, McQuaid D, Nowak N. Karyotypic changes detected by comparative genomic hybridization in a stillborn infant with chorioangioma and liver hemangioma. Birth Defects Res A Clin Mol Teratol. 2007;79(3):236–41.
20. Selmin A, Foltran F, Chiarelli S, Ciullo R, Gregori D. An epidemiological study investigating the relationship between chorangioma and infantile hemangioma. Pathol Res Pract. 2014;210(9):548–53.
21. Tai MH, Chang CC, Kiupel M, Webster JD, Olson LK, Trosko JE. Oct4 expression in adult human stem cells: evidence in support of the stem cell theory of carcinogenesis. Carcinogenesis. 2005;26(2):495–502.
22. Zangrossi S, Marabese M, Broggini M, Giordano R, D'Erasmo M, Montelatici E, et al. Oct-4 expression in adult human differentiated cells challenges its role as a pure stem cell marker. Stem Cells. 2007;25(7):1675–80.
23. Guo ZK, Guo K, Luo H, Mu LM, Li Q, Chang YQ. The expression analysis of nanog in the developing rat myocardial tissues. Cellular Physiology Biochemistry : InterJ Experimental Cellular Physiology, Biochemistry, Pharmacology. 2015;35(3):866–74.
24. Luo H, Li Q, Pramanik J, Luo J, Guo Z. Nanog expression in heart tissues induced by acute myocardial infarction. Histol Histopathol. 2014;29(10):1287–93.
25. Gibbs CP, Kukekov VG, Reith JD, Tchigrinova O, Suslov ON, Scott EW, et al. Stem-like cells in bone sarcomas: implications for tumorigenesis. Neoplasia. 2005;7(11):967–76.
26. Levings PP, McGarry SV, Currie TP, Nickerson DM, McClellan S, Ghivizzani SC, et al. Expression of an exogenous human Oct-4 promoter identifies tumor-initiating cells in osteosarcoma. Cancer Res. 2009;69(14):5648–55.
27. Wu C, Wei Q, Utomo V, Nadesan P, Whetstone H, Kandel R, et al. Side population cells isolated from mesenchymal neoplasms have tumor initiating potential. Cancer Res. 2007;67(17):8216–22.
28. Martins-Neves SR, Lopes AO, do Carmo A, Paiva AA, Simoes PC, Abrunhosa AJ, et al. Therapeutic implications of an enriched cancer stem-like cell population in a human osteosarcoma cell line. BMC Cancer. 2012;12:139.
29. Suva ML, Riggi N, Stehle JC, Baumer K, Tercier S, Joseph JM, et al. Identification of cancer stem cells in Ewing's sarcoma. Cancer Res. 2009;69(5):1776–81.
30. Salerno M, Avnet S, Bonuccelli G, Hosogi S, Granchi D, Baldini N. Impairment of lysosomal activity as a therapeutic modality targeting cancer stem cells of embryonal rhabdomyosarcoma cell line RD. PLoS One. 2014;9(10), e110340.
31. Riggi N, Suva ML, De Vito C, Provero P, Stehle JC, Baumer K, et al. EWS-FLI-1 modulates miRNA145 and SOX2 expression to initiate mesenchymal stem cell reprogramming toward Ewing sarcoma cancer stem cells. Genes Dev. 2010;24(9):916–32.
32. Gorden BH, Saha J, Khammanivong A, Schwartz GK, Dickerson EB. Lysosomal drug sequestration as a mechanism of drug resistance in vascular sarcoma cells marked by high CSF-1R expression. Vascular Cell. 2014;6:20.
33. Khammanivong A, Gorden BH, Frantz AM, Graef AJ, Dickerson EB. Identification of drug-resistant subpopulations in canine hemangiosarcoma. Vet Comp Oncol. 2014. doi:10.1111/vco.12114.
34. Kurisetty V, Bryan BA. Aberrations in Angiogenic Signaling and MYC Amplifications are Distinguishing Features of Angiosarcoma. Angiology: Open access. 2013;1.

35. Guo T, Zhang L, Chang NE, Singer S, Maki RG, Antonescu CR. Consistent MYC and FLT4 gene amplification in radiation-induced angiosarcoma but not in other radiation-associated atypical vascular lesions. Genes Chromosomes Cancer. 2011;50(1):25–33.

36. Mentzel T, Schildhaus HU, Palmedo G, Buttner R, Kutzner H. Postradiation cutaneous angiosarcoma after treatment of breast carcinoma is characterized by MYC amplification in contrast to atypical vascular lesions after radiotherapy and control cases: clinicopathological, immunohistochemical and molecular analysis of 66 cases. Modern Pathol : Off J US Canadian Acad Pathol, Inc. 2012;25(1):75–85.

37. Hadj-Hamou NS, Lae M, Almeida A, de la Grange P, Kirova Y, Sastre-Garau X, et al. A transcriptome signature of endothelial lymphatic cells coexists with the chronic oxidative stress signature in radiation-induced post-radiotherapy breast angiosarcomas. Carcinogenesis. 2012;33(7):1399–405.

38. Italiano A, Chen CL, Thomas R, Breen M, Bonnet F, Sevenet N, et al. Alterations of the p53 and PIK3CA/AKT/mTOR pathways in angiosarcomas: a pattern distinct from other sarcomas with complex genomics. Cancer. 2012;118(23):5878–87.

39. Tran D, Verma K, Ward K, Diaz D, Kataria E, Torabi A, et al. Functional genomics analysis reveals a MYC signature associated with a poor clinical prognosis in liposarcomas. Am J Pathol. 2015;185(3):717–28.

# 26

# Liver cancer with concomitant *TP53* and *CTNNB1* mutations

Juliane Friemel[1,2], Markus Rechsteiner[1], Marion Bawohl[1], Lukas Frick[1,4], Beat Müllhaupt[3], Mickaël Lesurtel[4] and Achim Weber[1*]

## Abstract

**Background:** In the spectrum of molecular alterations found in hepatocellular carcinoma (HCC), somatic mutations in the WNT/β-catenin pathway and the p53/cell cycle control pathway are among the most frequent ones. It has been suggested that both mutations occur in a mutually exclusive manner and they are used as molecular classifiers in HCC classification proposals.

**Case presentation:** Here, we report the case of a treatment-naïve mixed hepatocellular/cholangiocellular carcinoma (HCC/CCC) with morphological and genetic intratumor heterogeneity. Within the predominant part of the tumor with hepatocellular differentiation, a p.D32V mutation in exon 3 of the *CTNNB1* gene occurred concomitantly with a *TP53* intron 7/exon 8 splice site mutation.

**Conclusion:** Intratumor heterogeneity challenges the concept of *CTNNB1* and *TP53* gene mutations being mutually exclusive molecular classifiers in HCC, which has implications for HCC classification approaches.

**Keywords:** Hepatocellular carcinoma (HCC), Intratumor heterogeneity, *CTNNB1*, *TP53*, Next generation sequencing

## Background

Hepatocellular carcinoma (HCC) is the fifths most common cancer in men and the second most common cause for cancer-related death worldwide [1]. HCC mostly develop on the background of chronic liver diseases including chronic viral hepatitis due to infection with hepatitis B virus (HBV), or hepatitis C virus (HCV), alcohol-induced liver injury, fatty liver disease or exposure to toxic factors such as aflatoxin. The spectrum of somatic mutations related to liver carcinogenesis has been identified [2]. With marked geographic variation, *TP53* and *CTNNB1* represent two of the most common driver mutations in the African-Asian countries (*TP53*) and in the western world (*CTNNB1*). Several molecular classifications of HCC distinguish HCC with alterations in the p53/cell cycle control pathway from HCCs with alterations in the WNT/β-catenin pathway, including activating mutations of the *CTNNB1* oncogene, *AXIN1* or

*APC* [3, 4]. Mutations of *TP53* and *CTNNB1* are largely considered to occur in a mutually exclusive manner [5]. Phenotypical and genetic intratumor heterogeneity with variable mutational status (i.e. wild type among mutated tumor cell clones) of *TP53* and *CTNNB1* in different tumor regions within the same tumor is frequently found in HCC [6]. Here, we describe a *de novo*, hepatitis C-related combined cholangiocellular and hepatocellular carcinoma with marked intratumor heterogeneity on three levels: morphology, immunohistochemical marker profile and mutational status with 3/14 tumor regions of solely hepatocellular differentiation harboring concomitant mutations of *CTNNB1* and *TP53*.

## Case presentation

A liver tumor was detected in a 72 year old male patient with liver cirrhosis Child-Pugh Stage A, a history of type 2 diabetes and chronic hepatitis C virus infection (HCV, genotype 1B), initially diagnosed 13 years ago. Liver enzymes were slightly elevated with alanine aminotransferase 89 U/L (reference: 10–50 U/L) and aspartate aminotransferase 65 U/L (reference: <50 U/L). The 4 cm tumor was detected by routine sonography and removed by laparoscopic liver segment resection.

* Correspondence: achim.weber@usz.ch
[1]Institute of Surgical Pathology, University and University Hospital Zurich, Schmelzbergstrasse 12, 8091 Zurich, Switzerland
Full list of author information is available at the end of the article

Morphological analysis, immunohistochemistry and multiregional, next generation sequencing (NGS) was applied on representative tumor sections as described [6]. Table 1 and Fig. 1 illustrate histopathological and molecular findings in 14 individual tumor areas, which were grouped into three tumor regions (A, B and C) according to their predominant morphological and molecular characteristics. In summary, a multinodular, combined hepatocellular/cholangiocellular carcinoma, tumor stage T1 grade 2–3, was diagnosed. Intratumoral heterogeneous expression of five liver cell markers (CK7, CK19, glutamine synthetase, p53, β-catenin) was detected including a double positivity for glutamine synthetase, nuclear β-catenin and p53 in tumor region A.

Next generation sequencing was performed with a minimum coverage of 1329 (SD ± 725) reads per amplicon of every single tumor area. Sequencing results yielded a p.D32V (c.363 A > T) mutation and a TP53 ivs8-1 (c.783-1 G > A) splice site mutation in tumor region A. Comparing mutated allele frequencies, CTNNB1 and TP53 gene copies showed a similar range of both frequencies in area A1-3 (Fig. 1). All mutated and wild type tumor areas additionally displayed a SNP of exon 7 (rs17880604). Collectively, morphological and immunohistochemical findings together with sequencing results demonstrated that a tumor subclone with hepatocellular differentiation had concomitant CTNNB1 and TP53 gene mutations.

To date, after a follow-up time of 12 months, the patient had a local recurrence of a liver tumor which was inoperable and therefore treated by transarterial chemoembolization (TACE).

## Conclusion

In this case of a HCV infection -related liver cancer, a CTNNB1/TP53 double mutation was detected in a tumor region of hepatocellular differentiation, among TP53 and CTNNB1 wild type tumor areas. The analysis of mutated allele frequencies using next generation sequencing techniques corroborates that the double mutation is located in the same tumor cell population. To our knowledge, this is the first detailed description of a CTNNB1/TP53 double mutation in a single liver cancer lesion. TP53 and CTNNB1 both are molecular classifiers for hepatocellular carcinoma. For instance, in the transcriptome-analysis based classification proposal by Boyault et al. [4], six HCC subgroups are distinguished: two groups are characterized by TP53 and two independent groups by CTNNB1 alterations. A study by Laurent-Puig et al. [5] on genetic alterations in hepatocarcinogenesis describes TP53 and CTNNB1 mutations as mutually exclusive. In agreement, a study by Tornesello et al. [7] records mutations of the two driver genes as being mutually exclusive.

CTNNB1 mutations are reported to be associated with hepatitis C infections [8]. TP53 point mutations frequently are reported to occur specifically at codon 249 after aflatoxin exposition. The frequency and the causal link between TP53 and CTNNB1 mutations in HCC have not been systematically investigated. A study by Öztürk et al. [9] on HCC cell lines provides evidence that inactivation of TP53 could cause aberrant nuclear β-catenin accumulation, suggesting a link between the two genes. In the presented case study, the CTNNB1 mutation affected the GSK-3β phosphorylation site [10] which argues for a β-catenin accumulation independent

**Table 1** Morphology, immunohistochemistry and mutational status of individual tumor areas

| | Area | A1 | A2 | A3 | B | C1 | C2 | C3 | C4 | C5 | C6 | C7 | C8 | C9 | C10 |
|---|---|---|---|---|---|---|---|---|---|---|---|---|---|---|---|
| | Size in mm$^2$ | 7.8 | 5.54 | 31.3 | 65 | 73.2 | 16.5 | 34.5 | 82.2 | 20.2 | 18.9 | 17.4 | 28.5 | 1.94 | 17.5 |
| Morphology | Solid | + | + | + | | + | + | + | | + | + | | + | | |
| | Glandular (cholangiocellular) | | | | + | | | | | | | | | | |
| | Trabecular | | | | | | + | + | | | | + | | + | + |
| | Clear cell change | | + | | | + | | | | | | | | | + |
| | Fatty change | | | | | | | | | | | + | | | |
| | CK19 | | | | | >50 % | >50 % | | | | | | | | |
| IC | CK7 | | | | | 70 % | SC | 50 % | 20 % | SC | 40 % | SC | | SC | 50 % |
| | glutamine synthetase | + | + | + | | | | | | | | | | | |
| | β-catenin nuclear | + | + | + | | | | | | | | | | | |
| | p53 | + | + | + | | | | | | | | | | | |
| Mutation | CTNNB1 sanger seq | D32 | D32 | wt | wt | wt | wt | wt | wt | wt | wt | wt | wt | wt | wt |
| | CTNNB1 deep seq | D32 | D32 | D32$^a$ | wt | wt | wt | wt | wt | wt | wt | wt | wt | wt | wt |
| | TP53 sanger seq | IVS8-1 | IVS8-1 | wt | wt | wt | wt | wt | wt | wt | wt | wt | wt | wt | wt |
| | TP53 deep seq | IVS8-1 | IVS8-1 | IVS8-1$^a$ | wt | wt | wt | wt | wt | wt | wt | wt | wt | wt | wt |

*sanger seq* sanger sequencing, *deep seq* deep sequencing (NGS), *wt* wild type, *SC* single cells positive
[a]low frequency (<10 %)

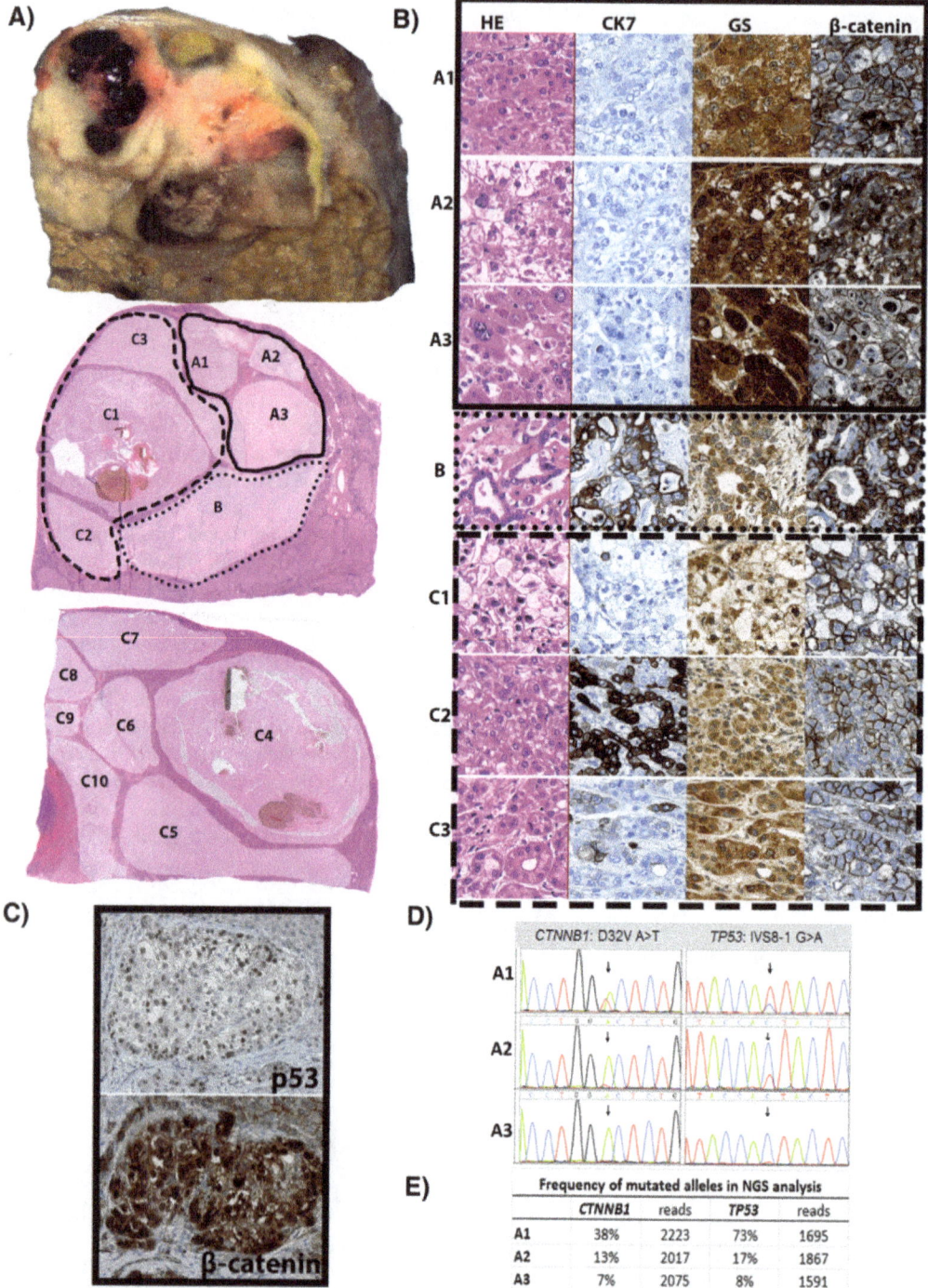

**Fig. 1** Combined HCC/CCC in a 72 year old male patient with history of hepatitis C and diabetes revealing morphological, immunohistochemical and genetic intratumor heterogeneity. **a** Gross morphology and slide overview (H&E staining) with annotations of defined tumor areas. **b** Microscopic images (40x) of different tumor areas (H&E staining, CK7, glutamine synthetase and β-catenin immunohistochemistry). **c** p53 and β-catenin nuclear positivity in consecutive slides of tumor area A2. **d** Nucleotide exchanges in *CTNNB1* and *TP53* genes (*TP53* depicted as reverse sequence). **e** Mutated allele frequencies of double mutated areas A1-3 with number of gene copies analyzed. Reference sequences: NM 1904.1 (*CTNNB1*) and NM 001126112.2 (*TP53*)

from the *TP53* mutation. The detected *TP53* mutation affects a splice site of exon 8. Although splice sites in *TP53* are not typical mutation sites, there is evidence that *TP53* splicing mutations lead to exon dropping indicating biological relevance [11]. Furthermore, the nuclear accumulation of the dysfunctional p53 protein in immunohistochemical analysis found in this case supports a functional significance of this splice site mutation. As has been reported, wild type p53 is rapidly degraded while mutations lead to nuclear accumulation of the p53 protein [12, 13].

In summary, the molecular, immunohistochemical and morphological diversity in the presented case indicates a high level of intratumor heterogeneity and challenges the concept that *TP53* and *CTNNB1* are mutually exclusive driver alterations in HCC. Distinct parts of the tumor reveal multinodularity, and differ with respect to their biomarker expression and mutational status, indicative of distinct tumor subpopulations [14]. This finding illustrates the challenge to molecularly characterize individual HCC. Routine pathological analysis is based on testing a small piece of a tumor, assuming that it represents the whole tumor. When analyzing distinct pathways of hepatocarcinogenesis such as the WNT/β-catenin pathway as a potential therapeutic target in HCC [15], it will be pivotal in the future to also take into account the level of intratumor heterogeneity.

## Abbreviations

CCC, cholangiocellular carcinoma; CTNNB1, Catenin β 1; HCC, hepatocellular carcinoma; TACE, transarterial chemoembolization; TP53, tumor protein 53

## Acknowledgements

We gratefully thank the patient and family members for allowing us to report this case.

## Funding

This work was supported by the following grants: A grant from the Theiler-Haag Stiftung, Zurich to AW and LF. Grants from the Krebsliga Schweiz (Oncosuisse) and from the "Kurt and Senta Herrmann Stiftung", Vaduz, Lichtenstein to AW.

## Authors' contributions

Conception: AW. Methods: JF, LF, MR, MB. Patient care and surgery: ML, BM. Writing of the manuscript: JF and AW. Critical revision of the manuscript: LF, ML, BM, AW, JF, MB. All authors read and approved the final manuscript.

## Authors' information

AW is Professor for Experimental and Molecular Pathology at the University (UZH) and University-Hospital (USZ) Zurich.

## Competing interests

The authors declare that they have no competing interests.

## Consent for publication

Written informed consent was obtained from the patient for publication of this case report and any accompanying images. A copy of the written consent is available for review by the Editor of this journal.

## Ethics approval and consent to participate

Ethical approval for the study was given by the local ethics commitee (StV 26–2005 and KEK-ZH-Nr. 2013–0382).

## Author details

[1]Institute of Surgical Pathology, University and University Hospital Zurich, Schmelzbergstrasse 12, 8091 Zurich, Switzerland. [2]Leibniz Institute for Prevention Research and Epidemiology (BIPS), Bremen, Germany. [3]Clinics of Hepatology and Gastroenterology, University and University Hospital Zurich, Zurich, Switzerland. [4]Swiss Hepato-Pancreato-Biliary Center, Department of Digestive and Transplant Surgery, University Hospital of Zurich, Zurich, Switzerland.

## References

1. Ferlay J, Soerjomataram I, Dikshit R, Eser S, Mathers C, Rebelo M, Parkin DM, Forman D, Bray F. Cancer incidence and mortality worldwide: sources, methods and major patterns in GLOBOCAN 2012. Int J Cancer. 2015;136(5): E359–86.
2. Nault JC, Mallet M, Pilati C, Calderaro J, Bioulac-Sage P, Laurent C, Laurent A, Cherqui D, Balabaud C, Zucman-Rossi J. High frequency of telomerase reverse-transcriptase promoter somatic mutations in hepatocellular carcinoma and preneoplastic lesions. Nat Commun. 2013;4:2218.
3. Guichard C, Amaddeo G, Imbeaud S, Ladeiro Y, Pelletier L, Maad IB, Calderaro J, Bioulac-Sage P, Letexier M, Degos F, et al. Integrated analysis of somatic mutations and focal copy-number changes identifies key genes and pathways in hepatocellular carcinoma. Nat Genet. 2012;44(6):694–8.
4. Boyault S, Rickman DS, de Reynies A, Balabaud C, Rebouissou S, Jeannot E, Herault A, Saric J, Belghiti J, Franco D, et al. Transcriptome classification of HCC is related to gene alterations and to new therapeutic targets. Hepatology. 2007;45(1):42–52.
5. Laurent-Puig P, Legoix P, Bluteau O, Belghiti J, Franco D, Binot F, Monges G, Thomas G, Bioulac-Sage P, Zucman-Rossi J. Genetic alterations associated with hepatocellular carcinomas define distinct pathways of hepatocarcinogenesis. Gastroenterology. 2001;120(7):1763–73.
6. Friemel J, Rechsteiner M, Frick L, Bohm F, Struckmann K, Egger M, Moch H, Heikenwalder M, Weber A. Intratumor heterogeneity in hepatocellular carcinoma. Clin Cancer Res. 2015;21(8):1951–61.
7. Tornesello ML, Buonaguro L, Tatangelo F, Botti G, Izzo F, Buonaguro FM. Mutations in TP53, CTNNB1 and PIK3CA genes in hepatocellular carcinoma associated with hepatitis B and hepatitis C virus infections. Genomics. 2013; 102(2):74–83.
8. Huang H, Fujii H, Sankila A, Mahler-Araujo BM, Matsuda M, Cathomas G, Ohgaki H. Beta-catenin mutations are frequent in human hepatocellular carcinomas associated with hepatitis C virus infection. Am J Pathol. 1999; 155(6):1795–801.
9. Cagatay T, Ozturk M. P53 mutation as a source of aberrant beta-catenin accumulation in cancer cells. Oncogene. 2002;21(52):7971–80.
10. de La Coste A, Romagnolo B, Billuart P, Renard CA, Buendia MA, Soubrane O, Fabre M, Chelly J, Beldjord C, Kahn A, et al. Somatic mutations of the beta-catenin gene are frequent in mouse and human hepatocellular carcinomas. Proc Natl Acad Sci U S A. 1998;95(15):8847–51.
11. Lai MY, Chang HC, Li HP, Ku CK, Chen PJ, Sheu JC, Huang GT, Lee PH, Chen DS. Splicing mutations of the p53 gene in human hepatocellular carcinoma. Cancer Res. 1993;53(7):1653–6.
12. Hsu HC, Tseng HJ, Lai PL, Lee PH, Peng SY. Expression of p53 gene in 184 unifocal hepatocellular carcinomas: association with tumor growth and invasiveness. Cancer Res. 1993;53(19):4691–4.
13. Chen GG, Merchant JL, Lai PB, Ho RL, Hu X, Okada M, Huang SF, Chui AK, Law DJ, Li YG, et al. Mutation of p53 in recurrent hepatocellular carcinoma and its association with the expression of ZBP-89. Am J Pathol. 2003;162(6): 1823–9.
14. Kanai T, Hirohashi S, Upton MP, Noguchi M, Kishi K, Makuuchi M, Yamasaki S, Hasegawa H, Takayasu K, Moriyama N, et al. Pathology of small hepatocellular carcinoma. A proposal for a new gross classification. Cancer. 1987;60(4):810–9.
15. Park JY, Park WS, Nam SW, Kim SY, Lee SH, Yoo NJ, Lee JY, Park CK. Mutations of beta-catenin and AXIN I genes are a late event in human hepatocellular carcinogenesis. Liver Int. 2005;25(1):70–6.

# 27

# Length of prostate biopsies is not necessarily compromised by pooling multiple cores in one paraffin block

Teemu T Tolonen[1,2]*, Jorma Isola[2], Antti Kaipia[3,4], Jarno Riikonen[4], Laura Koivusalo[3,5], Sanna Huovinen[1], Marita Laurila[1], Sinikka Porre[1], Mika Tirkkonen[1] and Paula Kujala[1]

## Abstract

**Background:** Individually submitted prostatic needle biopsies are recommended by most guidelines because of their potential advantage in terms of core quality. However, unspecified bilateral biopsies are commonly submitted in many centers. The length of the core is the key quality indicator of prostate biopsies. Because there are few recent publications comparing the quality of 12 site-designated biopsies versus pooled biopsies, we compared the lengths of the biopsies obtained by both methods.

**Methods:** The material was obtained from 471 consecutive subjects who underwent prostatic needle biopsy in the Tampere University Hospital district between January and June 2013. Biopsies from 344 subjects fulfilled the inclusion criteria. The total number of cores obtained was 4047. The core lengths were measured on microscope slides. Extraprostatic tissue was subtracted from the core length.

**Results:** The aggregate lengths observed were $129.5 \pm 21.8$ mm (mean $\pm$ SD) for site-designated cores and $136.9 \pm 26.4$ mm for pooled cores ($p = 0.09$). The length of the core was $10.8 \pm 1.8$ mm for site-designated cores and $11.4 \pm 2.2$ mm for pooled cores ($p = 0.87$). The median length for pooled cores was 11 mm (range 5 mm – 18 mm). For individual site-designated cores, the median length was 11 mm (range 7 mm –15 mm). The core length was not correlated with the number of cores embedded into one paraffin block ($r = 0.015$). There was no significant difference in cancer detection rate ($p = 0.62$).

**Conclusions:** Our results suggest that unspecified bilateral biopsies do not automatically lead to reduced core length. We conclude that carefully embedded multiple (three to nine) cores per block may yield cores of equal quality in a more cost-efficient way and that current guidelines favoring individually submitted cores may be too strict.

**Keywords:** Prostate cancer, Prostatic needle biopsies, Biopsy quality, Guidelines

## Background

The diagnosis of prostatic adenocarcinoma is based on the histopathological findings obtained from prostatic needle biopsies. There is a lot of debate on the best protocol for submitting and labeling of prostate biopsies. According to several current guidelines, individual site-designated biopsies submitted in separate vials are preferred, as they are thought to give better quality samples in terms of tissue fragmentation as well as core length [1,2]. However, it is a common practice to submit unspecified bilateral biopsies both in the U.S. and in Europe [3,4]. The length of the biopsy core is the key quality indicator of a successful biopsy, which influences cancer detection rates and the estimation of prognostic parameters [5-7]. Currently, the recommended procedure is to take five to six biopsies from each side [1,2]. Specifically, additional laterally targeted biopsies have been shown to detect 31% more cancers when compared to the sextant biopsy protocol [5]. The role of augmented biopsy protocols is still controversial. It has been suggested that there is no advantage to taking extended

* Correspondence: teemu.tolonen@fimlab.fi
[1]Department of Pathology, Fimlab Laboratories, Tampere University Hospital, Tampere, Finland
[2]Department of Cancer Biology, Institute of Biomedical Technology, University of Tampere, Tampere, Finland
Full list of author information is available at the end of the article

(20 cores) or saturation biopsies (24 cores) in the initial biopsy [8,9]. However, a recent meta-analysis has shown that initial diagnostic saturation biopsies may be warranted for patients with low PSA-values or high-volume prostates [10].

In terms of biopsy quality, it has been suggested that up to three cores could be safely embedded in one paraffin block without compromising the biopsy quality [11]. Currently, approximately half of the pathology laboratories in Europe receive unspecified bilateral biopsies together with individually submitted targeted biopsies from a distinct nodule, while only 40% of laboratories receive all biopsies in separate vials [4]. In the U.S., it is slightly more common to submit site-designated biopsies [3]. Compared to pooled biopsies, a submission of 12 site-designated biopsy cores by the urologist increases the workload for pathology laboratories. The advantage of site-designated biopsies is that localization information is spared, which is important for active surveillance follow-up protocols and helps the urologist to plan surgeries. The quality of needle biopsies is operator dependent, but the main result (i.e., how the tissue looks on a slide) is also dependent upon the pathology laboratory [12]. A recent guideline by the pathology committee of the European Randomized Study of Screening for Prostate Cancer (ERSPC) highlights the importance of special techniques in processing and (pre-)embedding for preserving the quality of the biopsy [13]. Such techniques include the use of sponges to flatten the cores during fixation and dehydration, and the use of metal tampers for the embedding process.

The aim of this study was to determine whether there is a quality difference between site-designated individually embedded and unspecified bilateral (pooled) biopsies, using core length as the main quality indicator and cancer detection rate as a secondary measure. It was hypothesized, that pooling samples in the same biopsy container and resulting paraffin block does not affect the quality of the biopsy. Pooling biopsies reduces the workload of laboratory technicians and pathologists, so if pooled samples are of similar quality than site-designated biopsies, it would be possible to get the same results with less effort.

## Methods

The study was approved by the Ethical Committee of Tampere University Hospital (TAUH), reference number R03203. The material was obtained from 471 consecutive prostate biopsies submitted to Fimlab Laboratories for evaluation during a half year period from January to June 2013. The biopsies were taken in the Tampere University Hospital (TAUH) district by several urologists under standard operating procedure. All the obtained prostate biopsies were evaluated with the following inclusion criteria: 1) the biopsy was reported by one of our five uropathologists (ML, MT, SH, PK, TT), 2) the biopsies were comprised of either 12 individually submitted cores or bilateral pooled biopsies submitted in two formalin vials (plus an extra vial containing one core from a distinct nodule in some cases), and 3) all cores were measured in millimeters and reported in a standardized manner (see later section). Biopsies from 344 subjects fulfilled the inclusion criteria and yielded a total number of 4047 biopsy cores. All of the accepted site-designated biopsies consisted of a set of 12 biopsy containers with a single biopsy inside, except for one case in which only 11 containers were submitted because there were erroneously two biopsies in one vial. A total of 127 cases were excluded. Although it met the inclusion criteria, one case with 12 individually processed cores containing only 20 mm intraprostatic tissue was excluded as a statistical outlier. The inclusion procedure is presented schematically in Figure 1.

All biopsies were taken transrectally with ultrasonography guidance using an 18-gauge needle biopsy gun with an 18-mm sample notch (Bard peripheral vascular, Temple, AZ, U.S.A., ref no. MC 1825) and a side-fire probe. Biopsies were put into vials containing 10% neutral-buffered formalin straight from the biopsy needle. Biopsies from a single patient were transported to our laboratory either in 12 separate vials or in two vials containing several biopsy cores (median number of cores per container was six). The number of submitted vials depended on how the urologist performed the prostate biopsy. All biopsies were processed in Fimlab Laboratories, Tampere University Hospital, in Tampere, Finland.

Site-designated individual biopsies were transferred to separate tissue cassettes in which they were straightened (not stretched) and flattened between sponges during standard dehydration and microwave processing. Pooled biopsies from one vial were treated equally but remained pooled (e.g., multiple straightened cores were sandwiched between sponges into one cassette). Two to four sections were cut from the individual cores and transferred to one slide, depending on the technologist's visual impression. Because pooled biopsies may have more planar variation inside the paraffin blocks, they were cut on four levels which resulted in the generation of two slides. The blocks were not cut through and step sections were not collected because our current protocol offers residual material for potential immunostaining in most cases.

The lengths of the biopsy cores were collected from pathology reports. For individually processed biopsies, the lengths were reported for each biopsy core in millimeters. The 12 loci of individual biopsies were standardized as follows: 1–3 were right lateral base, mid and apex, 4–6 were right medial base, mid and apex, 7–9

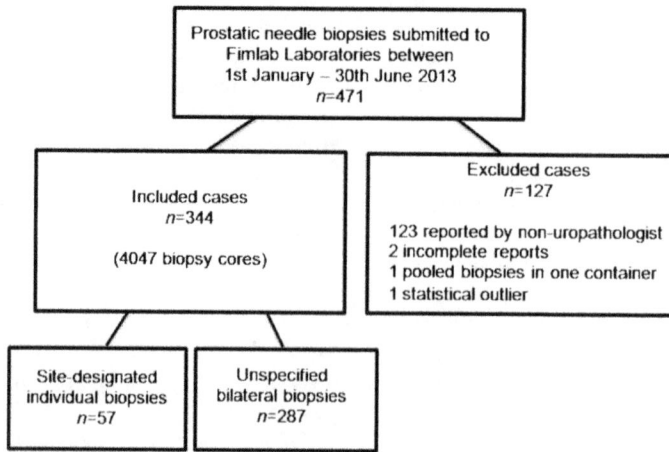

**Figure 1 Study flow chart.** The inclusion criteria were as follows: 1. the biopsy was reported by an uropathologist, 2. bilateral pooled biopsies in two formalin vials or 12 individually submitted cores, 3. the core lengths were measured and reported in millimeters in a standardized manner.

were left lateral base, mid and apex, and 10–12 were left medial base, mid and apex, respectively. The current scheme for site-specific needle biopsies in the TAUH district is presented in Figure 2. In the case of multiple biopsies per paraffin block, the information regarding the number of biopsies in the block and the total length of the biopsies in millimeters was required. Separately submitted additional cores targeting a region of palpable resistance were excluded from the length measurements but were included in the cancer detection rate. The length of the core and the possible length of the cancerous tissue were measured from hematoxylin-eosin (H&E) -stained slides either under a light microscope as multiples of 4x/10x objectives visual field diameter or by a liner, depending on the extent of the cancer. According to our standardized protocol, extraprostatic tissue was subtracted from the total core length to obtain the most

accurate percentage of cancer. Tissue was considered extraprostatic when containing obvious fat or loose mesenchymal tissue that was distinct from the (pseudo)capsule. For cancerous prostates, a standardized scoring table was applied. The recorded parameters included primary and secondary Gleason patterns, the number of positive cores/total number of cores, cancer length/total length, the percentage of cancer, high grade prostatic intraepithelial neoplasia, and perineural invasion. The microscopic appearance of slides with individually embedded and pooled biopsies are represented in Figure 3.

### Statistical analysis

Data were analyzed using a two-tailed Wilcoxon-Mann–Whitney test to compare aggregate and single biopsy length means and a two-tailed Fisher's exact test to compare cancer detection rates. The impact of the number of cores embedded in a single paraffin block on the mean length of cores in the corresponding block was tested using Pearson's correlation coefficient analysis. Statistical significance was considered at $p < 0.05$.

### Results

Individual site-designated biopsies were submitted to our laboratory in 57 (16.6%) cases, and non-specified (pooled) bilateral biopsies were submitted in 287 (83.4%) cases. Of the pooled biopsies, exactly six plus six cores from the right and left sides were obtained 188 (65.5%) times. More than 12 biopsies were submitted in 38 (13.2%) cases, and less than 10 biopsies were submitted in 18 (6.2%) cases. The minimum number of biopsy cores per subject was 6 (n = 1), and the maximum number was 15 (n = 7).

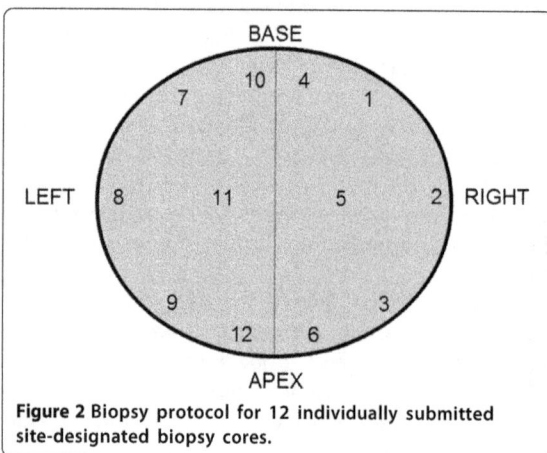

**Figure 2** Biopsy protocol for 12 individually submitted site-designated biopsy cores.

Length of prostate biopsies is not necessarily compromised by pooling multiple cores in one...

221

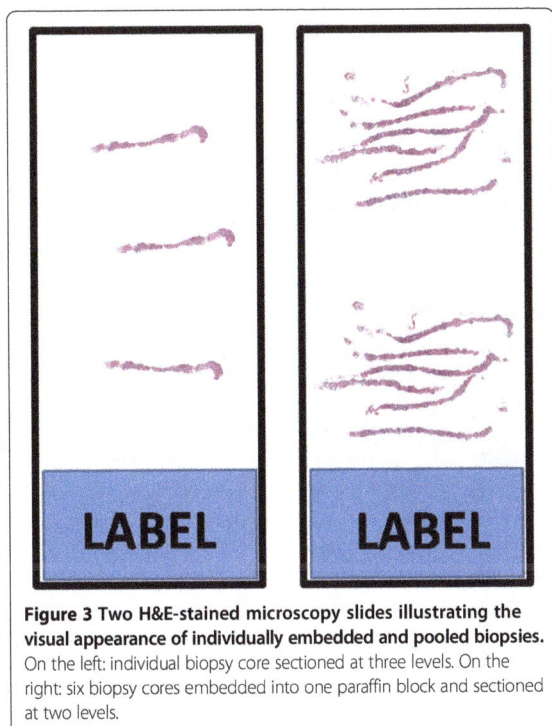

**Figure 3 Two H&E-stained microscopy slides illustrating the visual appearance of individually embedded and pooled biopsies.** On the left: individual biopsy core sectioned at three levels. On the right: six biopsy cores embedded into one paraffin block and sectioned at two levels.

The mean aggregate length of all biopsy cores from one subject was $133.6 \pm 29.9$ mm (mean ± SD). No statistically significant difference in the mean aggregate lengths was noted between site-designated and pooled (6 + 6) biopsies or between benign and malignant biopsies (Table 1).

The average core length was $11.4 \pm 2.2$ mm for pooled biopsies and $10.8 \pm 1.8$ mm for individually processed cores (p = 0.87). The median length for pooled cores was 11 mm (range 5 mm - 18 mm). For individual site-designated cores the median length was 11 mm (range 7 mm - 15 mm). Because the number of biopsy cores in the vials varied from 1 to 9, we also tested whether increasing the number of cores in a paraffin block would have an adverse effect on the mean length of the cores

**Table 1 Comparison of aggregate lengths of the biopsy cores**

|  | n | Aggregate length, mm (mean ± SD) |
|---|---|---|
| All | 344 | 133.6 ± 29.9 |
| Site-designated | 57 | 129.5 ± 21.8[1] |
| Pooled 6 + 6 | 188 | 136.9 ± 26.4[1] |
| Benign | 151 | 132.7 ± 29.3[2] |
| Malignant | 193 | 134.2 ± 30.4[2] |

[1]No statistically significant difference was noted between 12 site-designated cores and unspecified bilateral (6 + 6) cores, p = 0.09.
[2]No statistically significant difference was noted between benign and malignant cases, p = 0.25.

as one might expect. However, no correlation was noted (Table 2).

The overall cancer detection rate was 55.8%. Adenocarcinoma was detected in 28/57 (49.1%) cases with site-designated biopsies and in 164/287 (57.1%) cases with pooled biopsies (p = 0.62).

## Discussion

A recent survey regarding the handling of prostate biopsies by the European Network for Uropathologists (ENUP) showed that there is a wide diversity among European pathology centers in the handling of prostate biopsy specimens [4]. The number of biopsy cores taken, the number of cores in a formalin vial, and the (pre-)embedding methods are all variable. Multiple biopsies per vial (and paraffin block) were used in approximately half of the centers that participated in the survey, which is not recommended due to a presumption that tissue quality will be compromised. In our study, there was no difference in the lengths of biopsies regardless of whether they were processed individually or pooled. Furthermore, cancer detection rates were approximately equal between the groups. The slightly lower cancer detection rate noted in individually processed biopsies may be related to the different indications for a biopsy procedure between the groups. However, the observed overall cancer detection rate of 55.8% is quite high. Previously, in a Finnish prostate cancer screening study conducted as a part of the European Randomized Study of Screening for Prostate Cancer (ERSPC), the observed cancer detection rate at a PSA cutoff level of 4 µg/l was found to be 27% [14].

There are several possible reasons for the high cancer detection rate observed in this study. The population included in the study has a relatively high PSA screening frequency due to the prostate cancer screening trial.

**Table 2 The impact of the number of biopsy cores embedded into one paraffin block to the mean length of cores in the corresponding block[1]**

| No. of cores in paraffin block | n | Length of cores, mm (mean ± SD) |
|---|---|---|
| 1 | 684 | 10.8 ± 1.8 |
| 3 | 8 | 12.9 ± 2.1 |
| 4 | 20 | 10.6 ± 2.7 |
| 5 | 75 | 11.0 ± 2.9 |
| 6 | 417 | 11.5 ± 2.4 |
| 7 | 40 | 11.8 ± 2.5 |
| 8 | 10 | 11.5 ± 2.1 |
| 9 | 2 | 11.1 ± 1.2 |

[1]The length of biopsies was not correlated to the number of cores in the block, r = 0.015.

Some of the patients may have PSA data going back to the start of screening trial in 1996, which has lead to a higher threshold for taking biopsies. Also, the PSA value is no longer considered the only indication for taking a prostate biopsy; more significance is given to the value of free PSA per total PSA. Another reason for the high cancer detection rate may be that some of biopsies are taken from patients in an active follow-up. Finally, there might be skewness in the results due to the inclusion criteria. Benign biopsies are not always reported with the same accuracy as cancer cases, and this inaccuracy in reporting of biopsy length may have disqualified some benign cases from inclusion in this study. Also, urgent cases with a high suspicion of cancer are more likely to be reported by one of the uropathologists conducting the study, which may increase the overall cancer detection percentage.

Our results suggest that the problems encountered with multiple biopsies in one container can be overcome by special tissue pre-embedding methods, including straightening and flattening the cores between sponges before tissue processing and by paying attention to the laboratory technologist's education. According to the ERSPC pathology committee's newest guidelines, up to three cores can be safely embedded in a single paraffin block without significant tissue loss [13]. Our results suggest that the maximum number of cores that can safely be embedded in a single paraffin block may be a matter of technique – if one is able to embed single cores well enough, why would it not work for the core next to it? In fact, in one of our earlier experiments, we embedded twelve biopsies in one paraffin block and obtained a satisfactory visual appearance. However, the technique was abandoned because there were two obvious disadvantages: the orientation of the biopsies in the paraffin block needed to be diagonal instead of longitudinal which made sectioning more difficult, and the tips of the cores stayed outside of the staining area of the automated immunostaining system due to their marginal position.

According to Bostwick et al., the mean length of prostate biopsies in Western Europe was 13.1 mm at the entry level of their study [12]. In the present study, the mean length of the core was shorter (11.4 mm). However, the aforementioned values are not comparable because in our study extraprostatic tissue was subtracted to obtain the most accurate percentage of cancer tissue possible.

It is likely that the most important advantage of individually embedded biopsies is not the biopsy core quality but rather the spared locus information. This is an important issue in selected cases, and site-designated biopsies should be encouraged. On the other hand, the use of multiple biopsies per vial (and paraffin block) is

supported by less extensive laboratory loading and better facilities for immunohistochemistry. Our medium-sized laboratory receives biopsies from approximately 1000 patients per year. Widespread use of site-designated biopsies would annually increase the number of paraffin blocks by approximately 10,000, which increases the workload for the pathology laboratory throughout various steps including processing, embedding, sectioning and analyzing. Roughly estimated this would take approximately 80 working days for sectioning only and would increase the time pathologists spend analyzing and reporting prostate biopsies (Figure 4).

There are several limitations in the present study. First, the prostate biopsies, although taken with same equipment, may have variations due to different urologists who performed the biopsies. Second, the slides were not re-evaluated. Additionally, by digitizing all of the material and measuring core areas instead of the lengths of the biopsies, the quality indicator would have been more accurate. In the present study we preferred to use our current methods because at the moment there are no area-based prognostic nomograms available, and measuring the actual tissue from histological slides is the gold standard. Third, the subtraction of extraprostatic tissue is somewhat subjective. However,

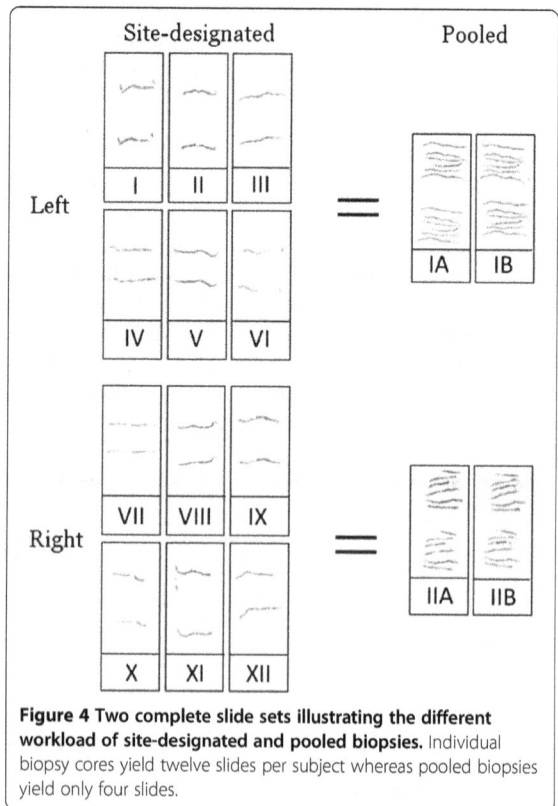

**Figure 4 Two complete slide sets illustrating the different workload of site-designated and pooled biopsies.** Individual biopsy cores yield twelve slides per subject whereas pooled biopsies yield only four slides.

Length of prostate biopsies is not necessarily compromised by pooling multiple cores in one...

223

this subjectivity should be equally transferred to both types of specimens. Finally, the amount of site-designated individual biopsies only represented 17% of the studied cases and the imbalance between the groups may cause unreliability in the final results. As a limitation of this study, it must be pointed out, that this study only shows the situation in our facility and to determine the real impact in a clinical context, a multicenter study would describe the overall situation of prostate biopsies better. Our aim was simply to determine whether there were fundamental differences in favor of either method.

## Conclusions

The number of submitted vials depends on how the urologist performs the prostate biopsy. We have received both individually submitted and pooled biopsies for several years without noticing an obvious difference in their quality. However, the workload for laboratory technologists and pathologists is substantially higher for site-designated individually embedded biopsy cores. In our material, we did not find evidence regarding the superior quality of the individually submitted and embedded biopsies. We conclude that the current recommendations favoring site-designated biopsies may be too strict - the guidelines should probably recommend a result rather than a process.

### Competing interests

The authors declare that they have no competing interests.

### Authors' contributions

TT was responsible for the conception, study design and implementation of the project and drafted the manuscript. JI, AK and JR participated in the conception and design of the study. JI, LK and AK helped to draft the manuscript. TT, SH, ML, SP, MT and PK participated in the analysis of the data. JI and TT performed the statistical analysis. All authors read and approved the final manuscript.

### Acknowledgements

The authors would like to thank Fimlab Laboratories, Tampere University Hospital, Satakunta Hospital and University of Tampere for enabling and funding parts of the research. The authors also thank the urologists of Tampere University Hospital district, who submitted the studied biopsies, and the skilful and dedicated laboratory personnel of pathology laboratory of Fimlab Laboratories.

### Author details

[1]Department of Pathology, Fimlab Laboratories, Tampere University Hospital, Tampere, Finland. [2]Department of Cancer Biology, Institute of Biomedical Technology, University of Tampere, Tampere, Finland. [3]Department of Surgery, Satakunta Hospital district, Pori, Finland. [4]Department of Urology, Tampere University Hospital, Tampere, Finland. [5]Department of Materials Science, Tampere University of Technology, Tampere, Finland.

### References

1. Epstein JI, Allsbrook Jr WC, Amin MB, Egevad LL. The 2005 International Society of Urological Pathology (ISUP) Consensus Conference on Gleason Grading of Prostatic Carcinoma. Am J Surg Pathol. 2005;29:1228–42.
2. Heidenreich A, Bellmunt J, Bolla M, Joniau S, Mason M, Matveev V, et al. EAU guidelines on prostate cancer. Part 1: screening, diagnosis, and treatment of clinically localised disease. Eur Urol. 2011;59:61–71.
3. Iczkowski KA, Bostwick DG. Sampling, submission, and report format for multiple prostate biopsies: a 1999 survey. Urology. 2000;55:568–71.
4. Varma M, Berney DM, Algaba F, Camparo P, Compérat E, Griffiths DFR, et al. Prostate needle biopsy processing: a survey of laboratory practice across Europe. J Clin Pathol. 2013;66:120–3.
5. Eichler K, Hempel S, Wilby J, Myers L, Bachmann LM, Kleijnen J. Diagnostic value of systematic biopsy methods in the investigation of prostate cancer: a systematic review. J Urol. 2006;175:1605–12.
6. Iczkowski KA, Casella G, Seppala RJ, Jones GL, Mishler BA, Qian J, et al. Needle core length in sextant biopsy influences prostate cancer detection rate. Urology. 2002;59:698–703.
7. Öbek C, Doğanca T, Erdal S, Erdoğan S, Durak H. Core length in prostate biopsy: size matters. J Urol. 2012;187:2051–5.
8. Jones JS, Patel A, Schoenfield L, Rabets JC, Zippe CD, Magi-Galluzzi C. Saturation technique does not improve cancer detection as an initial prostate biopsy strategy. J Urol. 2006;175:485–8.
9. Irani J, Blanchet P, Salomon L, Coloby P, Hubert J, Malavaud B, et al. Is an extended 20-core prostate biopsy protocol more efficient than the standard 12-core? A randomized multicenter trial. J Urol. 2013;190:77–83.
10. Jiang X, Zhu S, Feng G, Zhang Z, Li C, Li H, et al. Is an initial saturation prostate biopsy scheme better than an extended scheme for detection of prostate cancer? A systematic review and meta-analysis. Eur Urol. 2013;63:1031–9.
11. Bertaccini A, Fandella A, Prayer-Galetti T, Scattoni V, Galosi AB, Ficarra V, et al. Systematic development of clinical practice guidelines for prostate biopsies: a 3-year Italian project. Anticancer Res. 2007;27:659–66.
12. Bostwick DG, Qian J, Drewnowska K, Varvel S, Bostwick KC, Marberger M, et al. Prostate needle biopsy quality in reduction by dutasteride of prostate cancer events study: worldwide comparison of improvement with investigator training and centralized laboratory processing. Urology. 2010;75:1406–10.
13. Van der Kwast T, Bubendorf L, Mazerolles C, Raspollini MR, Van Leenders GJ, Phil C-G, et al. Guidelines on processing and reporting of prostate biopsies: the 2013 update of the pathology committee of the European Randomized Study of Screening for Prostate Cancer (ERSPC). Virchows Arch. 2013;463:367–77.
14. Mäkinen T. The Finnish population-based prostate cancer screening trial: a clinical perspective. Tampere: Tampere University Press; 2008.

# Permissions

All chapters in this book were first published in Clinical Pathology, by BioMed Central; hereby published with permission under the Creative Commons Attribution License or equivalent. Every chapter published in this book has been scrutinized by our experts. Their significance has been extensively debated. The topics covered herein carry significant findings which will fuel the growth of the discipline. They may even be implemented as practical applications or may be referred to as a beginning point for another development.

The contributors of this book come from diverse backgrounds, making this book a truly international effort. This book will bring forth new frontiers with its revolutionizing research information and detailed analysis of the nascent developments around the world.

We would like to thank all the contributing authors for lending their expertise to make the book truly unique. They have played a crucial role in the development of this book. Without their invaluable contributions this book wouldn't have been possible. They have made vital efforts to compile up to date information on the varied aspects of this subject to make this book a valuable addition to the collection of many professionals and students.

This book was conceptualized with the vision of imparting up-to-date information and advanced data in this field. To ensure the same, a matchless editorial board was set up. Every individual on the board went through rigorous rounds of assessment to prove their worth. After which they invested a large part of their time researching and compiling the most relevant data for our readers.

The editorial board has been involved in producing this book since its inception. They have spent rigorous hours researching and exploring the diverse topics which have resulted in the successful publishing of this book. They have passed on their knowledge of decades through this book. To expedite this challenging task, the publisher supported the team at every step. A small team of assistant editors was also appointed to further simplify the editing procedure and attain best results for the readers.

Apart from the editorial board, the designing team has also invested a significant amount of their time in understanding the subject and creating the most relevant covers. They scrutinized every image to scout for the most suitable representation of the subject and create an appropriate cover for the book.

The publishing team has been an ardent support to the editorial, designing and production team. Their endless efforts to recruit the best for this project, has resulted in the accomplishment of this book. They are a veteran in the field of academics and their pool of knowledge is as vast as their experience in printing. Their expertise and guidance has proved useful at every step. Their uncompromising quality standards have made this book an exceptional effort. Their encouragement from time to time has been an inspiration for everyone.

The publisher and the editorial board hope that this book will prove to be a valuable piece of knowledge for researchers, students, practitioners and scholars across the globe.

# List of Contributors

**Giorgio Perino**
Department of Pathology, Hospital for Special Surgery, 535 East 70th Street, New York, NY 10021, USA.

**Benjamin F Ricciardi and Seth A Jerabek**
Department of Orthopedic Surgery, Hospital for Special Surgery, New York, NY, USA.

**Guido Martignoni**
Department of Pathology and Diagnostics, University of Verona, Verona and Pederzoli Hospital, Peschiera, Italy

**Gabrielle Wilner, Dan Maass, Steven R Goldring and P Edward Purdue**
Division of Research, Hospital for Special Surgery, New York, NY, USA

**Ru-Xin Melanie Foong, Osvaldo Borrelli, Eleni Volonaki, Robert Dziubak, Rosan Meyer and Mamoun Elawad**
Paediatric Gastroenterology Department, Great Ormond Street Hospital, London WC1N 3JH, United Kingdom

**Neil J. Sebire**
Histopathology Department, Great Ormond Street Hospital, London, United Kingdom.

**Neil Shah**
Paediatric Gastroenterology Department, Great Ormond Street Hospital, London WC1N 3JH, United Kingdom
Institute of Child Health/ UCL, London WC1N 1EH, UK

**Joanna J Moser, Marvin J Fritzler and Jerome B Rattner**
Department of Biochemistry and Molecular Biology, Faculty of Medicine, University of Calgary, Calgary, AB, Canada

**Khaleel Al-Obaidy, Fatimah Alruwaii, Areej Al Nemer and Mohamed A Shawarby**
Pathology Department, College of Medicine, University of Dammam, P.O. Box 1982, Dammam 31441, Saudi Arabia

**Raed Alsulaiman**
Department of Internal Medicine, College of Medicine, University of Dammam, P.O. Box 1982, Dammam 31441, Saudi Arabia

**Zainab Alruwaii**
King Fahd Hospital of the University, University of Dammam, P.O. Box 2208, Al-Khobar 31952, Saudi Arabia

**Emma Gustbée, Andrea Markkula, Maria Simonsson, Björn Nodin, Karin Jirström and Helena Jernström**
Division of Oncology and Pathology, Department of Clinical Sciences, Lund, Lund University, Barngatan 2B, SE 22185 Lund, Sweden

**Helga Tryggvadottir and Signe Borgquist**
Division of Oncology and Pathology, Department of Clinical Sciences, Lund, Lund University, Barngatan 2B, SE 22185 Lund, Sweden
Department of Oncology, Skåne University Hospital, Lund, Sweden

**Carsten Rose**
CREATE Health and Department of Immunotechnology, Lund University, Medicon Village, Building 406, Lund, Sweden

**Christian Ingvar**
Department of Clinical Sciences, Division of Surgery, Lund, Lund University, Lund, Sweden and Skåne University Hospital, Lund, Sweden

**Joel E. Mortensen, Cindi Ventrola and Sarah Hanna**
Department of Laboratory Medicine, Cincinnati Children's Hospital, MLC1010, 3333 Burnet Ave, 45229 Cincinnati, OH, USA

**Adam Walter**
BD Diagnostics, Sparks, MD, USA

**Claudio A. Mastronardi and Gilberto Paz-Filho**
Department of Genome Sciences, The John Curtin School of Medical Research, The Australian National University, 131 Garran Rd, Canberra, Acton ACT 2601, Australia

**Belinda Whittle and Robert Tunningley**
Australian Phenomics Facility, The Australian National University, 117 Garran Rd, Canberra, Acton ACT 2601, Australia

**Teresa Neeman**
Statistical Consulting Unit, The Australian National University, 27 Union Lane, Canberra, Acton ACT 2601, Australia

**Takuto Nosaka, Katsushi Hiramatsu, Tomoyuki Nemoto, Yasushi Saito, Yoshihiko Ozaki, Kazuto Takahashi, Tatsushi Naito, Kazuya Ofuji, Hidetaka Matsuda, Masahiro Ohtani, Hiroyuki Suto and Yasunari Nakamoto**
Second Department of Internal Medicine, Faculty of Medical Sciences, University of Fukui, Fukui, Japan

**Yoshiaki Imamura**
Department of Pathology, University of Fukui Hospital, Fukui, Japan

**William H. Bradley and Janet S. Rader**
Department of Obstetrics and Gynecology, Medical College of Wisconsin, 8701 Watertown Plank Road, Milwaukee, WI 53226, USA

**Kevin Eng**
Department of Biostatistics and Medical Informatics, University of Wisconsin-Madison, Madison, WI 53792, USA

Current Address: Department of Biostatistics and Bioinformatics, Roswell Park Cancer Institute, Buffalo, NY, USA

**Christina Kendziorski**
Department of Biostatistics and Medical Informatics, University of Wisconsin-Madison, Madison, WI 53792, USA

**Min Le and A. Craig Mackinnon**
Department of Pathology, Medical College of Wisconsin, Milwaukee, WI 53226, USA

**Michael Majores, Anne Schindler, Angela Fuchs, Johannes Stein, Peter and Glen Kristiansen**
Institute of Pathology, University of Bonn, Sigmund-Freud-Str. 25, D-53127 Bonn, Germany

**Lukas Heukamp**
New Pathology, Cologne, Germany

**Altevogt**
Skin Cancer Unit, German Cancer Research Center (DKFZ), Heidelberg, Germany Department of Dermatology, Venereology and Allergology University Medical Center Mannheim, Ruprecht-Karl University of Heidelberg, Mannheim, Germany

**Ruza Arsenic, Denise Treue, Annika Lehmann, Michael Hummel, Manfred Dietel, Carsten Denkert and Jan Budczies**
Institute of Pathology, Charité University Hospital Berlin, Berlin, Germany

**Imogen Ptacek, Ainslie Garrod, Sian Bullough, Nicola Bradley, Colin P. Sibley, Rebecca L. Jones, Paul Brownbill and Alexander E. P. Heazell**
Institute of Human Development, Faculty of Medical and Human Sciences, University of Manchester, Oxford Rd, Manchester M13 9PL, UK
Maternal and Fetal Health Research Centre, 5th floor (Research), St Mary's Hospital, Oxford Road, Manchester M13 9WL, UK

**Gauri Batra and Anna Smith**
Department of Histopathology, Royal Manchester Children's Hospital, Central Manchester University Hospitals NHS Foundation Trust, Manchester Academic Health Science Centre, Manchester M13 9WL, UK

**Benjamin F. Ricciardi and Seth A. Jerabek**
Department of Orthopedic Surgery, Hospital for Special Surgery, New York, NY, USA

**Allina A. Nocon**
Healthcare Research Institute, Hospital for Special Surgery, New York, NY, USA

**Gabrielle Wilner, Elianna Kaplowitz, Steven R. Goldring and P. Edward Purdue**
Division of Research, Hospital for Special Surgery, New York, NY, USA

**Giorgio Perino**
Department of Pathology and Laboratory Medicine, Hospital for Special Surgery, 535 East 70th Street, New York, NY 10021, USA

**Lara Termini, Maria A Andreoli and Maria C Costa**
Santa Casa de São Paulo, INCT-HPV at Santa Casa Research Institute, School of Medicine, Rua Marquês de Itú, 381, 01223-001 São Paulo, Brazil

**José H Fregnani**
Teaching and Research Institute, Barretos Cancer Hospital, Rua Antenor Duarte Vilela, 1331, 14784-006 Barretos, Brazil

**Enrique Boccardo**
Department of Microbiology, Institute of Biomedical Sciences, University of São Paulo, Av. Prof. Lineu Prestes, 1374 - Ed. Biomédicas II, Cidade Universitária, 05508-900 São Paulo, Brazil

**Walter H da Costa, Ademar Lopes and Gustavo C Guimarães**
Pelvic Surgery Department, A. C. Camargo Cancer Center, Rua Prof. Antônio Prudente 211, 01509-010 São Paulo, Brazil

**Adhemar Longatto-Filho**
Laboratory of Medical Investigation (LIM) 14, Department of Pathology, School of Medicine, University of São Paulo, Av. Dr. Arnaldo 455, 01246-903 São Paulo, Brazil Life and Health Sciences Research Institute, School of Health Sciences, ICVS/3B's - PT Government Associate Laboratory, University of Minho, Braga, Guimarães, Portugal
Molecular Oncology Research Center, Barretos Cancer Hospital, Pio XII Foundation, Barretos, Rua Antenor Duarte Villela, 1331, 14784-400 Barretos, Brazil

**Isabela W da Cunha and Fernando A Soares**
Department of Anatomic Pathology, A. C. Camargo Cancer Center, Rua Prof. Antônio Prudente 109, 01509-900 São Paulo, Brazil

**Luisa L Villa**
Santa Casa de São Paulo, INCT-HPV at Santa Casa Research Institute, School of Medicine, Rua Marquês de Itú, 381, 01223-001 São Paulo, Brazil
Department of Radiology and Oncology, School of Medicine, University of São Paulo and Cancer Institute of the State of São Paulo, ICESP, Av Dr Arnaldo 250, 01246-000 São Paulo, Brazil

**Louis S. Nelson, Scott R. Davis, Robert M. Humble, Jeff Kulhavy and Matthew D. Krasowski**
Department of Pathology, University of Iowa Hospitals and Clinics, Iowa Melkamu Getinet1, Baye Gelaw2, Abinet Sisay1, Eiman A. Mahmoud3 and Abate Assefa2*City, IA 52242, USA

**Dean R. Aman**
Hospital Computing Information Services, University of Iowa Hospitals and Clinics, Iowa City, IA 52242, USA

**Melkamu Getinet and Abinet Sisay**
Debre Markos Referral Hospital, Debre Markos, Ethiopia

**Baye Gelaw and Abate Assefa**
Department of Medical Microbiology, School of Biomedical and Laboratory Sciences,

College of Medicine and Health Sciences, University of Gondar, Gondar, Ethiopia

**Eiman A. Mahmoud**
Department of Basic Sciences, College of Osteopathic Medicine, Touro University, Vallejo, CA, USA

**Bernard Seshie**
Department of Surgery, Tema General Hospital, Tema, Ghana

**Joe-Nat Clegg-Lamptey, Nii Armah Adu-Aryee and Florence Dedey**
Department of Surgery, School of Medicine and Dentistry, University of Ghana, Accra, Ghana

**Benedict Calys-Tagoe**
Department of Community Health, School of Public Health, University of Ghana, Accra, Ghana

**Emmanuel Kamgobe, Dismas Matovelo and Tito Chaula**
Department of Obstetrics and Gynecology, Catholic University of Health and Allied sciences, P.O.BOX 1464, Mwanza, Tanzania

**Anthony Massinde and Edgar Ndaboine**
Department of Obstetrics and Gynecology, Catholic University of Health and Allied sciences, P.O.BOX 1464, Mwanza, Tanzania
Department of Obstetrics and Gynecology, Bugando Medical Centre, P.O.BOX 1370, Mwanza, Tanzania

**Peter Rambau**
Department of Pathology, Catholic University of Health and Allied sciences, P.O.BOX 1464, Mwanza, Tanzania

**Mohamed Allaoui, Adil Boudhas, Mustapha Azzakhmam, Mohammed Boukhechba, Abderrahmane Al Bouzidi and Mohamed Oukabli**
Department of Pathology, Military General Hospital Mohammed V, Mohammed V Souissi University - Faculty of Medicine and Pharmacy of Rabat, Hay Riad, Rabat 10000, Morocco

**Ilias Benchafai**
Department of Clinical Haematology, Military General Hospital Mohammed V, Mohammed V Souissi University- Faculty of Medicine and Pharmacy of Rabat, Hay Riad, Rabat 10000, Morocco

**El Mehdi Mahtat and Safae Regragui**
Department of Otorhinolaryngology, Military General Hospital Mohammed V, Mohammed V Souissi University- Faculty of Medicine and Pharmacy of Rabat, Hay Riad, Rabat 10000, Morocco

**Mouna Khmou, Najat Lamalmi, Abderrahmane Malihy, Lamia Rouas and Zaitouna Alhamany**
Department of Pathology, Children's Hospital Faculty of Medicine and Pharmacy, Mohammed V University Ibn Sina University Hospital, Rabat, Morocco

**Margareta Heby, Jakob Elebro, Björn Nodin, Karin Jirström and Jakob Eberhard**
Department of Clinical Sciences Lund, Division of Oncology and Pathology, Lund University, Skåne University Hospital, 221 85 Lund, Sweden

**Xi Wang, Kirsten Woolf, David G. Hicks and Shuyuan Yeh**
Department of Pathology, University of Rochester Medical Center, Rochester, NY 14642, USA

**Brian Z. Ring**
Institute for Genomic and Personalized Medicine, School of Life Science and Technology, Huazhong University of Science and Technology, Wuhan, China

**Robert S. Seitz**
Insight Genetics Inc., Nashville, TN, USA

**Douglas T. Ross**
CardioDx, Inc., Redwood City, CA, USA

**Rodney A. Beck**
Conversant Biologics, Huntsville, AL, USA

**Mohamed Reda El Ochi, Mohamed Allaoui, Abderrahman Albouzidi**
and Mohamed Oukabli
Department of Pathology, Mohamed V military Hospital, Hay Riad, Faculty of Medicine, Mohamed V University, BP10000 Rabat, Morocco

**Mehdi Toreis and Mohamed Ichou**
Department of Medical Oncology, Mohamed V military Hospital, Hay Riad, Faculty of Medicine, Mohamed V University, Rabat, Morocco

**Mohamed Benchekroun**
Department of of Orthopaedics and Traumatology, Mohamed V military Hospital, Hay Riad, Faculty of Medicine, Mohamed V University, Rabat, Morocco.

**Zineb Benkerroum**
Department of of Gynecology and obstetrics, Mohamed V military Hospital, Hay Riad, Faculty of Medicine, Mohamed V University, Rabat, Morocco.

**Basma El Khannoussi**
Department of Pathology, National Institute of Oncology, Hay Riad, Faculty of Medicine, Mohamed V University, Rabat, Morocco

**Bjørn Westre, Anita Giske and Hilde Guttormsen**
Department of Pathology, Ålesund Hospital, Møre and Romsdal Health Trust, Ålesund, Norway

**Sveinung Wergeland Sørbye**
Department of Clinical Pathology, University Hospital of North Norway, 9038 Tromsø, Norway

**Finn Egil Skjeldestad**
Research Group Epidemiology of Chronic Diseases, Department of Community Medicine, UiT The Arctic University of Norway, Tromsø, Norway

**Clarissa N. Amaya and Brad A. Bryan**
Department of Biomedical Sciences, Paul L. Foster School of Medicine, Texas Tech University Health Sciences Center, El Paso, TX, USA

**Markus Rechsteiner, Marion Bawohl and Achim Weber**
Institute of Surgical Pathology, University and University Hospital Zurich, Schmelzbergstrasse 12, 8091 Zurich, Switzerland

**Juliane Friemel**
Institute of Surgical Pathology, University and University Hospital Zurich, Schmelzbergstrasse 12, 8091 Zurich, Switzerland.
Leibniz Institute for Prevention Research and Epidemiology (BIPS), Bremen, Germany

**Lukas Frick**
Institute of Surgical Pathology, University and University Hospital Zurich, Schmelzbergstrasse 12, 8091 Zurich, Switzerland
Swiss Hepato-Pancreato-Biliary Center, Department of Digestive and Transplant Surgery, University Hospital of Zurich, Zurich, Switzerland

**Beat Müllhaupt**
Clinics of Hepatology and Gastroenterology, University and University Hospital Zurich, Zurich, Switzerland

**Mickaël Lesurtel**
Swiss Hepato-Pancreato-Biliary Center, Department of Digestive and Transplant Surgery, University Hospital of Zurich, Zurich, Switzerland

**Sanna Huovinen, Marita Laurila, Sinikka Porre, Mika Tirkkonen and Paula Kujala**
Department of Pathology, Fimlab Laboratories, Tampere University Hospital, Tampere, Finland.

**Teemu T Tolonen**
Department of Pathology, Fimlab Laboratories, Tampere University Hospital, Tampere, Finland
Department of Cancer Biology, Institute of Biomedical Technology, University of Tampere, Tampere, Finland

**Jorma Isola**
Department of Cancer Biology, Institute of Biomedical Technology, University of Tampere, Tampere, Finland

**Antti Kaipia**
Department of Surgery, Satakunta Hospital district, Pori, Finland
Department of Urology, Tampere University Hospital, Tampere, Finland

**Laura Koivusalo**
Department of Surgery, Satakunta Hospital district, Pori, Finland
Department of Materials Science, Tampere University of Technology, Tampere, Finland

**Jarno Riikonen**
Department of Urology, Tampere University Hospital, Tampere, Finland

# Index

www.ingramcontent.com/pod-product-compliance
Lightning Source LLC
Chambersburg PA
CBHW061946190326
41458CB00009B/2794